IADVL Manual on Management of Dermatophytoses

2nd Edition

IADVL Manual on Management of Dermatophytoses

2nd Edition

Editor-in-Chief

Kabir Sardana
MD DNB MNAMS
Director–Professor and Head
Department of Dermatology and STD
Atal Bihari Vajpayee Institute of Medical Sciences and
Dr Ram Manohar Lohia Hospital, New Delhi
Professor of Dermatology, IP University, Delhi
Associate Professor, Delhi University
Former Professor
Department of Dermatology
Maulana Azad Medical College, New Delhi

Associate Editors

Ananta Khurana
MD DNB MNAMS FRCP (London)
Professor
Department of Dermatology
Atal Bihari Vajpayee Institute of Medical Sciences and
Dr Ram Manohar Lohia Hospital
New Delhi

Meghana Phiske
MD DNB DVD DDV
Associate Professor
Department of Dermatology
MGM Institute of Medical Sciences
Navi Mumbai

Assistant Editors

Dipali Rathod
DNB DDVL FIDD FIADVL MNAMS
Assistant Professor
Department of Dermatology
Seth GS Medical College and KEM Hospital, Mumbai

Mohammad Adil
MD (DVL)
Associate Professor
Department of Dermatology
Jawaharlal Nehru Medical College
Aligarh Muslim University, Aligarh

Preethi B Nayak
MD DNB FRGUHS (Dermatosurgery) MNAMS
Consultant Dermatologist
Dermatosurgeon and Hair Transplant Surgeon
Experia Advanced Skin and Hair Clinic, Bengaluru

CBS Publishers & Distributors Pvt Ltd
New Delhi • Bengaluru • Chennai • Kochi • Kolkata • Lucknow • Mumbai
Gujarat • Hyderabad • Jharkhand • Nagpur • Patna • Pune • Uttarakhand

IADVL
Manual on
Management of
Dermatophytoses
2nd Edition

ISBN: 978-93-49057-72-2

Second Edition: 2026
First Edition: 2018

Published by Satish Kumar Jain and produced by Varun Jain for
CBS Publishers & Distributors Pvt Ltd
4819/XI Prahlad Street, 24 Ansari Road, Daryaganj, New Delhi 110 002, India
Ph: 011-23289259, 23266838 Website: www.cbspd.com
e-mail: delhi@cbspd.com

Corporate Office: 204 FIE, Industrial Area, Patparganj, Delhi 110 092, India
Ph: 011-4934 4934 Fax: 011-4934 4935 e-mail: publishing@cbspd.com; publicity@cbspd.com

For Pharma queries, please write to
Mr SK Verma
Mob: +91-9810126251 Website: www.cbspd.com
e-mail: verma@cbspd.com; pharma@cbspd.com

Branches

- **Bengaluru:** Seema House 2975, 17th Cross, KR Road, Banasankari 2nd Stage, Bengaluru 560 070, Karnataka, India
  Ph: +91-80-26771678/79 Fax: +91-80-26771680 e-mail: bangalore@cbspd.com
- **Chennai:** 18/8B, Subbarayan Street, Shenoy Nagar, Chennai 600 030, Tamil Nadu, India
  Ph: +91-44-42032115, 26681266 e-mail: chennai@cbspd.com
- **Kochi:** 42/1325, 1326, Power House Road, Opposite KSEB, Power House, Ernakulam 682018, Kochi, Kerala, India
  Ph: +91-484-4059061–65, 67 Fax: +91-484-4059065 e-mail: kochi@cbspd.com
- **Kolkata:** 147, Hind Ceramics Compound, 1st Floor, Nilgunj Road, Belghoria, Kolkata 700056, West Bengal, India
  Ph: +91-33-25633055/56 e-mail: kolkata@cbspd.com
- **Lucknow:** Basement, Khushnuma Complex, 7 Meerabai Marg (behind Jawahar Bhawan), Lucknow 226001, UP, India
  Ph: +91-522-4000032 e-mail: tiwari.lucknow@cbspd.com
- **Mumbai:** PWD Shed, Gala No. 25/26, Ramchandra Bhatt Marg, Next JJ Hospital Gate No. 2, Opp. Union Bank of India, Noorbaug, Mumbai 400009, Maharashtra, India
  Ph: +91-22-66661880/89 e-mail: mumbai@cbspd.com

Representatives

• **Gujarat** • **Hyderabad** • **Jharkhand** • **Nagpur** • **Patna** • **Pune** • **Uttarakhand**

For trade terms please contact customercare@cbspd.com
For general enquiries please contact info@cbspd.com

Printed at: Printed in India

to

our parents, seniors and patients

Preface to the Second Edition

The second edition of the *IADVL Manual on Management of Dermatophytoses* comes 8 years after the first edition. While at the time of writing the first edition, the reasons for the sudden emergence of recalcitrance in dermatophytoses were still unknown, a lot of progress has been made in the past six years. The most prominent among these is the recognition of *T. indotineae* as the new species causing dermatophytosis of the glabrous skin. Within a short span of time, *T. indotineae* has become the predominant cause of glabrous tinea in the country. However, owing to the inability of culture based methods to reliably distinguish *T. indotineae* from closely related species—*T. mentagrophytes* and *T. interdigitale*, and unavailability of appropriate sequencing based identification in routine microbiology laboratories, the true extent of *T. indotineae* in the country may still be underestimated.

In addition to identification of the novel species, we also have significant data on epidemiology, clinical characteristics, treatment responses and relapses in the current scenario. Clinical trials on Itraconazole and Terbinafine have provided reasonable insights into the efficacy of these drugs against the novel species. In addition, synergy studies have added to our understanding of possible topical-systemic combinations of potential use in clinical settings.

However, several irrational treatment regimens have come to fore in the current context in a bid to achieve rapid results, although it is amply clear that "cure" now requires prolonged durations of treatment, even with the most effective antifungal against the species. The use of higher and higher doses of Itraconazole is unjustified as high cure rates have been documented with lower doses also. The trend of systemic antifungal combinations is unfortunate, not evidence based and strongly discouraged by the editors. Further, use of third generation azoles for dermatophytoses is discouraged, as firstly, these are reserve drugs for invasive mycoses and secondly, these have not shown clear superiority over Itraconazole in clinical studies.

The second edition of *IADVL Manual on Management of Dermatophytoses* elucidates these facets in various chapters, authored by authors with keen interest in the respective topics. The book provides a comprehensive coverage of dermatophytoses, effectively blending detailed explanations with up-to-date information from the latest literature. It delves into the epidemiology of dermatophytes in detail, comparing current context with past literature. The clinical presentations and established and newer diagnostic methods are discussed in depth in respective chapters. The existing literature on *T. indotineae* and what research is still lacking is covered effectively from both clinicians and mycologists' viewpoints. Drug treatment, including the details on pharmacodynamics and pharmacokinetics of antifungals to various formulations and preparations available and experimental molecules on the horizon are elucidated. Treatment guidelines cover the most up to date literature on various antifungals offering both depth and clarity. The illustrations in the form of high-quality clinical photographs depict varied typical and atypical clinical presentations and differential diagnoses while the schematic images aid make complex pathogenetic concepts easily understandable. The inclusion of recent research and treatment protocols ensures that the content reflects the latest advancements in dermatophytosis management, making it an invaluable resource for practitioners, academicians as well as postgraduates.

Kabir Sardana
Editor-in-Chief

Preface to the First Edition

The *IADVL Manual on Management of Dermatophytoses* comes at a very appropriate time, when dermatologists all over the nation are grappling with the issue of recalcitrant dermatophytic infections. Though the issue continues to perplex us and scientific reasoning for it is still awaited, we have made an attempt to bring out a comprehensive text covering all aspects of dermatophytoses, to update the reader of existing literature and possible directions for the future.

This project has many "creators" and we were the accidental editors. It was originally the brain child of Dr Yogesh S Marfatia and the ITART and was then handed over to the IADVL Academy who under Dr Ameet Valia, Dr Kolalapudi Seetharaman and Dr Deepika Pandhi invited nomination for the book and its team. We thank them for assigning us this task. The contents were largely their suggestions and the idea of scenarios was of Dr Yogesh S Marfatia.

The manual begins with a detailed analysis on the changing patterns of dermatophytoses both clinically and mycologically. It is evident that the clinical morphologies we are witnessing now reflect a shift in the host–pathogen relationship, with hitherto rare and unusual forms being commonly encountered. This is well illustrated by Dr Manjunath Shenoy M in the concerned chapter. A possible species-shift as a reason for the present situation is discussed at length by Dr Shital Poojary. The author puts forward numerous references, both old and new, from across the country, exploring this possibility. Dr Shukla Das, an accomplished mycologist, provides useful insights into the laboratory confirmation techniques and antifungal susceptibility testing. Dermoscopy, an upcoming tool in diagnostic assessment of dermatophytoses, is covered with ample illustrations by Dr Ananta Khurana and Dr Deepak Jhakar. Dr Namrata Chhabra has contributed a large part covering general measures, topical therapies and role of ancillary treatments. Chapter 8 by Dr Madhu Rengarajan, provides an in-depth knowledge of the various systemic drugs for dermatophytoses, covering pharmacokinetics, pharmacodynamics and adverse effects of each. This is taken further in Chapter 9 focussing specifically on the rationale of use of antifungal drugs based on skin pharmacokinetics. The topic has been succinctly covered by Dr Pooja Arora Mrig and Dr Kabir Sardana. An elaborate overview on steroid modified tinea has been presented by Dr Yogesh S Marfatia, bringing to forefront the ill effects of topical steroids and the ramifications thereof. An in-depth review of the possible causes of the present scenario of recalcitrant infections and treatment options is presented by Dr Kabir Sardana and Dr Ananta Khurana. Separate sections on management of dermatophytic infections of the hair and nail have been done full justice by Dr Taru Garg and Dr Chander Grover respectively. Treatment in certain special patient groups, an often ignored aspect, is covered in detail by Dr Ananta Khurana. In the last section, Dr Ananta Khurana covers the emerging, though yet lacking quality evidence backing, therapies for onychomycosis in the form of lasers and PDT.

The end of the book has clinical scenarios which is an important part as it gives views of various practitioners across India and also gives an idea of the different approaches to the problem. The one unique aspect is that clinicians have used various oral drugs, including fluconazole, terbinafine, griseofulvin and itraconazole with good results, which goes against the theory of *in vitro* resistance, which discredits all drugs except itraconazole. It has insights into novel interventions including ciclopirox olamine which certainly holds potential.

A big thanks to CBS Publishers & Distributors, Mr SK Jain CMD, and Mr YN Arjuna Senior Vice President—Publishing, Editorial and Publicity, and their team, Mrs Ritu Chawla Assistant General Manager—Production, Mr Vikrant Sharma, Mr Sanjay Chauhan, Mr Neeraj Prasad, Mr Prasenjit Paul, and Mr SK Verma, apart from the great support staff at their easily accessible office. Also as Chief Editor a big thanks to my team including Dr Shilpa Garg and Dr Shital Poojary, who took out time from their schedules to pay attention to this book. Needless to say a big thanks to Dr Ananta Khurana who manages to take out hidden energy and inexplicable time from her already over encumbered academic and personal schedules for her assigned tasks. And thanks to the academy for such great co-editors.

Hope the book and its contents are useful for the readers.

Kabir Sardana
Chief Editor

List of Contributors

Ananta Khurana
MD DNB MNAMS FRCP (London)
Professor
Department of Dermatology
Atal Bihari Vajpayee Institute of Medical Sciences and Dr Ram Manohar Lohia Hospital
New Delhi, India

Angoori Gnaneshwar Rao
MD (Derm) DD
Professor
Department of Dermatology
SVS Medical College
Mahabubnagar, Telangana

Atiya Yaseen
MD (DVL)
Sub-District Hospital, Pampore
Department of Health and Medical Education
Jammu and Kashmir, India

Bikash Ranjan Kar
MD
Department of Dermatology
Venereology and Leprosy
Institute of Medical Sciences and SUM Hospital
Bhubaneswar, Odisha

Dattatray Gopal Saple
MD FCPS Fellow John Hopkins (USA)
Consultant Dermatologist and Chief Director
La'Mer Skin Clinic
Dadar, Mumbai, Maharashtra

Dipali Rathod
DNB DDVL FIDD FIADVL MNAMS
Assistant Professor
Department of Dermatology
Seth GS Medical College and KEM Hospital
Mumbai

Jyothi Jayaraman
DVD DNB
Assistant Professor
Department of Dermatology
Father Muller Medical College
Mangaluru, Karnataka

Kabir Sardana
MD DNB MNAMS
Director-Professor and Head
Department of Dermatology and STD
Atal Bihari Vajpayee Institute of Medical Sciences and Dr Ram Manohar Lohia Hospital, New Delhi
Professor of Dermatology, IP University, Delhi
Associate Professor, Delhi University
Former Professor
Department of Dermatology
Maulana Azad Medical College
New Delhi, India

Konakanchi Venkata Chalam
MD (Dermatology)
Professor and Head
Department of Dermatology
Government Medical College
Srikakulam, Andhra Pradesh

Manjunath Shenoy M
MD DNB
Department of Dermatology
Venereology and Leprosy
Yenepoya Medical College
Deralakatte, Mangaluru, Karnataka

Meghana Phiske
MD DNB DVD DDV
Associate Professor
Department of Dermatology
MGM Institute of Medical Sciences
Navi Mumbai, Maharashtra

Mohammad Adil
MD (DVL)
Associate Professor
Department of Dermatology
Jawaharlal Nehru Medical College
Aligarh Muslim University
Aligarh, Uttar Pradesh

Nayankumar H Patel
MD (DVL)
Professor and Head
Department of DVL
GCS Medical College Hospital and Research Center
Ahmedabad, Gujarat

Nidhi Gupta
MD
Consultant Dermatologist
Skinaa Clinic
Jaipur, Rajasthan

Prachisingh Rajpoot
DNB (Dermatology)
Assistant Professor
Department of Dermatology
KJ Somaiya Medical College and Research Center
Mumbai, Maharashtra

Prakriti Shukla
MD (DVL)
Assistant Professor
Department of Dermatology
Maharshi Devraha Baba Autonomous
State Medical College
Deoria, Uttar Pradesh

Preethi B Nayak
MD DNB FRGUHS (Dermatosurgery) MNAMS
Consultant Dermatologist
Dermatosurgeon and Hair Transplant Surgeon
Experia Advanced Skin and Hair Clinic
Bengaluru, Karnataka

Rashmi Jindal
MD FRCP (Edinburgh)
Professor and Head
Department of Dermatology
Himalayan Institute of Medical Sciences
Dehradun, Uttarakhand

Richa Anjleen Tigga
MD (Microbiology)
Assistant Professor
Department of Microbiology
Chandulal Chandrakar Memorial
Government Medical College
Kachandur, Durg, Chhattisgarh

Ruchi Hemdani
MD (DVL)
Assistant Professor
Department of Dermatology
Himalayan Institute of Medical Sciences
Dehradun, Uttarakhand

Shaily Gupta
MD (DVL)
Consultant Dermatologist
Apollo Clinic, AB Road
Indore, Madhya Pradesh

Shashank Bhargava
MD FAHRS
Associate Professor
RD Gardi Medical College
Ujjain, Madhya Pradesh

Shital Poojary
MD DNB
Professor and Head
Department of Dermatology
KJ Somaiya Medical College and Research Centre
Mumbai, Maharashtra

Shukla Das
MD DNB MNAMS
Director-Professor
Department of Microbiology
University College of Medical Sciences and
Guru Teg Bahadur Hospital
Dilshad Garden, Delhi, India

Sinu Rose Mathachan
MD DNB EBDVD
Specialist Dermatologist
Asther DM Healthcare
Dubai

Sushrut N Save
DNB (Skin) MNAMS
Consultant Dermatologist
La'Mer Skin Clinic
Dadar, Mumbai, Maharashtra

Vivek M Pai
MD DNB FRGUHS (Dermatosurgery) MNAMS
Consultant Dermatologist
Dermatosurgeon and
Hair Transplant Surgeon
Experia Advanced Skin and Hair Clinic
Bengaluru, Karnataka

Contents

CHAPTER 1

Epidemiology of Dermatophytic Infections

• Manjunath Shenoy M • Bikash Ranjan Kar

INTRODUCTION

Dermatophytes thrive on keratin and commonly belong to *Trichophyton, Microsporum* and *Epidermophyton* genera, although recent taxonomical revision has recognized newer genera. According to the host it infects, it can be classified as Anthropophilic (Human), Zoophilic (animals) and Geophilic (soil). The target tissues of human infection include skin, hair and nail. In the last few years there has been an alarming increase in the incidence of this infection. The clinical manifestations of the disease has seen a lot of modifications and transformations over last few years. Extensive disease, atypical morphologies and more severe forms are common nowadays. There is also a multi-fold increase in the incidence of chronic, relapsing and recurrent cases.

Superficial dermatophytosis is a commonly encountered infection affecting 20–25% of the population worldwide.[1] According to recent studies, there has been an alarming increase in the incidence of dermatophytosis across the country in the past decade and especially so over the past 5–6 years.[2,3]

Dermatophytosis has been clinically classified based on the site of infection. There are differences in the epidemiology, triggers and species causing these infections. They are summarized in **Table 1.1**.

INCIDENCE AND PREVALENCE

It is difficult to calculate the exact incidence and prevalence of dermatophytosis because of paucity of community-based surveys. Over the last 7–8 years there has been a rising trend of dermatophytosis all over the country.[2,3] Most of this data comes from hospital-based studies over periods ranging from 1–2 years.[4–6] The current reported prevalence in India ranges between 2.41% and 61.5%[4–6] based on the hospital statistics.

Chronic dermatophytosis is defined as dermatophytosis occurring for more than 6 months with or without recurrence despite being treated.[3] ***Recurrent dermatophytosis*** refers to re-occurrence of the glabrous tinea after 4 weeks of stopping treatment following clinical cure. Chronic and recurrent dermatophytosis (CRD) has been a matter of serious concern in the current scenario in India.

GEOGRAPHIC AREA

Studies are from hospital statistics, and hence the true prevalence may not be clearly recognized. A prevalence of 4.1–27.6% has been reported in studies from south India,[4,6] while

TABLE 1.1: Clinical classification of dermatophytosis along with risk/trigger factors

Type	Site of infection	Common agents	Risk/trigger factors
Tinea capitis	Hair and skin on the scalp	*Trichophyton tonsurans, Trichophyton violaceum, Microsporum canis, Microsporum audouinii, Trichophyton mentagrophytes, Trichophyton schoenleinii*	Children, contact with pets, sharing combs, hats and other articles
Tinea barbae	Hair and skin in the beard and moustache area	*Trichophyton violaceum, Trichophyton schoenleinii, Trichophyton tonsurans, Microsporum canis*	Contact with pets, and domestic animals, diabetes mellitus, local trauma (barber shop), steroid use
Tinea faciei	Glabrous skin of the face	*Trichophyton mentagrophytes/ Trichophyton interdigitale species complex (including Trichophyton indotineae), Trichophyton verrucosum, Trichophyton rubrum, Trichophyton violaceum*	Humid environmental conditions, excessive sweating, poor hygiene, low socioeconomical status, overcrowding, sharing of clothes and soap
Tinea corporis	Glabrous skin of the body except face and groin/pubic area	*Trichophyton mentagrophytes/ Trichophyton interdigitale* species complex (including *Trichophyton indotineae*), *Trichophyton verrucosum, Trichophyton rubrum, Trichophyton violaceum*	Humid environmental conditions, excessive sweating, poor hygiene, low socioeconomical status, overcrowding, sharing of clothes and soap
Tinea manuum	Palm, fingers and other parts of hands	*Trichophyton rubrum, Trichophyton interdigitale, Epidermophyton floccosum, Microsporum canis*	Humid environmental conditions, excessive sweating, fungal infection in feet or groin
Tinea cruris	Groin, genital, pubic, perineal, and perianal skin	*Trichophyton mentagrophytes/ Trichophyton interdigitale species complex (including Trichophyton indotineae), Trichophyton verrucosum, Trichophyton rubrum, Trichophyton violaceum*	Humid environmental conditions, excessive sweating, poor hygiene, low socioeconomical status, overcrowding, sharing of clothes and soap, synthetic inner garments
Tinea pedis	Sole, toes, web spaces and other parts of feet	*Trichophyton rubrum, Trichophyton interdigitale, Epidermophyton floccosum, Microsporum canis*	Wearing occlusive shoes, using community baths, showers, and pools
Tinea unguium	Nail plate and nail bed	*Trichophyton rubrum, Trichophyton interdigitale, Epidermophyton floccosum*	Old age, diabetes, peripheral vascular disease, occlusive footwear, using community baths, showers, and pools

a high prevalence of 61.5% is reported from a study from north India.[5] CRD was more prevalent in Amritsar as compared to Mumbai as per the hospital survey,[6] however, there are no population studies that defines the true prevalence of the disease in different geographical regions of India.

AGE AND GENDER

Except for tinea capitis, which is commoner in pediatric age group, all other forms of dermatophytosis occur more frequently in post-pubertal age group. There may be an increase of pediatric glabrous dermatophytosis (tinea corporis, tinea cruris and tinea faciei) in the recent times which is in parallel to the increasing prevalence of dermatophytosis in general.[7] Approximately 20% of the infections seem to occur in children and adolescents under 18 years of age.[6]

Men are usually more frequently affected than women because of the outdoor work-related activities that predispose men to hot, humid and sweaty ambience. There is an increase in female cases recently as evidenced in literature. Earlier the ratio across various studies was 3–5:1 which has come down to <2 in last 3–4 years.[8, 9] Lately there are reports of men to women ratio reversal.[10, 11]

Chronic and recurrent dermatophytosis may be more common in the late middle age group, around fifth decade, which may be due to waning immunity, comorbidities like diabetes, use of topical steroid-antifungal creams and immunosuppressants intake.[12] A large multicentric study has reported high prevalence of CRD with a magnitude of 27.86% of the total dermatophytosis cases, of which approximately 78% and 22% were chronic dermatophytosis and recurrent dermatophytosis respectively.[6] CRD was reported at equal frequency in both genders.[6] The mean age of patients with chronic dermatophytosis was 32.5 years as reported by Pathania et al.[13]

FAMILY HISTORY

History of dermatophytosis in close contacts up to the extent of 50–82% has been reported recently across multiple studies.[6, 11, 13, 14] Prevalence is reported to be very high in people living in overcrowded homes, slums, hostel rooms and dormitories. Familial dermatophytosis is an important contributing factor to the increasing rates of treatment failure. Untreated cases of dermatophytosis might be associated with increased frequency of infection in a single family.[15] Patients of recurrent chronic dermatophytosis usually have more than one family member who is affected.[8] This imposes a financial burden on the entire family.

Fomites act as a medium of transfer of the organism. Soaking the clothes of all the family members together in cold water tub may be a factor favoring transfer of the infection.[16] Sharing of bath stool, soaps, towels or other articles while taking a bath is more prevalent in India compared to the West, and hence these articles may serve as fomites and promote transmission. Fomite sharing was common and accounted for up to 69% of the patients.[6, 13]

SOCIOECONOMIC FACTORS

Previous studies reported a rural predominance of various dermatophytosis probably because of the outdoor type of work people are engaged in and the resultant perspiration they have.[4, 17] However recent studies have focussed more on an urban background of the patients.[5, 18] Majority of patients (61–67%) belong to a poor socioeconomic background.[4,18,19] Overcrowding, linen sharing, lack of hygiene and poor nutrition promote the growth of dermatophytes.

OCCUPATION

People engaged in various sweat inducing physical activities in hot and humid environments are at a higher risk of infection. Manual laborers are more commonly affected.[10, 18, 20] Farmers have an additional risk due to increased exposure to fungal pathogens from the environment and frequent contact with soil and animals.[7] Housewives who work near a fire source are prone to dermatophytosis.[6, 21] Student community is affected possibly due to tight-fitting shoes and synthetic clothes, especially with the use of denims.[6, 10]

MIGRATION

Migration has a major role in demographic changes of dermatophytosis as exemplified by *Trichophyton tonsurans* and *Trichophyton soudanense*. *T. tonsurans* originated from Southeast Asia and Australia, it spread to Latin America and from there with work immigrants to North America and to other parts of the globe, including the African continent.[22–24] *Trichophyton rubrum* accounted for the majority of the infections in the 1980s and 90s.[24]

Trichophyton tonsurans was first reported in the early 2000s in Japan, and its number increased among the Judo-club members and school age children. *T. tonsurans* is a major cause of pediatric tinea capitis (95% of cases) in US.[25] Two other dermatophytes: *T. violaceum* and *T. soudanense* are also significant causes of tinea capitis in children in association with migration, specifically in African immigrants. A tinea capitis outbreak was also reported in children of African immigrants in Israel in 2016.[26]

There are not many studies related to the migration from India. Higher incidence of dermatophyte infections has been reported from north east Bihar, an area which shares border with West Bengal and Nepal and has a lot of migratory population.[27]

TOPICAL STEROID ABUSE

This is a problem specific to India and certain other countries where potent corticosteroids are rampantly used by layman because of lack of federal control. Easily available topical steroid formulations are prone to abuse and is one of the most important contributory factor of the current outbreak of chronic and recalcitrant dermatophytosis. India has seen a huge increase in the caseload of recalcitrant dermatophytosis over last 10 years parallel to the easy availability of cheap and potent topical steroid containing combination creams. Over the last 1–2 years studies have revealed that the frequency of prior application of topical steroid-containing combination creams is very high among patients accounting up to 80%.[2, 6]

Epidemiology of Tinea Incognito

Ive and Mark[28] first described tinea incognito in 1968 for various atypical clinical presentations of tinea due to prior use of topical or systemic steroids or other topical immunomodulators like topical calcineurin inhibitors. Atzori et al.[29] suggested *tinea atypica* for the same and proposed that it could be due to variable dermatophyte invasiveness, the site of invasion, excessive washing and sun exposure.

Tinea incognito most commonly affects females as per various studies probably due to the skin lightening effect of the steroid based creams which are being inadvertently marketed as fairness creams. This also explains face as the most common site of involvement though other studies have shown trunk as the most common site of involvement. *Trichophyton* group is the most common species isolated from the lesions followed distantly by *Microsporum* species. The various clinical morphologies described as a part of tinea incognito are eczema-like, psoriasis-like, lupus erythematosus-like, rosacea-like, etc.

Last few years have seen an exponential increase in the case load of tinea incognito. This reflects the proportionate increase in the sale of over the counter irrational steroid containing creams. A whopping 42–81%[30, 31] of patients who present to the dermatologist with tinea incognito have history of topical steroid abuse whereas use of only topical antifungal is present in only 6–47%.[2, 32]

CLIMATE CHANGE

Though dermatophytosis is expected to be more prevalent in the hot and humid climates of south India and less so in north India, no such association was apparent across various Indian literature in the current scenario. In fact, higher prevalence has been reported from north India.[5, 6] Statistically significant increased prevalence of dermatophytosis in rainy season as compared to the dry season has been observed in a multicentric study from India, however the prevalence of CRD was higher in dry season.[6]

Superficial fungal infections, particularly tinea corporis, have been reported to occur more frequently following flooding; e.g. after the Indian Ocean Tsunami (2004) and Hurricane Katrina in the US (2005).[33, 34] In the last two decades, the epidemiology of dermatophytosis in India has shifted substantially. First, its overall prevalence is rising, and it has been hypothesized that increasing average ambient temperature and humidity in India, where there have been especially severe heat waves recently, may be a causative factor.[35] Now, it is amply clear that the species variations is the cause and climate change as a factor is not important.

DERMATOPHYTE SPECIES

Trichophyton mentagrophytes has emerged as the predominant organism of late, surpassing *Trichophyton rubrum*. Various factors have been implicated including the belief that the zoophilic *Trichophyton mentagrophytes* has acclimatised itself and has undergone anthropization leading to this epidemiological shift among humans.[2] In the past decade, more so in the last 5–7 years, the reported prevalence of *Trichophyton mentagrophytes* has not only increased,[4,5,18–20] but it has even replaced *Trichophyton rubrum* in a few studies.[7,19,36] In a multicentric study from India, *Trichophyton mentagrophytes* isolates amounted to 93.2%, whereas, *Trichophyton rubrum* was isolated in only 6.8%.[2] Yet another study recently demonstrated 97.2% of isolated dermatophytes to be *Trichophyton mentagrophytes* complex with the most significant species being *Trichophyton interdigitale*.[12]

Earlier studies from India have described *Trichophyton rubrum* as the most common agent causing dermatophytosis.[37, 38] It was the most prevalent dermatophyte in central and northern Europe where it accounted for 80–90% of the strains isolated.[24] A similar epidemiological situation was also seen in America.[24] Studies from Rajasthan, Tamil Nadu and Goa published approximately in 2010 have shown higher isolation of *Trichophyton rubrum*.[39, 40] However, studies from Karnataka, Sikkim and central India published after 2014 have mostly shown high isolation of *Trichophyton mentagrophytes*.[41, 42] The causes for the shift of causative organisms are not known, but it can be postulated due to multiple factors, including changing agent, indiscriminate use of oral and topical antifungals, host immune factors as well as environmental changes.

Few studies done in India utilizing the molecular diagnostic techniques (genomic sequencing) have been published.[2, 21, 43, 44] All these studies have shown that *Trichophyton mentagrophyte* complex as the most common species with very low isolation of *Trichophyton rubrum*. There has been a confusion regarding the nomenclature of the identified species, however, recently the species prevailing in India has been identified as a new species and has been named as *Trichophyton indotineae*.[45] Culture is inadequate to correctly identify *T. indotineae*, and differentiate it from *T. mentagrophytes*, and studies based on culture identification alone thus label it as *T. mentagrophytes*. Currently, its isolation has also been reported from Bahrain, Canada, Denmark, Finland, France, Germany, Iran, Japan, Vietnam, Russia, and Switzerland due to travel and migration.[46–48] This accounts for the existence of pandemic of recalcitrant tinea infection that has not been able to draw sufficient attention of the health authorities across the world.

Various factors proposed for the shift include the increasing environmental temperature due to global warming, prevalence of diabetes, increased use of immunosuppressives, indiscriminate use of topical steroids, use of tight fitting synthetic clothes and shoes and sharing of fomites, though no good answer is there for this problem.

ANTIFUNGAL RESISTANCE

Current epidemic of dermatophytosis has also seen an antifungal resistance, especially, squalene epoxidase gene mutation-related terbinafine resistance.[2, 21, 43, 44] It has now been understood that the new agent has high *in vitro* terbinafine resistance that has transformed into therapeutic failure of terbinafine.

FUTURE DIRECTIONS

Broad classification of dermatophytes on the basis of ecological and clinical parameters leads to three types of dermatophytes namely geophilic, zoophilic and anthropophilic. Both the geophilic and zoophilic produce inflammatory lesions that may culminate into self-limiting infections and epidemics. Recent taxonomical revisions based on multilocus gene sequencing such as internal transcribed spacer region (ITS) and partial β-tubulin (BT) sequences has led to identification of newer genera of dermatophytosis.[48] Hence, new genera have been identified and added to the existing three genera namely *Trichophyton, Microsporum* and *Epidermophyton*. They include *Arthroderma, Lophophyton, Paraphyton* and *Nannizzia.*[49] Nearly all anthropophilic dermatophytes belong to the *Trichophyton* and *Epidermophyton*, along with some zoophilic species that regularly infect humans. *Microsporum* is restricted to some species around *Microsporum canis*, while the geophilic species and zoophilic species that are more remote from the human sphere are included in the *Arthroderma, Lophophyton* and *Nannizzia.*[48, 49]

There is increasing data looking at reasons for failure of Itraconazole which includes efflux mechanisms and transporters apart from mutations and there is a need for proteonomic data on the prevalent species to modulate therapy in difficult cases of Tinea in India.[50, 51]

Table 1.2 shows some of the clinico-mycological studies conducted in India depicting the important epidemiological characteristics of dermatophytosis in the current scenario (after 2014). Future epidemiological studies and information is likely to be based on identifying the species by genomic sequencing of the dermatophytes. Molecular diagnosis will also find a place in the surveillance of dermatophytosis which is essential to determine the likely changes in etiological trends and distribution profile of this infection.

CONCLUSION

Defining epidemiology of dermatophytosis in India has become more important than ever before due to the pandemic of recalcitrant dermatophytosis that has silently affected entire India and many other countries. Defining various epidemiological factors and identifying the causative agent by conventional and molecular methods are the important measures to tackle this current burden of dermatophytosis. There is a need for identifying host immune factors that may contribute to recurrent dermatophytosis.

TABLE 1.2: Clinico-mycological studies on dermatophytosis conducted after 2014 in India

Author	Place	Time line	Study population	Number	Age	M:F	Positive family history	TCS misuse	Clinical type	Culture positivity	Isolated agent
Mahajan S et al. 2017[14]	Varanasi (UP)	Jan to Oct 2014	All patients	265	20–40 years	3:1	–	71%	Mixed type (46.8%)	139 (52%)	*T. mentagrophytes* (104, 75.9%), *T. rubrum* (30, 21.9%), *T. tonsurans* (1, 0.7%)
Rudramurthy SM et al. 2018[21]	Chandigarh	Jul to Dec 2014	Consecutive patients	195	Median age – 33.5 years	3:1	–	–	Tinea corporis (59, 30.2%)	133 (6%)	*T. interdigitale* (88, 66.1%), *T. rubrum* (35, 26.3%), *T. tonsurans* (4, 3%), *M. gypseum* (4, 3%), *M. canis* (2, 1.5%)
Sharma R et al. 2017[41]	Sikkim	Jan to Dec 2015	All patients	192	16–30 years (55%)	1.8:1	–	NA	Tinea corporis (54%)	60 (31%)	*T. mentagrophytes* (24, 40%), *T. schoenleinii* (20, 33.33%), *T. tonsurans* (10, 16.66%), *T. rubrum* (4, 6.66%)
Pathania S et al. 2018[13]	Chandigarh	Jan to Dec 2015	Recurrent dermatophytosis	150	Mean age– 32.5 years	3:2	72%	53%	Multiple sites (97, 64.6%)	90 (60%)	*T. mentagrophytes* (36, 40%), *T. rubrum* (29, 32.2%), *T. interdigitale* (10, 11.1%)
Tigga et al. 2018[12]	New Delhi	Nov 2015 to Apr 2017	All cases	300	15–30 year (66.33%)	2:1	–	–	Tinea corporis and tinea cruris (53.0%)	212 (71%)	*T. mentagrophytes* (206, 97.2%), *T. rubrum* (5, 2.3%), *T. violaceum* (1,0.5%)
Nenoff P et al. 2019[2]	Many cities	Aug 2017 to Jan 2018	–	199	–	2:1	–	81.3%	Tinea corporis *(65.6 %)*	149 (75%)	*T. mentagrophytes* (138, 92.62%) *T. rubrum* 11 (7.38%)

(Contd.)

TABLE 1.2: Clinico-mycological studies on dermatophytosis conducted after 2014 in India *(Contd.)*

Author	Place	Time line	Study population	Number	Age	M:F	Positive family history	TCS misuse	Clinical type	Culture positivity	Isolated agent
Saxena V et al. 2020[42]	Mangalore	May to Jul 2017	All cases	154	20–30 years (41%)	2:1	–	–	–	96 (62%)	*T. Mentagrophytes* (55, 57.3%), *Trichophyton spp* (17, 17.7%), *M. gypseum* (15, 15.6%), *T. rubrum* (6, 6.3), *M. canis* (2, 2.1%)], *E. floccosum* (1, 1%)
Singh BS et al. 2020[31]	Bhubaneswar	Jan to Jun 2018	All cases	340	Mean age-31.35 year	1.2:1	48.8%	21.7%	Multiple site (77.17%)	221 (74%)	*T. mentagrophytes* (79.91%), *T. rubrum* (13.53%), *T. tonsurans* (4.36%), *T. verrucosum* (0.9%), *E. floccosum* (0.9%), *M. audouinii* (0.4%)
Das S et al. 2022[52]	Kolkata	Apr to Sep 2018	All naïve cases	103	18–40 years	2:1	50.4%	–	*T. corporis*	55 (53%)	*T. verrucosum* (26, 47%), *T. rubrum* (15, 27%), *T. mentagrophytes* (8, 15%), Microsporum (1, 2%), *E. floccosum* (5, 9%)
Vanapalli S et al. 2022[53]	Vizianagaram	Jan 2018 to Jun 2019	Extensive dermato-phytosis	150	18 to 40 years (64%)	1.0: 0.8	43%	–	Tinea corporis et cruris (62.7%)	78 (52%)	*T. mentagrophytes* (78, 92.8%), *M. gypseum* (6, 7.2%)
Amin N et al. 2022[54]	Mangalore	Jul to Dec 2019	Therapy resistant tinea	190 screened, 64 analysed	18–45 years (79.68)	1:1	78.2%	71.8%	*T. corporis* (100%), *Tinea cruris* (78%)	64	*T. mentagrophytes* (55, 85.9%), *T. rubrum* (7, 10.9%); *Nannizzia gypsea* (2, 3.1%)
Das D et al. 2022[27]	Kishanganj	Jan to Dec 2021	All cases	198	21–30 years (40%)	1.0: 0.8	–	–	92 (54.76)	68 (34%)	*T. mentagrophytes* 36 (52.9%), *T. rubrum* (16 (23.5%), *T. verrucosum* 10 (14.7%), *Epidermophyton* (6 (8.8%)

Key Points

- There is a rise in the prevalence of dermatophytosis and recalcitrant dermatophytosis in India. Majority of the data is collected from the hospital-based studies. Face of dermatophytosis may also be changing in the world.
- There may be some variation in the prevalence based on the region, climate, socioeconomical factors and migration, however, current scenario of dermatophytosis has shown a consistent rise in the prevalence from all parts of India.
- There is a high incidence of spread among close contacts probably due to high contagious nature and fomite transmission of the infecting agent.
- There is a near complete dominance of *T. indotineae* in the country, and this has largely replaced *T. rubrum* and *T. mentagrophytes* as the most common cause of dermatophytic skin infections.[55]
- Terbinafine resistance due to squalene epoxidase gene mutations is widely prevalent in *T. indotineae*, resulting in need of higher drug doses.[56]
- Recent high quality proteonomic data from India has shown that there is a combination of mutation of *Erg 11* gene and increased efflux pumps that can explain failures of itraconazole.

REFERENCES

1. Havlickova B, Czaika VA, Friedrich M. Epidemiological trends in skin mycoses worldwide. Mycoses 2008;51 (Suppl 4):2–15.
2. Nenoff P, Verma SB, Vasani R, Burmester A, Hipler UC, Wittig F, et al. The current Indian epidemic of superficial dermatophytosis due to *Trichophyton mentagrophytes*: A molecular study. Mycoses 2019;62:336–56.
3. Rengasamy M, Shenoy MM, Dogra S, Asokan N, Khurana A, Poojary S, et al. Indian Association of Dermatologists, Venereologists and Leprologists (IADVL) task force against recalcitrant tinea (ITART) consensus on the management of glabrous tinea (INTACT). Indian Dermatol Online J 20204:502–19.
4. Hanumanthappa H, Sarojini K, Shilpashree P, Muddapur SB. Clinicomycological study of 150 cases of dermatophytosis in a tertiary care hospital in South India. Indian J Dermatol 2012;57:322–3.
5. Kaur R, Panda PS, Sardana K, Khan S. Mycological pattern of dermatomycoses in a tertiary care hospital. J Trop Med 2015:157828.
6. Shenoy MM, Rengasamy M, Dogra S, Kaur T, Asokan N, Sarveswari KN, et al. A multicentric clinical and epidemiological study of chronic and recurrent dermatophytosis in India. Mycoses 2022;65(1):13–23.
7. Mishra N, Rastogi MK, Gahalaut P, Yadav S, Srivastava N, Aggarwal A. Clinico-mycological study of dermatophytoses in children: Presenting at a tertiary care center. Indian J Paediatr Dermatol 2018;19:326–30.
8. Bhatia VK, Sharma PC. Epidemiological studies on dermatophytosis in human patients in Himachal Pradesh, India. Springerplus 2014;3:134. 25.
9. Bhagra S, Ganju SA, Kanga A, Sharma NL, Guleria RC. Mycological pattern of dermatophytosis in and around Shimla hills. Indian J Dermatol 2014;59:268–70.
10. Vineetha M, Sheeja S, Celine MI, Sadeep MS, Palackal S, Shanimole PE, et al. Profile of dermatophytosis in a tertiary care center. Indian J Dermatol 2018;63:490–5.
11. Patro N, Panda M, Jena AK. The menace of superficial dermatophytosis on the quality of life of patients attending referral hospital in Eastern India: A cross-sectional observational study. Indian Dermatol Online J 2019;10:262–6.
12. Tigga RA, Das S, Bhattacharya SN, Saha R, Pandhi D, Datt S, et al. Burden of chronic dermatophytosis in a tertiary care hospital: Interaction of fungal virulence and host immunity. Mycopathologia 2018;183:951–9.
13. Pathania S, Rudramurthy SM, Narang T, Saikia UN, Dogra S. A prospective study of the epidemiological and clinical patterns of recurrent dermatophytosis at a tertiary care hospital in India. Indian J Dermatol Venereol Leprol 2018;84:678–84.

14. Mahajan S, Tilak R, Kaushal SK, Mishra RN, Pandey SS. Clinico- mycological study of dermatophytic infections and their sensitivity to antifungal drugs in a tertiary care center. Indian J Dermatol Venereol Leprol 2017;83:436–40.
15. Verma S, Madhu R. The great Indian epidemic of superficial dermatophytosis: an appraisal. Indian J Dermatol 2017:62(3):227–36.
16. Amichai B, Grunwald MH, Davidovici B, et al. The effect of domestic laundry processes on fungal contamination of socks. Int J Dermatol 2013;52(11):1392–4.
17. Vyas A, Pathan N, Sharma R, Vyas L. A clinicomycological study of cutaneous mycoses in Sawai Man Singh Hospital of Jaipur, North India. Ann Med Health Sci Res 2013;3:593–7.
18. PoluriL V, Indugula JP, Kondapaneni SL. Clinicomycological study of dermatophytosis in South India. J Lab Physicians 2015;7:84–9.
19. Noronha TM, Tophakhane RS, Nadiger S. Clinico-microbiological study of dermatophytosis in a tertiary-care hospital in North Karnataka. Indian Dermatol Online J 2016;7:264–71.
20. Hazarika D, Jahan N, Sharma A. Changing trend of superficial mycoses with increasing nondermatophyte mold infection: A clinicomycological study at a tertiary referral center in Assam. Indian J Dermatol 2019;64:261–5.
21. Rudramurthy SM, Shankarnarayan SA, Dogra S, Shaw D, Mushtaq K, Paul RA, et al. Mutation in the squalene epoxidase gene of *Trichophyton interdigitale* and *Trichophyton rubrum* associated with allylamine resistance. Antimicrob Agents Chemother 2018;62:e02522–17.
22. Rippon JW. The changing epidemiology and emerging patterns of dermatophyte species. New York, NY: Springer Verlag, Curr Topin Medi Mycol 1985;1:208–34.
23. Rippon JW. "Dermatophytosis and dermatomycosis," in *Medical Mycology. The Pathogenic Fungi and the Pathogenic Actinomycetes*, 3rd edn, ed. JW Rippon (Philadelphia, PA: Saunders), 1988;169–275.
24. Seebacher C, Bouchara JP, Mignon B. Updates on the epidemiology of dermatophyte infections. *Mycopathologia* 2008;166:335–52.
25. Grigoryan KV, Tollefson MM, Olson MA, Newman CC. Pediatric tinea capitis caused by *Trichophyton violaceum* and *Trichophyton soudanense* in Rochester, Minnesota, United States. Int J Dermatol 2019;58:912–5.
26. Mashiah J, Kutz A, Ben Ami R, Savion M, Goldberg I, Gan Or T, et al. Tinea capitis outbreak among paediatric refugee population, an evolving healthcare challenge. Mycoses 2016;59:553–7.
27. Das D, Mondal H, Deb Roy A, Anand A, Matti P, Ray A, et al. A Cross-sectional clinicomycological study on dermatophytosis: A report from a single tertiary healthcare center in eastern India. Cureus 2022;14(11): e31728.
28. Ive FA, Marks R. Tinea incognito. Br Med J 1968;3(5611):149–52.
29. Atzori L, Pau M, Aste N. Tinea atypica. G Ital Dermatol Venereol 2013;148(6):593–601.
30. Dutta B, Rasul ES, Boro B. Clinico-epidemiological study of tinea incognito with microbiological correlation. Indian J Dermatol Venereol Leprol 2017;83:326–31.
31. Singh S, Verma P, Chandra U, Tiwary NK. Risk factors for chronic and chronic-relapsing tinea corporis, tinea cruris and tinea faciei: Results of a case-control study. Indian J Dermatol Venereol Leprol 2019;85:197–200.
32. Agarwal US, Saran J, Agarwal P. Clinico-mycological study of dermatophytes in a tertiary care centre in northwest India. Indian J Dermatol Venereol Leprol 2014;80(2):194.
33. Jablecki J, Keller R, DeGraw C, Ratard R, Straif-Bourgeois S, Holcombe JM, et al. Infectious disease and dermatologic conditions in evacuees and rescue workers after Hurricane Katrina–multiple states, JAMA 2005;294(17) 2158–60.
34. Tempark T, Lueangarun S, Chatproedprai S, Wananukul S. Flood-related skin diseases: a literature review. International Journal of Dermatology 2013;52(10):1168–76.
35. Gadre A, Enbiale W, Andersen LK, Coates SJ. The effects of climate change on fungal diseases with cutaneous manifestations: A report from the International Society of Dermatology Climate Change Committee. The Journal of Climate Change and Health 2022;6;100–56.
36. Singh BS, Tripathy T, Kar BR, Ray A. Clinicomycological study of dermatophytosis in a tertiary care hospital in eastern India: A cross-sectional study. Indian Dermatol Online J 2020;11:46–50.

37. Gupta CM, Tripathi K, Tewari S, Rathore Y, Nema S, Dhanvijay AG. Current trends of clinicomycological profile of dermatophytosis in central India. J Appl Dent Med Sci 2014;13:23–6.
38. Naglot A, Shrimali DD, Nath BK, Gogoi HK, Veer V, Chander J, et al. Recent trends of dermatophytosis in northeast India (Assam) and interpretation with published studies. Int J Curr Microbiol App Sci 2015;4:111–20.
39. Jain N, Sharma M, Saxena VN. Clinico-mycological profile of dermatophytosis in Jaipur, Rajasthan. Indian J Dermatol Venereol Leprol 2008;74:274–5.
40. Lakshmanan A, Ganeshkumar P, Mohan SR, Hemamalini M, Madhavan R. Epidemiological and clinical pattern of dermatomycoses in rural India. Indian J Med Microbiol 2015;33(Suppl S1):134.
41. Sharma R, Adhikari L, Sharma RL. Recurrent dermatophytosis: A rising problem in Sikkim, a Himalayan state of India. Indian J Pathol Microbiol 2017;60:541–5.
42. Saxena V, Shenoy MM, Devrari JC, Pai V, Agrawal V. A mycological study of tinea corporis: A changing epidemiological trend from *Trichophyton rubrum* to *Trichophyton mentagrophytes* in India. Indian J Dermatol Venereol Leprol 2020;86(5):607.
43. Singh A, Masih A, Khurana A, Singh PK, Gupta M, Hagen F, et al. High terbinafine resistance in *Trichophyton interdigitale* isolates in Delhi, India harbouring mutations in the squalene epoxidase gene. Mycoses 2018;61(7):477–84.
44. Ebert A, Monod M, Salamin K, Burmester A, Uhrlaß S, Wiegand C, et al. Alarming India-wide phenomenon of antifungal resistance in dermatophytes: A multicentre study. Mycoses 2020;63(7):717–728.
45. Uhrlaß S, Verma SB, Gräser Y, Rezaei-Matehkolaei A, Hatami M, Schaller M, et al. *Trichophyton indotineae*–An Emerging Pathogen Causing Recalcitrant Dermatophytoses in India and Worldwide-A Multidimensional Perspective. J Fungi (Basel) 2022;8(7):757.
46. Jabet A, Brun S, Normand AC, Imbert S, Akhoundi M, Dannaoui E, et al. Extensive dermatophytosis caused by terbinafine-resistant *Trichophyton indotineae*, France. Emerg Infect Dis 2022;28(1):229–33.
47. Gupta AK, Venkataraman M, Hall DC, Cooper EA, Summerbell RC. The emergence of *Trichophyton indotineae*: Implications for clinical practice. Int J Dermatol 2022 Jul 22.
48. de Hoog GS, Dukik K, Monod M, Packeu A, Stubbe D, Hendrickx M, et al. Toward a novel multilocus phylogenetic taxonomy for the dermatophytes. Mycopathologia 2017;182 (1–2):5–31.
49. Baert F, Stubbe D, D'hooge E, Packeu A, Hendrickx M. Updating the taxonomy of dermatophytes of the BCCM/IHEM collection according to the new standard: A phylogenetic approach. Mycopathologia 2020;185(1):161–8.
50. Bhattacharyya A, Sadhasivam S, Sinha M, Gupta S, Saini S, Singh H, et al. Treatment recalcitrant cases of tinea corporis/cruris caused by *T. mentagrophytes-interdigitale* complex with mutations in ERG11 ERG 3, ERG4, MDR1 MFS genes & SQLE and their potential implications. Int J Dermatol. 2023 May;62(5):637–648.
51. Sardana K, Sharath S, Khurana A, Ghosh S. An update on the myriad antifungal resistance mechanisms in dermatophytes and the place of experimental and existential therapeutic agents for *Trichophyton* complex implicated in tinea corporis and cruris. Expert Rev Anti Infect Ther. 2023;21(9):977–991.
52. Das S, De A, Saha R, Sharma N, Khemka M, Singh S, et al. The current Indian epidemic of dermatophytosis: A study on causative agents and sensitivity patterns. Indian J Dermatol 2020;65:118–22.
53. Vanapalli S, Turpati NR, Gopal KVT, Krishnam Raju PV, Devi BG. A clinico-mycological, antifungal drug sensitivity and therapeutic study of extensive dermatophytosis in coastal Andhra Pradesh. Indian Dermatol Online J 2022;13(6):747–53.
54. Amin N, Shenoy MM, Keekan KK, Pai V, Halady DK, Kanavu NS, et al. Therapy: Resistant dermatophyte infection in Indiaclinico mycological study. APIK J Int Med 2022;10:263–7.
55. Khurana A, Sharath S, Sardana K, Chowdhary A. Clinico-mycological and therapeutic updates on cutaneous dermatophytic infections in the era of *Trichophyton indotineae*. J Am Acad Dermatol. 2024 Aug;91(2):315–323.
56. Khurana A, Masih A, Chowdhary A, Sardana K, Borker S, Gupta A, et al. Correlation of *In Vitro* Susceptibility Based on MICs and Squalene Epoxidase Mutations with Clinical Response to Terbinafine in Patients with Tinea Corporis/Cruris. Antimicrob Agents Chemother. 2018;62(12):e01038–18.

CHAPTER 2

Etiopathogenesis of Dermatophytic Infections and Mechanisms of Drug Tolerance and Resistance

• *Prakriti Shukla*

INTRODUCTION

Dermatophytes are a group of filamentous primary pathogenic fungi with an affinity for keratin found in skin, hair, and nails for their survival. The three genera responsible for infections in humans are *Trichophyton*, *Epidermophyton*, and *Microsporum*. They are classified based on their mode of transmission as zoophilic (from animals), geophilic (from soil), and anthropophilic (from humans). Globally, *Trichophyton rubrum*, an anthropophilic dermatophyte, is the most common causative agent. However, since 2017, there has been a surge in recalcitrant infections, initially observed in India and subsequently worldwide, attributed to a new species, *T. indotineae*.

Conventional methods face limitations in accurately identifying species, compounded by initial inaccuracies in genetic databases, leading to misidentifications such as *T. interdigitale* or *T. mentagrophytes* by various authors.[1-4]

PATHOGENESIS

Pathogenesis of dermatophytosis involves a complex interplay between the agent, host and environment **(Fig. 2.1)**.

1. ***The agent factors:*** The dermatophytes grow only within the stratum corneum, where it exists as mycelium and arthroconidia. They invade epidermis starting with adherence,

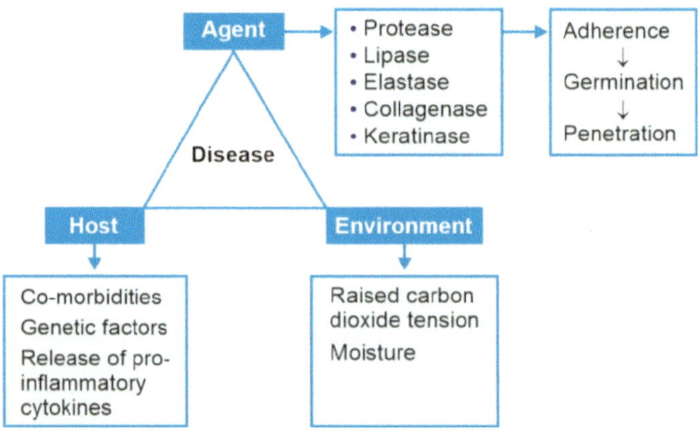

FIGURE 2.1: A depiction of the interplay of factors that lead to dermatophytosis

followed by penetration of corneocytes and later host response.[5] *In vitro* studies show that within 1–2 hours of contact, the infective arthroconidia of dermatophytes adhere to the keratinocytes. Germination of arthroconidia follows soon after, and for the next 24–72 hours the hyphae spread to deeper layers of epidermis for better adhesion and nutrient supply.

Penetration through and into the corneocytes is facilitated by release of several proteases, lipases, elastases and collagenases by the dermatophyte, that also contribute to its nutrition. *Trichophyton* have shown high keratinase activity that leads to adaptation to human skin referred to as "anthropization".[6] The initial keratin utilization is promoted by the genes upregulated at acidic pH, and maintenance of dermatophytic infection by those that function at alkaline pH, where the PacC/Pal signal transduction pathway is responsible for the adaptive pH regulatory mechanism.[7] Several toxins with immunosuppressive activity are secreted such as xanthomegnin by *T. megninii, T. rubrum, T. violaceum,* and hemolysins by *T. rubrum, T. interdigitale*.[8, 9] Further, various heat shock proteins have been found to be over-expressed.[5] Also, mannan in the cell wall inhibit keratinocyte proliferation, thus preventing shedding of the organism.[10]

2. ***The host factors:*** Extensive dermatophytosis is observed in patients with other co-morbidities such as atopic dermatitis, leukemia/lymphoma, diabetes, liver cirrhosis due to hepatitis B/C, alcoholic liver disease, hemodialysis for renal failure, congenital adrenal hyperplasia, Cushing disease, and those on immunosuppressants.[11–13] A few genetic factors are also associated with increased susceptibility of dermatophytic infections, such as HLA-DR8 for onychomycosis, mutations in the *STAT1* gene and *CARD9* gene for unusual or deep dermatophytosis, mutations in gene *CLEC7A* and gene *DEFB4* for increased incidence of dermatophytosis and a genetic susceptibility factor inherited as autosomal recessive for tinea imbricata (**Box 2.1**).[7, 14–16]

   Various pro-inflammatory cytokines such as IL-8, TNF-α, IFN-γ, IL-1β, IL-22 and IL-16 are secreted on exposure to dermatophytes.[17] Classically, zoophilic species elicit larger inflammatory response due to release of several cytokines as compared to anthropophilic species that generate relatively lesser inflammatory response.[18, 19] Antimicrobial peptides such as cathelicidins and defensins are also secreted by keratinocytes that have some antifungal activity as well.[20] Langerhan's cells contain pattern recognition receptors (PRP) like toll-like receptors (TLR), C-type lectin receptors (CLR) and galectins, that identify the pathogen- associated molecular patterns (PAMPs) on the fungi and so when reduced,

BOX 2.1: Risk factors for extensive dermatophytosis

- Atopic dermatitis
- Leukemia/lymphoma
- Diabetes mellitus
- Hepatitis B/hepatitis C
- Alcoholic liver disease
- Renal failure
- Congenital adrenal hyperplasia
- Cushing disease
- Immunosuppressant drugs
- HLA-DR8
- Mutation in genes-*STAT1, CARD9, CLEC7A, DEFB4*

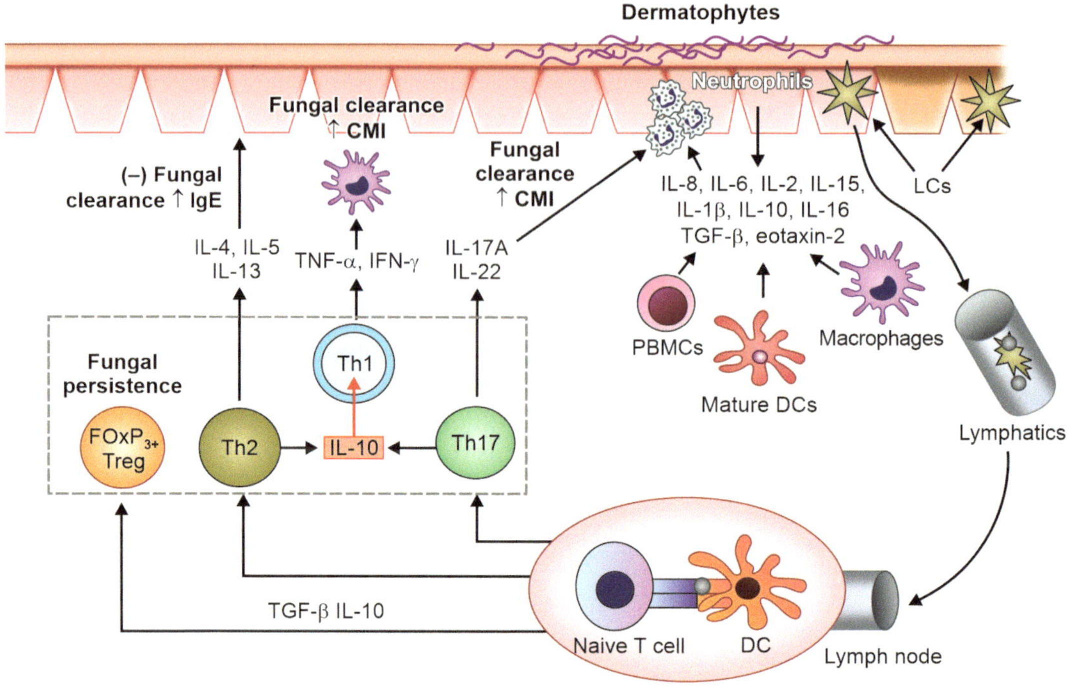

FIGURE 2.2: A depiction of the immune responses to dermatophyte infection. The antigenic presentation of the fungi lead to a host tissue response wherein Th1/Th2 and its related cytokines mediate the inflammation with ancillary role of Th 17. The IL-10 and TGF beta mediated Treg response has been implicated in chronic infection. The immune response elicited also varies with the dermatophyte species involved. While zoophilic dermatophytes such as *Arthroderma benhamiae* induce a wide range of cytokines, anthropophilic dermatophytes such as *Trichophyton mentagrophyte* and *T. rubrum* induce the production of a limited array of mediators. Note that the cytokine milieu is not the cause but the effect of the *Trichophyton* invasion (Indian Dermatol Online J. 2021 May 12;12(3):389–99)

increases the risk for dermatophytosis.[21] Dectins-1, 2 and CLRs recognize β-glucan in the fungal cell wall, thereby causing activation of TLR 2 and 4.[22, 23] This leads to production of pro-inflammatory cytokines like IL-6, 10, 12, 17 and TNF-α, that in turn stimulate the adaptive immunity. Neutrophils and macrophages release TNF-α and stimulate the oxidative pathway causing fungal lysis.[24, 25] Furthermore, IL-17 expression has been demonstrated by three days of dermatophyte infection, suggesting its role in innate immune response **(Fig. 2.2)**.[26]

Recurrent and chronic cases of dermatophytosis have reduced expression of IFN-γ, Th1, IL-17 and Th17 cells population, as well as impaired delayed type hypersensitivity response.[27, 28] Overall, elimination of dermatophytoses is mediated by Th1 type of cell-mediated immunity while Th2 response predisposes to infection or results in an allergic response. Th1 cells stimulate phagocytosis by releasing cytokines like IFN-α, whereas Th2 cells cause the release of immunoglobulins and IL-4, 5, 13.[26, 29–31] Initially, IFN-γ level is low along with high levels of IL-10, which inhibit Th1 response. Subsequently, IL-10 production reduces, while the levels of IFN-γ increase. Key factor in this dysfunction is the elevation of IL-10, contributing to persistent infection.[32] This cycle of elevated IL-10 and IL-17 can further exacerbate the infection and lead to chronicity. Recent studies have also shown IL-17A to mobilize neutrophils and stimulate defensins' secretion, contributing to the rapid and effective control of infection.[33, 34]

Here it must be noted that the cytokine milieu is the effect and not the cause of the dermatophyte infection.

3. ***The environment factors:*** Dermatophytes grow poorly at the normal human body temperature of 37°C and it partially explains the lack of deep invasive dermatophytosis. Raised carbon dioxide tension can facilitate arthroconidial formation, in addition to aiding in adhesion and penetration. Also, moisture is essential for the germination of arthroconidia.[5]

MECHANISMS OF DRUG TOLERANCE AND RESISTANCE

The ideal antifungal agent would be a compound that inhibits potential virulence factors, affects fungi physiology, and also acts on specific fungal cellular targets. The overlapping mechanisms of action of the commonly used drugs may contribute to the multidrug resistance (MDR) phenotypes observed for several pathogenic fungi.[35] Moreover, patients commonly show poor drug compliance.

Clinical resistance is defined as the failure of infection clearance even with the administration of drugs that display *in vitro* activity, whereas ***microbial resistance*** is due to molecular mechanisms used by the fungus to overcome the inhibitory effects of the antifungal drugs.[36] These mechanisms can act alone or in combination. They involve overexpression of efflux pumps or detoxification enzymes, along with target and drug modification.[35, 37–39] Fungal survival in adverse environments, such as in the presence of antifungal agents, relies on the stress responses and involves a global modulation of gene expression, resulting in the synthesis of specific proteins that are fundamental to counteract stress **(Fig. 2.3)**. These genes may act as potential therapeutic targets in future owing to their crucial role in the survival of the fungus.

1. ***Drug efflux:*** Efflux cell membrane transporters are proteins capable of binding to different compounds (for example, antifungal agent), and subsequently extruding them from

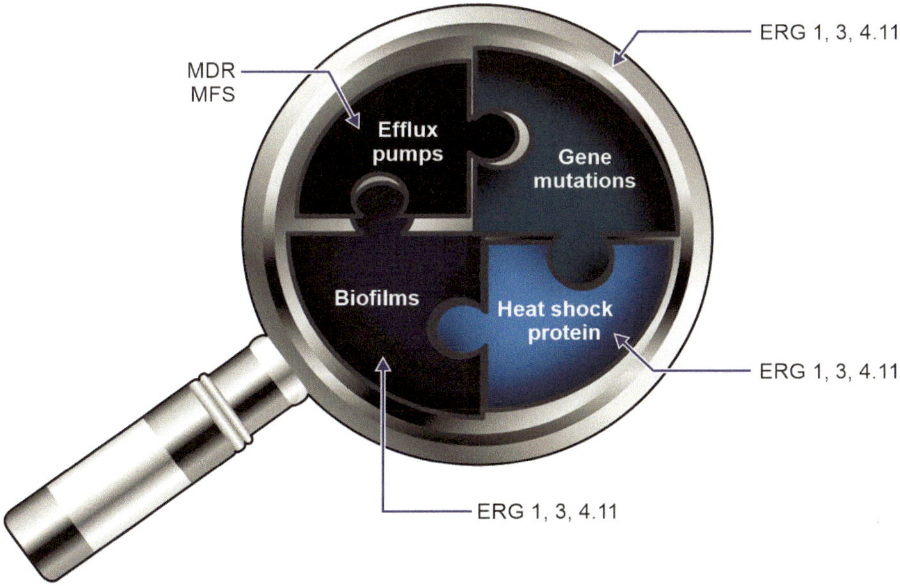

FIGURE 2.3: A depiction of the salient and possibly complimentary mechanisms of dermatophyte resistance

the cell. The expression of these molecular pumps is one of the most important causes for treatment failure, as it reduces the cytotoxic effects of the drug by hampering the accumulation of toxic products.[40–42] The resultant decreased effectiveness of the drug leads to a gradual increase in resistance. This has been demonstrated in azole resistance strains of *T. rubrum* through over expression of TruMDR3, a newly identified transporter of ABC family.[43] Also, major facilitator superfamily (MFS)-type transporter (TruMFS1) has been identified to confer resistance to dermatophytes against chloramphenicol, as well as higher minimum inhibitory concentration for fluconazole.[44] Mutations in *MDR1* and *MFS* have been found in treatment recalcitrant dermatophytoses caused by *T. mentagrophytes – interdigitale complex*, in addition to other mutations (discussed later), that could explain the rising incidences of multi-drug failure in such cases.[45] The implications are that novel agents can help by inhibition or modulation of these transporters to prevent the drug efflux. However, as multidrug transporter genes are also relatively conserved from microorganisms to humans, such agent must therefore be capable of chemosensitizing cells to existing effective antifungal agents while also shielding human orthologs.

2. ***Drug detoxification:*** When fungi are exposed to cytotoxic drugs at sub-inhibitory concentrations, several genes involved in cellular detoxification are activated that aggravate drug tolerance. As catalase protects the cells from oxidative stress, increased expression of catalase genes occurs as a compensatory mechanism to maintain the intracellular level of this enzyme, so as to protect the cells from cytotoxic effects of drugs. It was found in a study that terbinafine resistant *T. rubrum* occurred due to multiple copies of the *salA* gene.[46]
3. ***Transcriptional modulation of kinase genes:*** Under adverse conditions, fungal elements exhibit stress responses for survival mediated via some cellular proteins that are phosphorylated. Protein kinases are involved in the above that may represent a potential target for antifungal drug therapy.[47]
4. ***Fungal heat shock proteins:*** Exposure to sub-lethal doses of cytotoxic drugs to dermatophytes leads to modulation of several *Hsp* genes.[7] There is up-regulation of genes encoding proteins belonging to the Hsp70 family and the small Hsp family as a stress response. Furthermore, it has been shown that Hsp90 inhibition impairs fungal growth as well as alters gene modulation for several other *Hsp* genes along with the *PacC* gene responsible for adaptive pH regulatory mechanism. Thus, Hsp90 can be implicated in both pathogenicity and drug susceptibility in *T. rubrum.*[48] Future efforts in anti-fungal therapy may focus on targeting Hsp90 for the above role.
5. ***Mutations affecting drug target genes:*** The enzyme lanosterol 14-α demethylase is encoded by *ERG11*, point mutation of which has been attributed to the fluconazole resistance encountered in dermatophytes.[49] Target enzyme for terbinafine is squalene epoxidase (SQLE) that catalyses the conversion of squalene to 2–3-Oxidosqualene in the ergosterol biosynthesis. Non-competitive inhibition of this enzyme by terbinafine leads to accumulation of squalene and depletion of ergosterol. Mutation in SQLE causes amino acid substitutions that end up in structural changes in the protein and thereby reduced binding of terbinafine, though the ergosterol synthesis continues unhampered.[50,51] Point mutations in *ERG1* at position 397 (Phe397Leu) have been previously described that is responsible for terbinafine resistance, and is the most common substitution in *T. indotineae* strains reported worldwide, followed by Leu393Phe, and Leu393Ser.[51] The latter substitutions were found to confer higher terbinafine resistance in *T. mentagrophytes*,

TABLE 2.1: Mechanisms of drug resistance in dermatophytes

Mechanism	Clinical implication
Drug efflux	Azole resistance in dermatophytes
Drug detoxification	Terbinafine resistance in *T. rubrum*
Mutations affecting drug target genes	*SQLE* gene mutation; *ERG4, ERG11, ERG3* gene mutation–terbinafine and azole resistance in dermatophytes, respectively
Structural elements influencing drug resistance	Biofilm production
Transcriptional modulation of kinase genes	–
Fungal heat shock proteins	–

T. interdigitale, T. indotineae, and *T. rubrum*. Furthermore, a large part of the double mutants at ERG1 exhibit resistance to both terbinafine and fluconazole, although this hypothesis remains unfounded.[52, 53] Multi-drug resistance observed in *T. mentagrophytes – interdigitale complex* is attributed to mutations in SQLE causing resistance to terbinafine, and in *ERG4, ERG11, ERG3* causing resistance to azoles, in addition to drug efflux pumps.[45]

6. ***Structural elements influencing drug resistance:*** Biofilms are comprised of complex, surface-associated cell populations embedded in an extracellular matrix. Dermatophytes have been shown to form biofilms *in vitro*.[54] Recently, the formation of biofilms in nail has also been demonstrated in an *in vitro* model of onychomycosis.[55] Furthermore, the production of arthroconidia by dermatophytes has also been proposed to contribute to drug resistance, as these are more resistant to antifungal drugs than hyphae **(Table 2.1)**.[56]

LACUNAE IN KNOWLEDGE

Our understanding of dermatophyte pathogenesis is relatively new and still evolving. Meanwhile, the organism is constantly exhibiting changes in epidemiological trends, mechanisms of drug tolerance, and treatment outcomes. The knowledge of host immune responses elicited by dermatophytes and the various mechanisms they employ to develop drug tolerance remains in its early stages.

FUTURE DIRECTIONS

The current anti-fungal therapy targets only a few key elements in pathogenesis of dermatophytes, leaving various others that can be exploited in future. As our knowledge grows about the several drug resistance mechanisms employed by these organisms, so should our chances for exploring newer treatment options as well as to reflect upon the ways our present treatment strategies could be made foolproof.

CONCLUSION

Dermatophytic infections are turning into a menace in the tropics. A better understanding of its pathogenesis and the ever-increasing drug tolerance mechanisms would open new doors into the future for anti-fungal therapy before it turns into a bigger threat. The present therapeutic options are a far cry from what needs to be achieved and an improved insight into the dermatophytes' way of working would help achieve an outcome that is in favor of the human host.

Key Points

- The three genera of dermatophytes that cause infection in humans are *Trichophyton, Epidermophyton* and *Microsporum*. They are classified as zoophilic, geophilic and anthropophilic on the basis of their mode of transmission from soil, from animals and from humans, respectively.
- *Trichophyton rubrum* is the most common causative agent world-wide. However, in India, *T. indotineae* is being increasingly isolated.
- Arthroconidia are the virulent form of dermatophytes, and their pathogenicity involves adherence, penetration and elicitation of host innate along with adaptive immune responses.
- Elimination of dermatophytoses is mediated by Th1 type of cell-mediated immunity, and Th2 response predisposes to infection as well as results in an allergic response.
- Drug tolerance and resistance in dermatophytes occur mainly due to mutation in the drug target genes and other mechanisms such as over-expression of efflux pumps or detoxification enzymes.

REFERENCES

1. Chowdhary A, Singh A, Kaur A, Khurana A. The emergence and worldwide spread of the species *Trichophyton indotineae* causing difficult-to-treat dermatophytosis: A new challenge in the management of dermatophytosis. PLoS Pathog 2022;18(9): e1010795.
2. Singh A, Masih A, Khurana A, Singh PK, Gupta M, Hagen F, et al. High terbinafine resistance in *Trichophyton interdigitale* isolates in Delhi, India harbouring mutations in the Squalene epoxidase (SQLE) gene. Mycoses 2018;61:477–84.
3. Rudramurthy SM, Shankarnarayan SA, Dogra S, Shaw D, Mushtaq K, Paul RA, et al. Mutation in the squalene epoxidase gene of *Trichophyton interdigitale* and *Trichophyton rubrum* associated with allylamine resistance. Antimicrob Agents Chemother 2018; 62:e02522–17.
4. Dabas Y, Xess I, Singh G, Pandey M, Meena S. Molecular identification and antifungal susceptibility patterns of clinical dermatophytes following CLSI and EUCAST guidelines. J Fungi 2017;3:E17.
5. Hay RJ, Ashbee HR. Fungal infections. In: Griffiths CE, Barker J, Bleiker J, Chalmers R, Creamer D (editors). Rook's Textbook of Dermatology, 9th ed. Chichester: Wiley Blackwell; 2016. pp. 32–7.
6. Sharma A, Chandra S, Sharma M. Difference in keratinase activity of dermatophytes at different environmental conditions is an attribute of adaptation to parasitism. Mycoses 2012;55:410–5.
7. Martinez-Rossi NM, Peres NT, Rossi A. Pathogenesis of dermatophytosis: Sensing the host tissue. Mycopathologia 2017;182:215–27.
8. Gupta AK, Ahmad I, Borst I, Summerbell RC. Detection of xanthomegnin in epidermal materials infected with *Trichophyton rubrum*. J Invest Dermato 2000;115:901–5.
9. Lopez-Martinez R, Manzano-Gayosso P, Mier T, Mendez-Tovar LJ, Hernandez-Hernandez F. Exoenzymes of dermatophytes isolated from acute and chronic tinea. Rev Latinoam Microbiol 1994;36:17–20.
10. Peres NT, Maranhão FC, Rossi A, Martinez-Rossi NM. Dermatophytes: host-pathogen interaction and antifungal resistance. An Bras Dermatol 2010;85:657–67.
11. Marconi VC, Kradin R, Marty FM, Hospenthal DR, Kotton CN. Disseminated dermatophytosis in a patient with hereditary hemochromatosis and hepatic cirrhosis: Case report and review of the literature. Med Mycol 2010; 48:518–27.
12. Hay RJ, Baran R. Deep dermatophytosis: Rare infections or common, but unrecognised, complications of lymphatic spread? Curr Opin Infect Dis 2004; 17:77–9.
13. Rouzaud C, Hay R, Chosidow O, Dupin N, Puel A, Lortholary O, et al. Severe dermatophytosis and acquired or innate immunodeficiency: A review. J Fungi 2015;2:4.
14. García-Romero MT, Granados J, Vega-Memije ME, Arenas R. Analysis of genetic polymorphism of the HLA-B and HLA-DR loci in patients with dermatophytic onychomycosis and in their first-degree relatives. Actas Dermosifiliogr (English Edition). 2012;103(1):59–62.
15. Glocker EO, Hennigs A, Nabavi M, Schäffer AA, Woellner C, Salzer U, et al. A homozygous CARD9 mutation in a family with susceptibility to fungal infections. N Engl J Med 2009;361:1727–35.

16. Jaradat SW, Cubillos S, Krieg N, Lehmann K, Issa B, Piehler S, et al. Low DEFB4 copy number and high systemic hBD-2 and IL-22 levels are associated with dermatophytosis. J Invest Dermatol 2015;135:750–58.
17. Sardana K, Gupta A, Mathachan SR. Immunopathogenesis of Dermatophytoses and Factors Leading to Recalcitrant Infections. Indian Dermatol Online J. 2021;12(3):389-399. doi: 10.4103/idoj.IDOJ_503_20. PMID: 34211904; PMCID: PMC8202482.
18. Nakamura Y, Kano R, Hasegawa A, Watanabe S. Interleukin-8 and tumor necrosis factor alpha production in human epidermal keratinocytes induced by *Trichophyton mentagrophytes*. Clin Diagn Lab Immunol 2002;9:935–7.
19. Shiraki Y, Ishibashi Y, Hiruma M, Nishikawa A, Ikeda S. Cytokine secretion profiles of human keratinocytes during *Trichophyton tonsurans* and Arthroderma benhamiae infections. J Med Microbiol. 2006;55:1175–85.
20. Mignon B, Tabart J, Baldo A, Mathy A, Losson B, Vermout S. Immunization and dermatophytes. Curr Opin Infect Dis 2008;21:134–40.
21. Reis APC, Correia FF, Jesus TM, Pagliari C, Sakai-Valente NY, Belda Júnior W, et al. In situ immune response in human dermatophytosis: Possible role of Langerhans cells (CD1a+) as a risk factor for dermatophyte infection. Rev Inst Med Trop Sao Paulo. 2019;61:e56.
22. Tainwala R, Sharma YK. Pathogenesis of dermatophytoses. Indian J Dermatol. 2011;56: 259–61.
23. Dahl MV. Dermatophytosis and the immune response. J Am Acad Dermatol. 1994;3 Pt 2: S34–S41.
24. Bressani VO, Santi TN, Domingues-Ferreira M Almeida A, Duarte AJ, Moraes-Vasconcelos D. Characterization of the cellular immunity in patients presenting extensive dermatophytoses due to *Trichophyton rubrum*. Mycoses 2013;56:281–8.
25. Brasch J. Current knowledge of host response in human tinea. Mycoses 2009;52:304–12.
26. Verma AH, Gaffen SL. Dermatophyte Immune Memory is Only Skin-Deep. J Investig Dermatol. 2019; 139: 517–9.
27. Patel N, Padhiyar J, Singh R, Bloch A, Babaria S. Comparative evaluation of host immune response and cytokine signature pertaining to Th1 and Th2 immune arms in serum and tissue among patients of acute localised vs. chronic disseminated dermatophytosis. Mycoses. 2022; 65(9):877–86.
28. Jha K, Shaw D, Karim A, Narang T, Saikia B, Rudramurthy SM, Saikia UN, Dogra S. Immunological response and clinical profile in patients with recurrent dermatophytosis. Mycoses. 2021;64(11):1429–41.
29. Waldman A, Segal R, Berdicevsky I, Gilhar A. CD4+ and CD8+ T cells mediated direct cytotoxic effect against *Trichophyton rubrum* and *Trichophyton mentagrophytes*. Int J Dermatol. 2010; 49:149–57.
30. Traynor TR, Huffnagle GB. Role of chemokines in fungal infections. Med Mycol. 2001;39:41–50.
31. Al HM, Fitzgerald SM, Saoudian M, Krishnaswamy G. Dermatology for the practicing allergist, Tinea pedis and its complications. Clin Mol Allergy 2004;2:5.
32. Dev PP, Bansal S, Bhargava A. Revisiting the pathogenesis of dermatophytosis: A cross-sectional analytic study of serum levels of interleukins-2, 8, 10 and 17. Mycoses. 2023 Oct;66(10):876-881. doi: 10.1111/myc.13625. Epub 2023 Jun 13. PMID: 37309232.
33. Gaffen SL, Hernandez-Santos N, Peterson AC. IL-17 signaling in host defense against *Candida albicans*. Immunol Res 2011;50:181–7.
34. Huppler AR, Conti HR, Hernandez-Santos N, Darville T, Biswas PS, Gaffen SL. Role of neutrophils in IL-17 dependent immunity to mucosal candidiasis. J Immunol 2014;192: 1745–52.
35. Martinez-Rossi NM, Peres NTA, Rossi A. Antifungal resistance mechanisms in dermatophytes. Mycopathologia 2008;166:369–83.
36. Kanafani ZA, Perfect JR. Antimicrobial resistance: resistance to antifungal agents: mechanisms and clinical impact. Clin Infect Dis 2008;46:120–8.
37. Cowen LE, Sanglard D, Howard SJ, Rogers PD, Perlin DS. Mechanisms of antifungal drug resistance. Cold Spring Harb. Perspect Med 2015; 5:a019752.
38. Pianalto KM, Alspaugh JA. New horizons in antifungal therapy. J Fungi 2016; 2:E26.
39. Kano R. ATP-binding cassette (ABC) transporter proteins in highly Terbinafine-resistant Strains of *Trichophyton indotineae* (Former Species Name: *Trichophyton interdigitale*). Med Mycol J 2021;62(1):21–5.
40. Putman M, Van-Veen HW, Konings WN. Molecular properties of bacterial multidrug transporters. Microbiol Mol Biol Rev. 2000; 64: 672–93.

41. Cervelatti EP, Fachin AL, Ferreira-Nozawa MS, Martinez-Rossi NM. Molecular cloning and characterization of a novel ABC transporter gene in the human pathogen *Trichophyton rubrum*. Med Mycol. 2006; 44: 141–7.
42. El-Awady R, Saleh E, Hashim A, Soliman N, Dallah A, Elrasheed A, et al. The role of eukaryotic and prokaryotic ABC transporter family in failure of chemotherapy. Front Pharmacol. 2016;7:535.
43. Monod M, Feuermann M, Salamin K, Fratti M, Makino M, Alshahni MM, et al. *Trichophyton rubrum* Azole Resistance Mediated by a New ABC Transporter, TruMDR3. Antimicrob Agents Chemother 2019;63(11):e00863–19.
44. Yamada T, Yaguchi T, Salamin K, Guenova E, Feuermann M, Monod M. MFS1, a pleiotropic transporter in dermatophytes that plays a key role in their intrinsic resistance to chloramphenicol and fluconazole. J Fungi (Basel) 2021;7(7):542.
45. Bhattacharyya A, Sadhasivam S, Sinha M, Gupta S, Saini S, Singh H, et al. Treatment recalcitrant cases of tinea corporis/cruris caused by *T. mentagrophytes–interdigitale* complex with mutations in ERG11, ERG 3, ERG4, MDR1, MFS genes & SQLE and their potential implications. Int J Dermatol 2023;62(5):637–48
46. Santos HL, Lang EAS, Segato F, Rossi A, Martinez-Rossi NM. Terbinafine resistance conferred by multiple copies of the salicylate 1-monooxygenase gene in *Trichophyton rubrum*. Med Mycol 2018; 56: 378–81.
47. Garaizar J, Brena S, Bikandi J, Rementeria A, Ponton J. Use of DNA microarray technology and gene expression profiles to investigate the pathogenesis, cell biology, antifungal susceptibility and diagnosis of *Candida albicans*. FEMS Yeast Res 2006; 6: 987–98.
48. Jacob TR, Peres NT, Martins MP, Lang EA, Sanches PR, Rossi A. Heat shock protein 90 (Hsp90) as a molecular target for the development of novel drugs against the dermatophyte *Trichophyton rubrum*. Front Microbiol 2015; 6:1241.
49. Gnat S, Lagowski D, Dylag M, Ptaszynska A, Nowakiewicz A. Modulation of ERG gene expression in fluconazole-resistant human and animal isolates of *Trichophyton verrucosum*. Braz J Microbiol. 2021;52(4):2439–46.
50. Khurana A, Sardana K, Chowdhary A. Antifungal resistance in dermatophytes: Recent trends and therapeutic implications. Fungal Genet Biol 2019;132:103255.
51. Khurana A, Masih A, Chowdhary A, Sardana K, Borker S, Gupta A, et al. Correlation of in vitro susceptibility based on MICs and squalene epoxidase mutations with clinical response to terbinafine in patients with tinea corporis/cruris. Antimicrob Agents Chemother 2018;62(12):e01038–18.
52. Burmester A, Hipler UC, Elsner P, Wiegand C. Point mutations in the squalene epoxidase Erg1 and sterol 14-α demethylase Erg11 gene of *T. indotineae* isolates indicate that the resistant mutant strains evolved independently. Mycoses 2022;65(1):97–102.
53. Burmester A, Hipler UC, Uhrlaß S, Nenoff P, Singal A, Verma SB, et al. Indian *Trichophyton mentagrophytes* squalene epoxidase Erg1 double mutants show high proportion of combined fluconazole and terbinafine resistance. Mycoses 2020.
54. Costa-Orlandi CB, Sardi JC, Santos CT, Fusco-Almeida AM, Mendes-Giannini MJ. In vitro characterization of *Trichophyton rubrum* and *T. mentagrophytes* biofilms. Biofouling 2014; 30:719–27.
55. Brilhante RSN, Correia EEM, Guedes GMM, Pereira VS, Oliveira JS, Bandeira SP, et al. Quantitative and structural analyses of the in vitro and ex vivo biofilm-forming ability of dermatophytes. J Med Microbiol. 2017; 66:1045–52.
56. Arrese JE, Pierard-Franchimont C, Pierard GE. A plea to bridge the gap between antifungals and the management of onychomycosis. Am J Clin Dermatol 2001;2:281–4.

CHAPTER 3

Clinical Features of Dermatophytoses

• Angoori Gnaneshwar Rao • Atiya Yaseen

INTRODUCTION

The clinical features of dermatophytic infection are variable and result from a combination of keratin destruction and inflammatory host response. Symptoms of skin inflammation are frequently less, but can become very noticeable, mainly when zoophilic dermatophytes cause it. Dermatophytic infections can be classified based on the area of involvement as mentioned in (**Table 3.1**).

CLINICAL FEATURES IN ADULT PATIENTS

Tinea Corporis (Ringworm of the Body)

The characteristic lesion is a circular, usually sharply marginated pink to slightly erythematous patch with a raised margin. As the lesion progresses, central clearing occurs, and the lesion takes an annular shape (**Fig. 3.1a and b**). The advancing border is scaly but, inflammatory forms, in general, caused by zoophilic or geophilic dermatophytes exhibit crusts, vesicles, papules or even pustules.

Follicular tinea occurs when a dermatophyte infection, such as tinea corporis, is exposed to occlusion or repeated superficial trauma, such as shaving. It clinically presents as an erythematous plaque with follicular papules or pustules. Erythema tends to be deeper than with classical tinea corporis (ringworm).

Majocchi's granuloma is typically situated on the legs and is caused by *Trichophyton rubrum*. The application of topical corticosteroid on a dermatophyte infection, such as tinea corporis may promote a deep follicular invasion by the fungus.[1] Thus, they are now commonly seen as a part of tinea incognito (**Fig. 3.1c**).

TABLE 3.1: Classification of dermatophytoses according to the area of involvement

Area of involvement	Clinical presentation
Glabrous skin	Tinea corporis, tinea cruris, tinea faciei
Highly keratinized skin (palms and soles)	Tinea manuum, tinea pedis
Skin rich in terminal hair follicles	Tinea capitis, tinea barbae
Nail infection	Tinea unguium

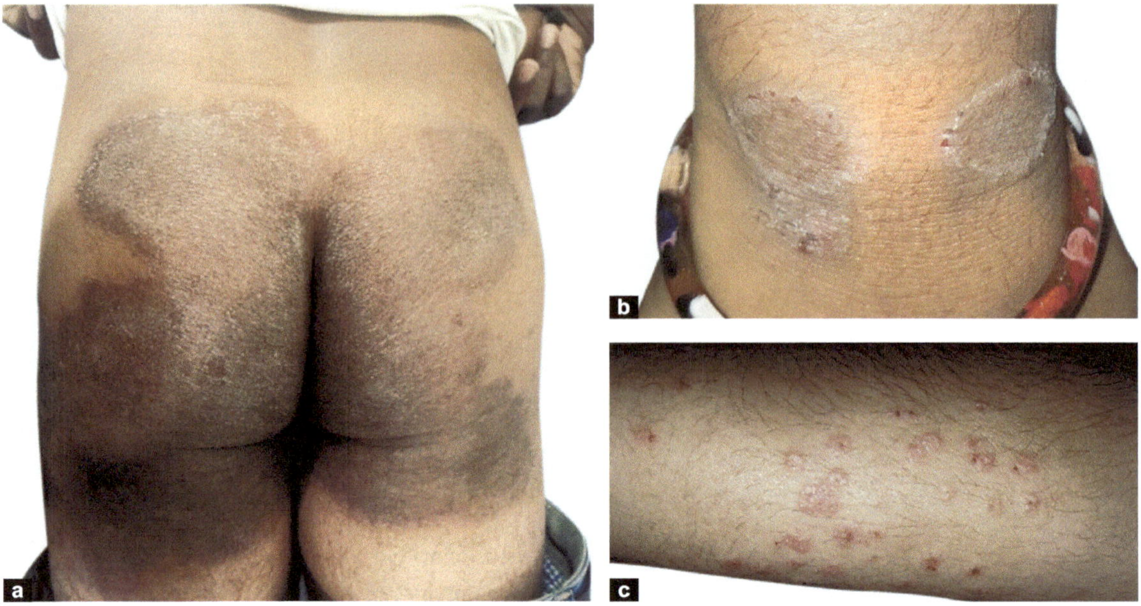

FIGURE 3.1a to c: (a) Tinea corporis/cruris in a young male; (b) Tinea corporis in a female; (c) Majocchi's granuloma in a young patient due to application of topical corticosteroids

Tinea imbricata and pseudoimbricata (Tokelau) is a superficial fungal infection limited to southeast Asia, India, Central America and southwest Polynesia. The causative agent is *Trichophyton concentricum*. The patches are characteristically concentric with lamellar plaques of scales, resembling erythema gyratum repens.[2] Of late, a more common cause is steroid abuse. Thus, the morphology of concentric rings is not restricted to *Trichophyton concentricum*, but can occur with other species depending on the clinical scenario **(Fig. 3.2a and b)**.

Tinea corporis gladiatorum is commonly seen among wrestlers where skin-to-skin contact transmits the infection.[3] The common sites of involvement in tinea corporis gladiatorum are the head and neck region and arms.

Tinea incognito is a type of tinea infection modified by steroids. It is also referred to a ***tinea atypica,*** and can mimic other dermatoses; hence posing diagnostic challenges for dermatologists. In most cases, the annular scaling and the circumscribed margins are absent. Instead, there is diffuse erythema with follicular papules and pustules, which is caused by intrafollicular invasion by the fungus. The varied patterns described include eczema-like, psoriasis-like, parapsoriasis-like, rosacea-like and pyoderma-like lesions.[4]

Tinea Cruris

Tinea cruris is an acute to chronic inflammatory reaction of the skin of the inguinal region caused by dermatophytes **(Fig. 3.3)**. *Trichophyton rubrum* was the most common etiologic agent until 2015 with a sudden change in the disease spectrum towards *T. mentagrophytes/ T. interdigitale spp.* complex (now identified as *T. indotineae*) since then.[5] Interestingly, *Epidermophyton inguinale* was the most common causative agent of tinea cruris during the last century.[6] Tinea cruris is more common among adults than in children, and compared to women, three times more common among men. Tight-fitting, sweaty or tight clothing or

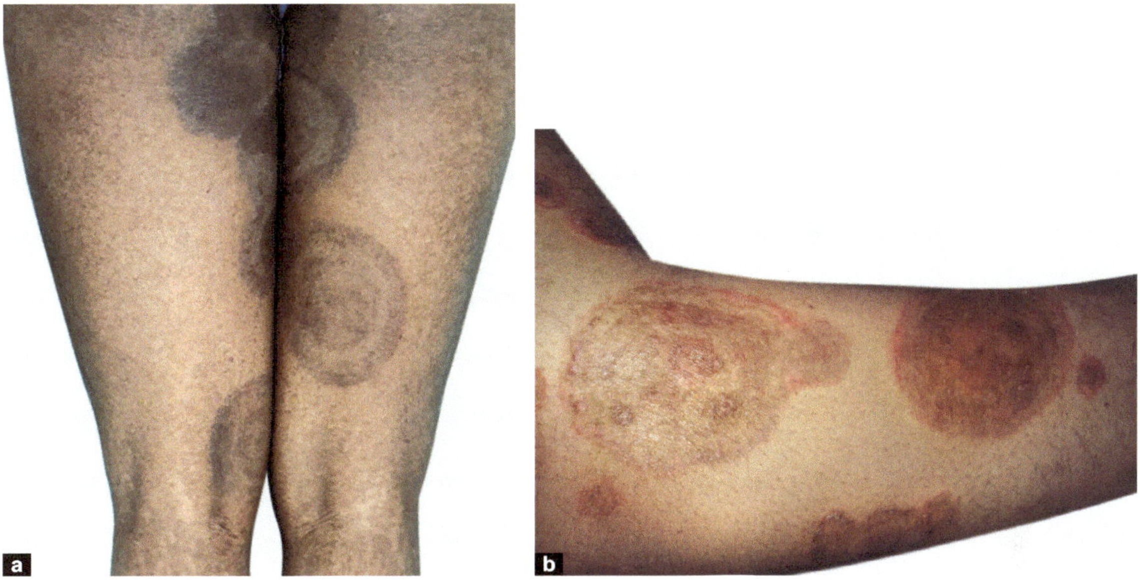

FIGURE 3.2a and b: Tinea imbricata in a young male

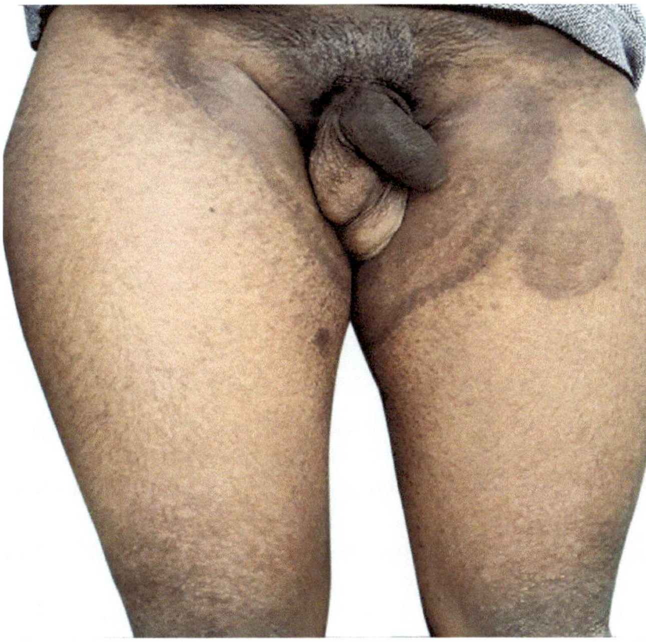

FIGURE 3.3: Tinea cruris in a 27-year-old male

undergarments favor the growth of fungus.[7] An acute inflammatory reaction is often associated with *Trichophyton mentagrophytes var. interdigitale.* Conversely, infection with *Trichophyton rubrum* and *T. indotineae,* in general, is less inflammatory and tends to become chronic.

In acute forms, the patch may be moist and exudative and can present as eczema (eczema marginatum of Hebra). In the chronic condition, the lesions are dry with an annular or arciform margin. Occasionally, some papules or small follicular nodules may develop.

Tinea Faciei

Tinea faciei is dermatophytic infection of the glabrous skin of the face. Although the lesions can have the typical features of a tinea corporis, more often, the redness and the scaly border are less pronounced **(Fig. 3.4)**. The causative agents vary according to geographic region. *T. indotineae* tends to affect the face more commonly than older species, and often presents with atypical morphologies at this site.

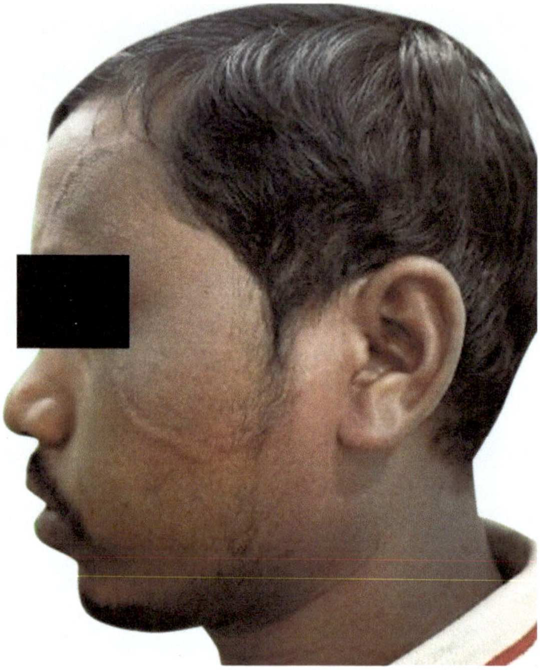

FIGURE 3.4: Tinea faciei in a young male

Tinea Pedis (Foot Ringworm, Athlete's Foot)

Tinea pedis is the most common form of dermatophyte infection in developed countries. The anatomical characteristics of keratinized skin are very important in understanding the clinical manifestations of fungal infections.[4] The skin of the palms and soles has a thick horny layer and is rich in eccrine sweat glands, although hair follicles and sebaceous glands are absent. The clinical manifestations are also influenced by external conditions such as hot, moist climate, hyperhidrosis and wearing of shoes. These factors predispose to more inflammatory lesions. The causative fungi will also affect the clinical presentation of infection. *T. indotineae* seems to have less propensity to involve palms and soles. *Trichophyton rubrum* is often associated with chronic, non-inflammatory, erythemato-squamous reaction. Infections due to *Trichophyton mentagrophytes var. interdigitale* often lead to vesicular or bullous inflammatory lesions. *Epidermophyton floccosum* may produce both types of reactions but infect significantly fewer toenails. Indeed, nail involvement is very common due to *Trichophyton rubrum*. In tinea manuum, *T. rubrum* is by far the commonest cause.[6] Genetic susceptibility to the condition may exist for tinea pedis caused by *T. rubrum*. Moreover, genetic factors are known to predispose to "two feet-one hand syndrome",[6] indicating that not only are both feet infected by *T. rubrum* but also the skin of one hand and, in many cases the toenails and fingernails.

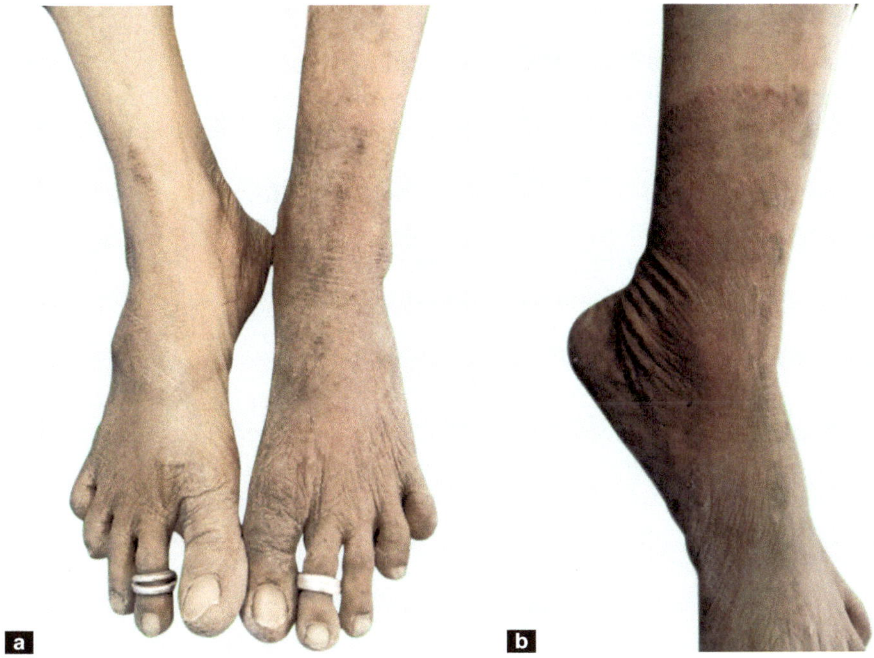

FIGURE 3.5a and b: (a) Tinea pedis (interdigital) over both legs in a female; (b) Tinea pedis extending to the dorsal surface of foot and distal leg

Interdigital Tinea Pedis

Interdigital tinea pedis commonly referred to as "athlete's foot", is a dermatophytic infection involving the web spaces of the feet. It is the most common subtype of tinea pedis. Some or all web spaces are involved, with the web space separating the fourth and fifth toes being most commonly affected **(Fig. 3.5a)**.

Simplex type of interdigital tinea pedis[6]

The clinical presentation may be characterized by dryness, scaling and fissuring or by white, moist maceration. Irritation and itching are often present.

Complex type of interdigital tinea pedis

Features of simplex type along with secondary maceration with overgrowth of the bacterial flora commonly complicate the eruption leading to an inflammatory "mixed" infection.[8]

When significant maceration is present in the web spaces, it becomes difficult to identify the fungal organisms on KOH preparation. In some cases, the dermatophytic infection may extend onto the dorsal surface of the foot, presenting as a typical tinea corporis with chronic, dry, annular eruption with an advancing, scaly, demarcated border **(Fig. 3.5b)**.

Vesicular Type of Tinea Pedis (Dyshidrotic Type)

A vesicular or dyshidrotic reaction of the sole often appears in patients suffering for months or years with interdigital tinea pedis. Hot, humid climatic conditions may be the inciting factor. The vesicular reaction may be limited, vesicles may rupture, leaving a fine collarette scaling and then healing spontaneously. When new vesicles appear, vesicular lesions can take an eczematous appearance. An acute inflammatory vesicular tinea pedis may be accompanied by a vesicular allergic reaction (fungid) of the hands. This pompholyx-like reaction is only seen in severe, acute inflammatory tinea.

Chronic Erythemato-squamous Tinea Pedis (Moccasin Type)

The mild form presents with a few, small, scaly collarettes, and severe form presents with diffuse, dry, silvery-white scaly patches, covering a mild pink to red, inflamed skin. In most severe cases, the soles, heels and sides of the feet are affected. The patients complain of dry, scaly skin, resistant to emollients. Occasionally, the lesions may become hyperkeratotic. In most cases, both feet are affected. Involvement of the dorsum of the foot is rare, but onychomycosis is a common association. The tinea pedis on the dorsal aspect of the foot is mainly situated above the interdigital spaces. In children, chronic tinea pedis is rare. The contact surface of the big toe and the weight-bearing parts of the sole and heel are affected.

Tinea Manuum (Dry Type, Inflammatory Type)

Ringworm of the palms (tinea manuum) is rare and typically affects only one hand.[4] *Trichophyton rubrum* is the commonest causative dermatophyte.[6] T-cell immunodeficiency against *T. rubrum* has been suggested in these patients. Clinically, it presents as diffuse dry, scaly patches with accentuation of the flexural creases of the palms (**Fig. 3.6a and b**). While *T. rubrum* is the most common causative agent, a chronic reaction can follow (vesicular or pustular) when other dermatophytes are involved.

Tinea Barbae

It is an infection of the beard region of adult men caused by zoophilic ectothrix fungi, *Trichophyton verrucosum* and *Trichophyton mentagrophytes,* which clinically presents with highly inflammatory pustular folliculitis or kerion.

Nail Infections (Tinea Unguium, Onychomycosis)

Infection of the nail by dermatophytes (tinea unguium), yeasts, or moulds, is usually indistinguishable clinically and, therefore, the general term of onychomycosis is often used.[6] Toenails are more often affected, with involvement of all or a few nails. *T. rubrum* accounts for 70% of onychomycosis, and the remaining is caused by *T. mentagrophytes var. interdigitale* (20%) and other species (10%). *T. indotineae* is not as prevalent in nail dermatophytic infections with only upto 20% cases of tinea unguium being attributable to this species.

Tinea unguium (onychomycosis) can be divided into five subtypes:

Distal Lateral Subungual Onychomycosis (DLSO)

This is the most common subtype of onychomycosis. The fungus invades the horny layer of the hyponychium, the nail bed, and under the surface of the nail plate. This causes thickening of the horny layer, which leads to raised free edge of the nail plate, which in turn leads to secondary onycholysis (**Fig. 3.7a and b**).

Proximal Subungual Onychomycosis

Proximal subungual onychomycosis (PSO) is a very rare subtype caused by *Trichophyton rubrum.* The infection begins in the proximal nail fold, spreads to the matrix, invades the lower portion of the nail plate and can involve all nails. A rapidly growing form can be a marker of immunodeficiency state (HIV infection).[6, 9]

Superficial White Onychomycosis (SWO)

Superficial white onychomycosis is usually confined to the toenails, and the causative agent is *Trichophyton mentagrophytes var. interdigitale* which is responsible for more than 90% of the

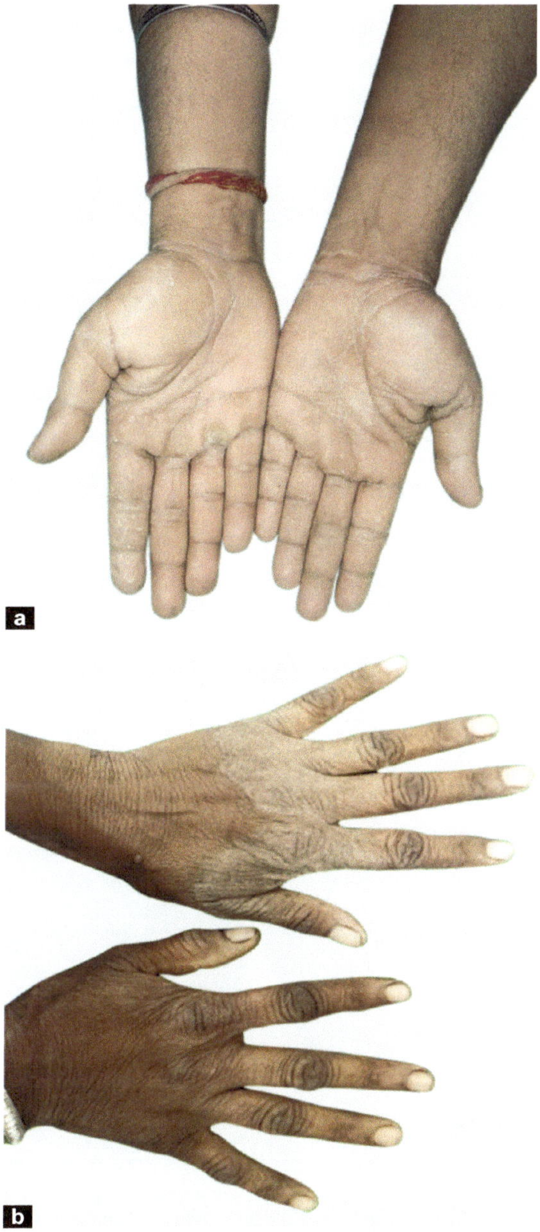

FIGURE 3.6a and b: (a) Tinea manuum involving both the palms and accentuation of scales over the palmar creases; (b) Tinea manuum extending to the dorsal surface of left hand

cases.[6] It clinically presents with white patches with distinct edges on the dorsal nail plate, which coalesce and eventually cover the whole nail. The surface becomes rough, and the texture becomes softer.

Endonyx Onychomycosis

Endonyx onychomycosis has been described as a rare subtype of onychomycosis. The causative agent is *Trichophyton soudanense*,[10] which clinically presents with diffuse milky-white discoloration.

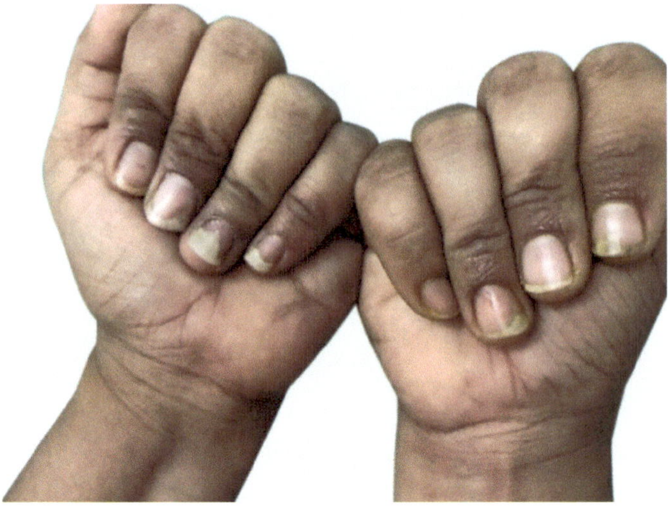

FIGURE 3.7a: Onychomycosis of the nails of both hands in a young lady

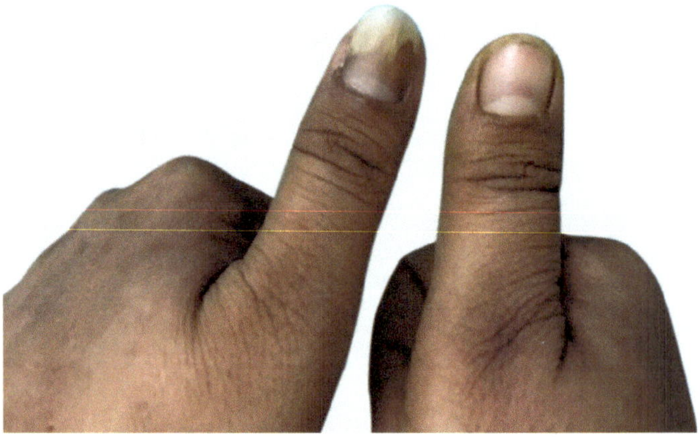

FIGURE 3.7b: Onychomycosis of thumbnails of both hands in the same patient

Total Dystrophic Onychomycosis (TDO)

Total dystrophic onychomycosis represents the most advanced form of onychomycosis. It is caused by *Candida spp.* or due to progression to the end-stage dermatophytic infection of the other four types of onychomycosis and is usually seen in immunodeficient and chronic mucocutaneous candidiasis patients. The nail crumbles and disappears, leaving a thickened, abnormal nail bed retaining keratotic nail debris.

Mixed infections: Bacteria, yeasts or moulds can complicate tinea unguium. The clinical features, including the color, can then be modified due to mixed infections. The treatment of these infections is not easy.

EMERGING SPECIAL/ATYPICAL FORMS

The epidemiology of dermatophytes has undergone a huge change since 2015/16 with reducing prevalence of *T. rubrum*.[1,2,4,11,12] Interestingly, all recent culture based studies form the country report predominance of *T. mentagrophytes*, but studies utilizing sequencing based identification report most isolates as *T. indotineae*.[13–15] This is as the accurate identification of *T. indotineae* cannot be done on culture methods alone.[16] *Trichophyton indotineae*, (previously *Trichophyton mentagrophytes* genotype VIII) is a new species of dermatophytes, which has become a significant concern in treating dermatophytosis due to the high level of terbinafine resistance reported in India and even worldwide.[17]

Changes in the Clinical Behavior of Dermatophytic Skin Infections Since the Advent of *T. indotineae*

With the rise of *T. indotineae*, the dermatophytoses have become more aggressive and atypical in their clinical behavior. A summary of the changes in the clinical presentation of superficial dermatophytosis in the current epidemic like situation in India is summarized in **Box 3.1**.

BOX 3.1: Summary of the changes seen in the clinical presentation of superficial dermatophytosis in the current epidemic like situation in India[14]

Changes in the distribution of lesions in dermatophytosis
- Tinea corporis et cruris–the most common presentation
- Tinea faciei–more common than earlier
- Multiple lesions are seen and multiple body sites are involved
- No concomitant increase in tinea unguium, tinea pedis or tinea capitis reported
- Erythrodermic variants seen–not infrequently

Changes in the clinical behavior of dermatophytosis
- Rapid spread of lesions to form large, bizarre-shaped patches
- Early involvement of distant areas
- Varying degrees of inflammation
- Easy spread to other family members often causing the entire family to suffer
- Post tinea eczema/dryness leading to persistence of itch
- Flare of lesions with increased inflammation within the lesions of tinea after initiation of oral potent antifungal, with occasional systematization
- Chronic dermatophytosis, recurrences, relapses common

Changes in morphology
- Steroid-modified tinea
- Varying morphology–arcuate, dumb-bell shaped, bizarre geographic lesions
- Double-edged tinea
- Tinea pseudoimbricata
- Tinea incognita–ill-defined borders, unclear borders–difficult to recognize tinea
- Eczematous lesions
- Tinea mimicking other dermatoses
- Bullous tinea
- Tinea recidivans-appearance of new lesions at the periphery of healed lesions[14]

Involvement of unusual locations
- Genital dermatophytosis of males and females-tinea pubogenitalis
- Superficial dermatophytosis of scalp skin
- Tinea auricularis
- Tinea labialis

(Contd.)

(*Contd.*)

- Tinea blepharitis and ciliaris
- Tinea of vellus hair
- Tinea in immunocompromised geographical areas affected by tinea being recognized as immunocompromised districts

Signs of topical/oral/injectable steroid abuse and irritant applications

Characteristics of itch in dermatophytosis

- Often disabling itch, frequent nocturnal aggravation
- Persistent itch after the resolution of lesions

Impact of disease on society

- Distressing to the patient and family; high impact on quality of life
- Major financial burden
- Production of unscientific combination of topical and oral antifungal agents by pharmaceutical companies

Quick Evolution

Lesions now often arise suddenly and progress rapidly, sometimes within days, unlike in the past.

Early Involvement of Distant Sites

There is early involvement of tinea at distant sites, which leads to patients presenting with multiple lesions at multiple anatomical locations.

Atypical Presentations

These are seen commonly with *T. indotineae* now: facial involvement with subtle signs, extension into the scalp, prominent pigmentary changes in darker patients, absence of central clearing, minimally inflammatory lesions.

Exacerbation of Inflammation after Starting Treatment

Signs of inflammation have been observed following antifungal therapy. Many of them have been on fixed-dose combinations of topical steroids. It results in the sudden emergence of many papules, plaques, and occasionally disseminated eczematous lesions with itching and burning in areas other than those with pre-existing tinea. Such lesions can lead to a diagnostic dilemma between dermatophytid and an adverse reaction to the antifungal medication, as it manifests shortly after initiation of oral antifungal therapy.

Chronicity, Recurrence and Relapse

Chronic dermatophytosis may be defined as a disease lasting for more than six months in a patient who has been adequately treated.[18] It is common in patients with long-standing infections who have received sub-optimal oral and topical antifungal therapy.

Recurrent dermatophytosis is defined as the disease in which there is a recurrence of the lesions within six weeks after the completion of treatment.[18]

Relapse refers to lesions that occur after a clinical cure has been achieved. Relapse rates between 33 to 65% have been reported following treatment with different drugs, thus largely ruling out drugs as a factor affecting relapse rates.[19, 20] Khurana et al. found no association of occurrence of relapse following itraconazole treatment with extent of lesions, dose of itraconazole used, duration of treatment with itraconazole, previous topical steroid usage, family history of tinea or presence of other skin or systemic diseases.[20]

Post Treatment Itch

Patients sometimes complain of itch despite having completed treatment. The probable causes are xerosis, impairment of skin barrier due to scratching and topical steroid abuse. Some dermatologists are of the opinion that the use of topical agents like luliconazole may produce xerosis and aggravate itching.[18] Khurana et al. reported that 43% patients in their RCT trial did not achieve a VAS zero by the time of achieving complete cure with varied doses of itraconazole.[20] This finding may be attributed to a barrier defect produced by the fungus and may be amenable to treatment with emollients and antihistamines.[21]

Morphological Variations

The morphological forms that have been observed are:

Steroid-modified tinea or tinea incognito: Morphologically, the typical tinea lesion is altered due to the application of steroid cream.[22] It is common to see lesions of varying shapes that are extremely large, either as a result of centrifugal spread or the coalescence of several lesions. Circular or annular lesions with an arcuate or dumbbell shape merge and form unusual geographic pattern. Both immunocompetent and immunosuppressed patients can present with erythrodermic dermatophytosis.[23]

The term "eczematous tinea" refers to patches of erythema with or without scaling that is irregularly shaped, and is frequently caused by partial clearance. Abuse of topical steroids reduces helpful pro-inflammatory mediators and delays cell turnover, which helps the fungus to survive.

Double edged tinea and Tinea pseudoimbricata: Intermittent application of steroid creams leads to periods of varying levels of inflammation producing the 'double edged tinea'. Concentric rings may similarly form when such cycles of inflammation persist for long periods, which has been described as 'tinea pseudoimbricata'.

Involvement of Unusual Anatomic Sites

Involvement of genitalia is rare in dermatophytic infections. However, recently, many cases with involvement of genitalia in males is being seen. Most cases are males with involvement of the base or shaft of the penis. The scrotum may be involved less commonly. It is important to examine these sites as they may be the focus of infection producing recurrence. 'Tinea auricularis' refers to isolated involvement of the ear. Involvement of scalp skin in immunocompetent adults is now commonly seen. Tinea blepharociliaris, dermatophytic infection of eyebrows and eyelashes have been reported. Similarly, there are reports of tinea over immunocompromised districts such as over plaques of psoriasis and healed herpes zoster site.

CLINICAL FEATURES IN PEDIATRIC AGE GROUP

Tinea in Neonates and Infants

An increased incidence of tinea corporis/cruris/faciei has been observed in small children, infants and even neonates in the current context. One must always look for infection in the caregiver in such cases. Dermatophyte infections in infants occur most commonly on the scalp and face.[24] Tinea capitis often presents as erythematous, scaly patches with partial alopecia.[25,26]

Clinical manifestations vary from non-inflammatory "black dot" to a scaly dermatitis-like eruption without apparent hair loss.[26, 27] Pustules may be present.[24] Kerion consists of pustules, nodules, and crusting, with underlying bogginess of the scalp. The inflammatory nature mimics a bacterial infection and often leads to unsuccessful therapy with antibacterial agents. Kerion has been reported in a neonate.[28] Posterior cervical lymphadenopathy is usually present.

Tinea infection on other body parts usually presents with annular plaques and superficial scaling with tiny pustules, which can be mistaken for dermatitis. Tinea faciei may mimic neonatal lupus. Cases of tinea faciei and tinea corporis have been reported in neonates.[29] Cases of resistant diaper dermatitis in infants due to dermatophytes have also been described.[30] In tinea presenting as diaper dermatitis, the presence of an annular margin with a scaly peripheral border is a clue to the diagnosis.

Tinea in Children

Tinea corporis and tinea cruris are common infections among children. Interestingly, there has been a decrease in the trend of tinea capitis in recent times. The shift in the etiological agent from the more common *T. rubrum* to the virulent *T. mentagrophytes* observed among adults has been reflected in children too.[31,32]

Tinea Capitis (Scalp Ringworm)

T. capitis is still a common disease in some urban areas in North America, Central, and South America, parts of Africa and India. The infection may be localized to the scalp, eyebrows, or eyelashes. The causative agents belong to *Trichophyton* and *Microsporum* genera. Inflammation is generally more pronounced when zoophilic fungi are responsible.

Fungal infection affecting the scalp may be classified based on the formation of spores by dermatophytes in the hair shaft.

Tinea capitis can be divided into:[6]

Grey patch *(Microsporosis):* The infection is more common in young boys than in girls. The source of infection, in most cases, is sick or asymptomatic cats and kitten. The infection is transmitted after short contact with an infected person or via fomites. The primary lesion is a small erythematous papule that encircles the hair shaft. Later, it becomes paler and scaly, with the destruction of the hair. Surrounding area presents as typical non-inflammatory or dry type tinea capitis, and the hair break off 1–3 millimeters above the scalp. Wood's lamp examination of microsporosis tinea capitis reveals a greenish fluorescence **(Fig. 3.8)**.

Black dot: *(Trichophytosis of the scalp):* Trichophytosis of the scalp can be caused by endothrix or ectothrix fungi. The causative agents can be anthropophilic or zoophilic. Zoophilic agents cause more inflammatory lesions. The anthropophilic endothrix, *T. tonsurans*, is the most common pathogen in the United States of America. *T. violaceum* is common in eastern Europe, Africa and the Indian subcontinent. In most cases, they cause dry non-inflammatory patches. Black dots can be seen as the hair break off at the opening of the follicle. Some folliculitis lesions may be present. In very severe forms, a frank kerion may be seen.

Secondary bacterial infection with *Staphylococcus aureus* may present with swollen lymph nodes in the neck and scarring alopecia. The zoophilic ectothrix species *T. verrucosum* and *T. mentagrophytes* cause more inflammatory forms (kerion).

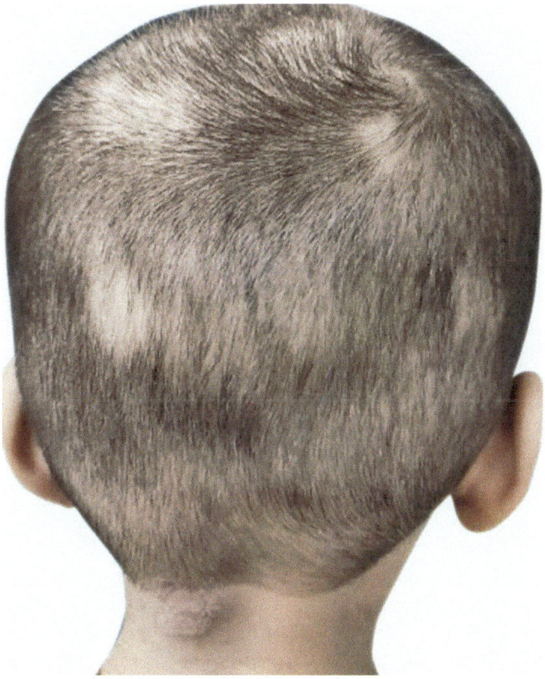

FIGURE 3.8: Grey patch type of tinea capitis in a 6-year-old child

Favus: Favus is a unique infection caused by *T. schoenleinii* and is characterized by cup-shaped crusts (known as scutula) consisting of hyphae and spores, which develop around follicular openings. It frequently leads to considerable scarring and alopecia.

Kerion: Kerion is an inflammatory type of tinea capitis and is often seen with zoophilic ectothrix dermatophytes such as *Microsporum canis*, but it is increasingly caused by endothrix infections such as *T. tonsurans*, especially in urban areas. Kerion is a T cell-mediated hypersensitivity reaction to the causative dermatophyte. It is characterized by a tender, erythematous, boggy swelling with associated alopecia and regional lymphadenopathy and is often misdiagnosed as a furuncle **(Figs 3.9 and 3.10)**.

Tinea Faciei

The face is an unusual site of fungus infection except when representing spread from another site, particularly the scalp. Lesions are similar to those found in other parts of the body.

Tinea Corporis

Tinea corporis is a superficial fungal infection of the trunk and limbs, characterized by circular patches with an active border. In contrast to zoophilic fungi, *T. rubrum* or *T. tonsurans* cause scaly, erythematous patches. *M. canis* produces erythematous scaly circinate lesions, frequently with a raised border and pustules.

Tinea Incognito

Tinea incognito is a dermatophyte infection altered by the application of potent topical steroid. The active margin of the patch may disappear with a loss of scaling **(Fig. 3.11)**. Papules and pustules may be noticeable.

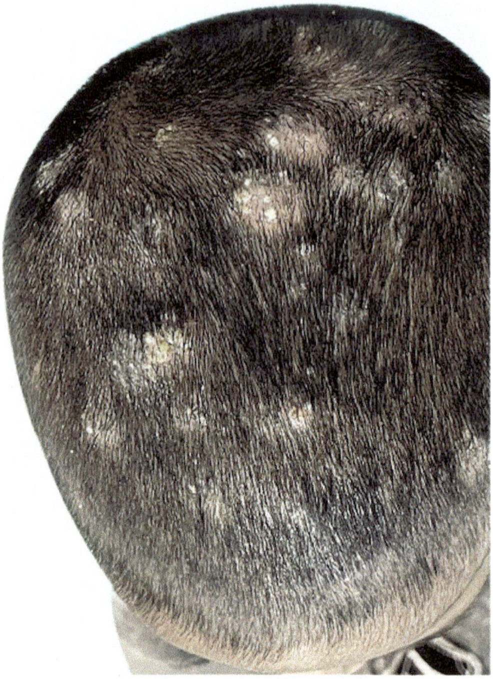

FIGURE 3.9: Inflammatory type of tinea capitis (Kerion) in a 4-year-old child

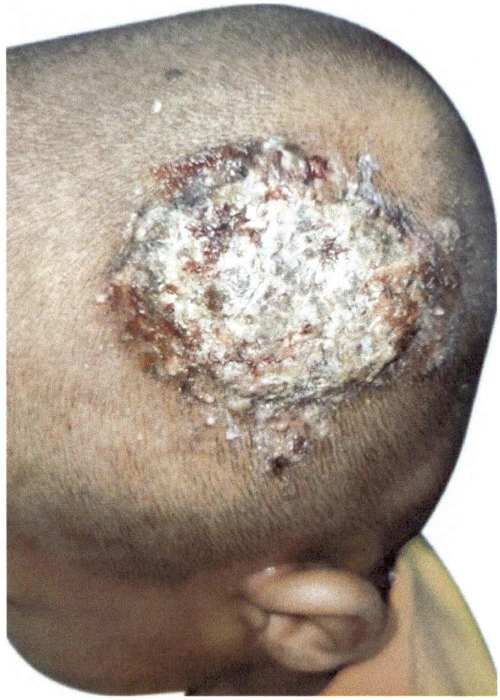

FIGURE 3.10: Inflammatory type of tinea capitis (Kerion) in a 5-year-old child

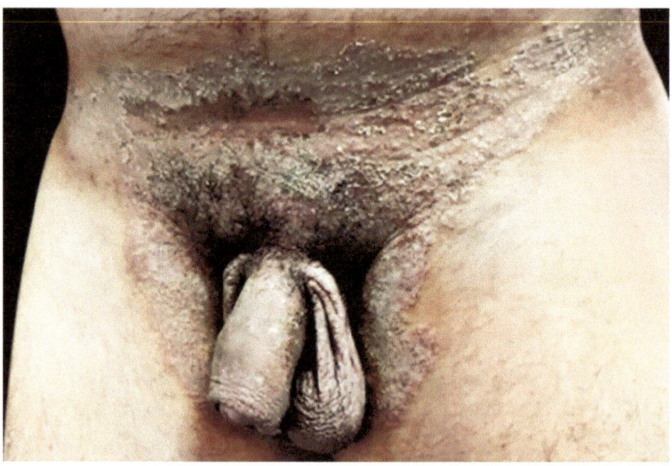

FIGURE 3.11: Tinea incognito (lesion modified post application of topical salicylic acid) in a 15-year-old child

Tinea Imbricata

The existence of numerous small, concentric scaly rings around the perimeter of the body is indicative of an infection.

Tinea Cruris

Tinea cruris is a superficial fungal infection involving the crural region. Clinical features of Tinea cruris in children are similar to adults **(Fig. 3.12a and b)**.

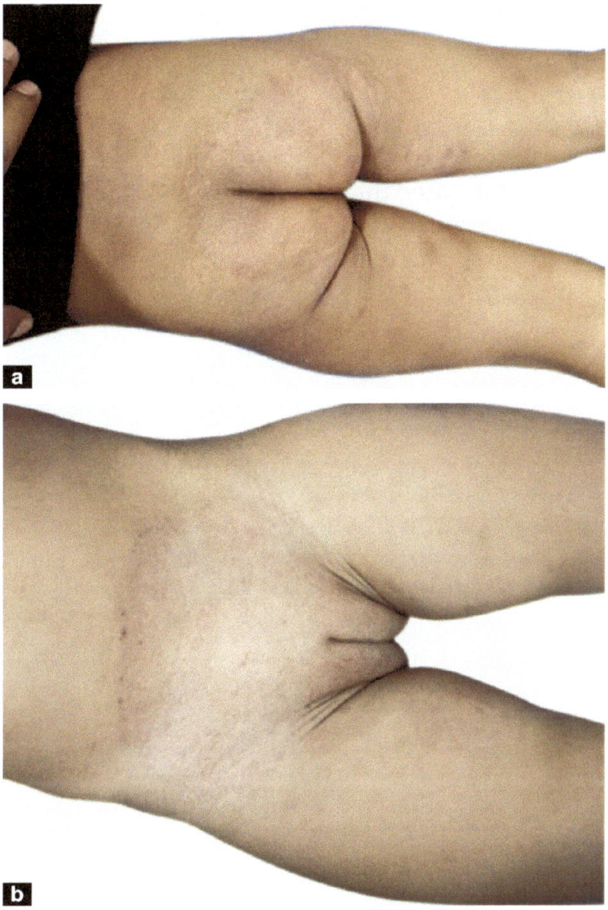

FIGURE 3.12a and b: Tinea cruris in a 7-year-old child

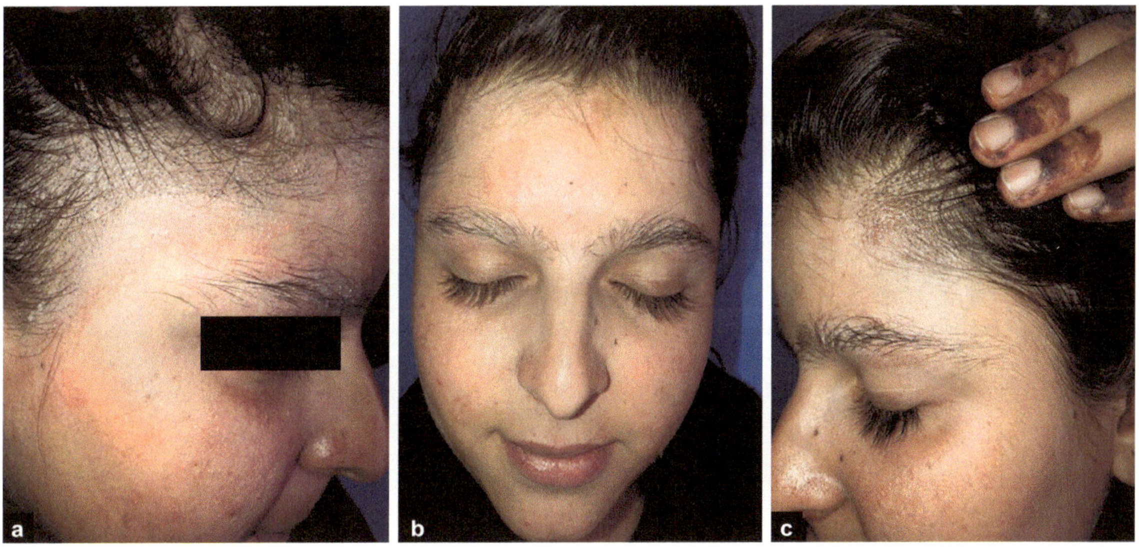

FIGURE 3.13a to c: Extensive tinea capitis in an adolescent girl with loss of scalp hair (a and c) and eyebrows (b)

DERMATOPHYTOSIS IN INSTITUTIONALIZED INDIVIDUALS

The incidence of nosocomial mycoses has increased world over, which can mainly be attributed to the use of intensive therapeutic regimens especially in those admitted in intensive care units and partly because of the epidemiological transformation of dermatophytosis.[33] Hospitalized immunocompromised patients are more susceptible to dermatophytosis. Fungi can enter the body through cuts and wounds, interventional devices or procedures like central venous catheters leading to fungal blood stream infection or fungemia.[34] Although invasive Aspergillosis and invasive Candidiasis is the most widely reported nosocomial fungal infections and is an increasing cause of mortality and morbidity in institutionalized patients, we need to appreciate the fact that there is paucity of data and documentation on superficial dermatophytosis in this population. A study from a rehabilitation facility has shown transmission of *Trichophyton tonsurans* tinea corporis from 6 years old child who had sustained burns to four health care workers after 9 weeks of hospitalization.[35] The reverse was observed in a newborn infant who contracted *Microsporum canis* infection of the occipital region during bottle feeding from the attending nurses. With use of long sleeve aprons for all the nurses, further outbreak was prevented.[36] Severe forms include invasive/extensive dermatophytosis such as deep dermatophytosis and Majocchi's granuloma. Atypical clinical manifestations are common. Diagnosis is based on histological and mycological findings.

COMPLICATIONS OF DERMATOPHYTOSIS

1. **Alopecia:** *Microsporum* and *Trichophyton* are dermatophyte species that invade hair follicles. Clinically they can cause inflammatory and non-inflammatory lesions. Tinea capitis usually results in non-cicatricial hair loss.[37] The inflammatory type, most prominently kerion, is complicated by scarring alopecia. Although it is more common in children, but any age group can be affected. Apart from scalp, eyebrows and eyelashes too can be involved **(Fig. 3.13)**.[38] The hair colonization gets easier in the presence of immunosuppressive conditions like diabetes, prolonged topical or systemic corticosteroid usage, anaemia and immunosuppressant medications. Poor hygiene and sharing of hair care tools are contributory factors. The hair loss can further be complicated by loss of self-esteem in adults and emotional impairment in children.
2. **Superadded bacterial infections:** A normal and healthy skin is resistant to the entry of microorganisms. The cutaneous site of dermatophytosis causes a breach in the skin and serves as entry point for opportunistic bacteria. Dermatophytes cause a change in normal skin morphology and bacterial flora resulting in severe infection. Diabetic individuals with tinea pedis and toenail onychomycosis have been identified as a risk factor for developing lower limb cellulitis, especially when the infection is localized to the web spaces.[39]
3. **Bullous lesions:** Bullous lesions in dermatophytosis have been reported to be caused by *Trichophyton rubrum* and *Trichophyton mentagrophytes*. Bullous and vesicular lesions can also occur as dermatophytid/Id reactions distant from the primary infection.[40]
4. **Erythema nodosum:** Erythema nodosum is a reaction pattern to a variety of microbial and non-microbial antigens. Kerion celsi has been rarely reported to be associated with erythema nodosum affecting the pre-tibial regions.[41]
5. **Urticaria and angioedema:** Infections are well documented causes of urticaria. Dermatophytosis have been shown to have a triggering role in urticaria and angioedema.

Urticaria occurs as an Id reaction to dermatophytosis.[42] Id reactions to dermatophytosis can also present as vesicles, papules, erysipelas-like plaques and erythema nodosum.

6. **Erythema multiforme:** Erythema multiforme is an immune mediated, self-limiting mucocutaneous condition that is associated with herpes simplex virus in most of the cases. It has also been described occurring secondary to *Trichophyton rubrum* infection.[43] In some cases it has been identified as an Id reaction to a distant focus of dermatophyte infection.
7. **Lymphangitis:** Although bacterial infections are the common cause of lymphangitis, but fungal infections too have been reported to cause recurrent lymphangitis.[44] The complication is commonly seen in gardeners.
8. **Nail deformities:** Dermatophytes can affect the nail apparatus resulting in crumbling, discolouration and scaling of nails. If left untreated the nails become thickened, hard and deformed.
9. **Deep dermatophytosis:** Deep dermatophytosis occurring secondary to dermatophytosis has been described in both immunocompetent and immunocompromised hosts.[45] Commonly involved tissues and organs include hair follicles, the dermis, subcutaneous tissue, and even internal organs such as lymph nodes, bone and the brain. Invasive dermatophytosis has been revealed as an important presentation of caspase recruitment domain family member 9 (CARD9) mutation, that plays an important role in the downstream regulation of pattern recognition receptor signaling and antifungal immunity.[46] Clinically, deep dermatophytosis manifests usually as multiple papules, plaques, and nodules, most frequently located on the lower extremities. It has been classified into four subtypes: Majocchi's granuloma associated with *T. mentagrophytes* and *T. tonsurans*, deeper dermal dermatophytosis mostly caused by *T. rubrum*, pseudomycetoma associated with *M. canis* and disseminated dermatophytosis.

CONCLUSION

The clinical presentation of dermatophytoses depends on the combination of host inflammatory response and keratin destruction. The classical tinea corporis and cruris is characterized by a sharply marginated, circular, erythematous plaque which shows central clearing and peripheral scaling and sometimes papules, vesicles, pustules and crusts. Infection caused by *Trichophyton indotineae* is becoming increasingly common and is responsible for the current epidemic-like situation of dermatophytosis in India and is causing great concern worldwide. Dermatophytic infections with this new species is considered responsible with the current scenario with dermatophytosis showing quick evolution, involvement of unusual sites, change in clinical behavior, distribution and morphology. There is an urgent need to raise awareness among general practitioners and the public at large about the need for adequate therapy and role of steroids in this menace. Dermatophytoses can sometimes involve deeper tissues or become invasive, particularly in immunosuppressed patients.

Key Points

- Clinical features of a dermatophytic infection are determined by the keratin destruction and inflammatory host response. Zoophilic species produce severe inflammation than anthropophilic dermatophytes.
- *T. indotineae* is an emerging species which has, in a short period, become the predominant cause of tinea of the glabrous skin in India.

(Contd.)

(*Contd.*)

- Changes observed in clinical patterns of dermatophytoses since the advent of *T. indotineae* include change in distribution (more facial involvement, tinea at unusual locations such as genitals, pinna, etc.), change in clinical behavior (rapid spread, early spread to distant sides, recalcitrant dermatophytoses, easy spread to contacts, etc.), prominent pigmentation after cure, persistent pruritus after cure and change in morphology (unusual shape of lesions, double edged lesions, tinea pseudoimbricata, eczematous lesions, bullae, tinea recidivans, etc.).
- Dermatophytosis in infants usually involves the head and neck area. Tinea at other body sites may be mistaken for dermatitis. Tinea cruris in groin may present as diaper rash in infants. Though tinea capitis is common in children, studies have shown a decline in its incidence.
- Dermatophytosis can cause a number of complications such as alopecia, superadded bacterial infections, erythema nodosum, erythema multiforme, urticaria and fungemia.
- Although invasive fungal infections like Aspergillosis and Candidiasis are common nosocomial infections, superficial fungal infections too are seen in institutionalized patients.

REFERENCES

1. Degreef H, De Doncker P, editors. Fighting fungal infections around the globe. Itraconazole in perspective. Kent: Wells medical holdings; 2000. p.71.
2. Bhagyashree M, Shilpashree P. A Clinico mycological study of tinea pseudoimbricata. Indian Dermatol Online J. 2022 Jan 24;13(1):73–77.
3. Kermani F, Moosazadeh M, Hosseini SA, Bandalizadeh Z, Barzegari S, Shokohi T. Tinea gladiatorum and dermatophyte contamination among wrestlers and in wrestling halls: A systematic review and meta-analysis. Curr Microbiol. 2020;77:602–11.
4. Ghaderi A, Tamimi P, Firooz A, Fattahi M, Ghazanfari M, Fattahi M. Updates on tinea incognita: Literature review. Curr Med Mycol. 2023;9(2):52–63. 10.22034/cmm.2023.345069.1425. PMID: 38375520; PMCID: PMC10874480.
5. Kumar P, Ramachandran S, Das S, Bhattacharya SN, Taneja B. Insights into changing dermatophytes spectrum in India through analysis of cumulative 161,245 cases between 1939 and 2021. Mycopathologia 2023;188:183–202.
6. Degreef H. Clinical forms of dermatophytosis (ringworm infection). Mycopathologia 2008;166:257–65.
7. Degreef H, De Doncker P, editors. Fighting fungal infections around the globe. Itraconazole in perspective. Kent: Wells medical holdings; 2000.p. 67.
8. Leyden JJ. Progression of interdigital infections from simplex to complex. J Am Acad Dermatol. 1993;28[5 Pt 1]:S7–11.
9. Choudhary SV, Koley S, Mallick S, Bose S, Basak S. Proximal subungual onychomycosis caused by Aspergillus flavus in a HIV-positive patient. Indian J Dermatol, Venereol Leprol. 2009 ;75:410.
10. Piraccini BM, et al. Onychomycosis: A review. J Fungi 2015;1:30–43.
11. Sharma R, Adhikari L, Sharma RL. Recurrent dermatophytosis: Arising problem in Sikkim, a Himalayan State of India. Indian J Pathol Microbiol 2017;60:541–5.
12. Verma S, Madhu R. The great Indian epidemic of superficial dermatophytosis: An appraisal. Indian J Dermatol 2017;62:227–36.
13. Singh A, Masih A, Monroy-Nieto J, et al. A unique multidrug-resistant clonal *Trichophyton* population distinct from *Trichophyton mentagrophytes/Trichophyton interdigitale* complex causing an ongoing alarming dermatophytosis outbreak in India: Genomic insights and resistance profile. Fungal Genet Biol 2019;133:103266.
14. Khurana A, Sardana K, Chowdhary A. Antifungal resistance in dermatophytes: Recent trends and therapeutic implications. Fungal Genet Biol 2019;132:103255.

15. Chowdhary A, Singh A, Singh PK, et al. Perspectives on misidentification of *Trichophyton interdigitale/ Trichophyton mentagrophytes* using internal transcribed spacer region sequencing: Urgent need to update the sequence database. Mycoses 2019;62:11–5.
16. Chowdhary A, Singh A, Kaur A, et al. The emergence and worldwide spread of the species *Trichophyton indotineae* causing difficult-to-treat dermatophytosis: A new challenge in the management of dermatophytosis. PLoS Pathog 2022;18:e1010795.
17. Kong X, Mei H, Zheng H, Song G, Tang C, De Hoog S, et al. First isolation of the terbinafine-and itraconazole-resistant *Trichophyton indotineae* in China. DOI: https://doi.org/10.21203/rs.3.rs-2504512/v1.
18. Verma SB, Panda S, Nenoff P, Singal A, Rudramurthy SM, Uhrlass S, et al. The unprecedented epidemic-like scenario of dermatophytosis in India: I. Epidemiology, risk factors and clinical features. Indian J Dermatol Venereol Leprol 2021;87:154–75.
19. Khurana A, Sharath S, Sardana K, et al. Therapeutic updates on the management of tinea corporis or cruris in the era of *Trichophyton indotineae*: Separating evidence from hype—A narrative review. Ind J Dermatol 2023;68:525–40.
20. Khurana A, Agarwal A, Agrawal D, Panesar S, Ghadlinge M, Sardana K, et al. Effect of different itraconazole dosing regimens on cure rates, treatment duration, safety, and relapse rates in adult patients with tinea corporis/cruris: A Randomized Clinical Trial. JAMA Dermatol. 2022;158(11):1269–78.
21. Sardana K, Gupta A, Mathachan SR. Immunopathogenesis of dermatophytoses and factors leading to recalcitrant infections. Indian Dermatology Online Journal 2021;12(3): 389–99.
22. Dhaher S. Tinea incognito: Clinical perspectives of a new imitator. Dermatol Reports. 2020;12(1):8323.
23. Naik SM, Kamoji SG, Nayak J. The rising menace of steroid abuse cascading from Tinea incognito to erythroderma. J Evol Res Dermatol Venereol 2016;2:4–6.
24. Song G, Zhang M, Kong X, Liu W, Liang G, Kong X, et al. Tinea capitis in children younger than two years old: a retrospective study and treatment recommendations. Mycopathologia. 2023;188:461–78.
25. Gilaberte Y, Rezusta A, Gil J, Sáenz-Santamaría MC, Coscojuela C, Navarro M, et al. Tinea capitis in infants in their first year of life. Br J Dermatol 2004;151:886–90.
26. Romano C, Gianni C, Papini M. Tinea capitis in infants less than 1 year of age. Pediatr Dermatol 2001;18:465–8.
27. Virgili A, Corazza M, Zampino MR. Atypical features of Tinea in newborns. Pediatr Dermatol 1993;10:92
28. Dogra S, Narang T. Emerging atypical and unusual presentations of dermatophytosis in India. Clin Dermatol Rev 2017;(Suppl 1) S1:12–8.
29. Alden ER, Chernila SA. Ringworm in an infant. Pediatrics 1969;44:261–2.
30. Bonifaz A, Rojas R, Tirado-Sánchez A, Chávez-López D, Mena C, Calderón L, et al. Superficial mycoses associated with diaper dermatitis. Mycopathologia. 2016;181(9-10):671–9.
31. Khurana A, Sardana K, Gupta A. Superficial Fungal Infections. In: Long SS, Prober CG, Fischer M, eds. Principles and Practice of Pediatric Infectious Diseases. Elsevier; USA: 2018.
32. Rengasamy M. The changing scenario of dermatophytosis in children. Indian Dermatology Online Journal. 2022;13(3):305–9.
33. Alangaden GJ. Nosocomial fungal infections: Epidemiology, infection control, and prevention. Infect Dis Clin North Am 2011;25:201–25.
34. Perlroth J, Cho B, Spellberg B. Nosocomial fungal infections: epidemiology, diagnosis, and treatment. Med Mycol 2007;45:321–46.
35. Lewis SM, Lewis BG. Nosocomial transmission of *Trichophyton tonsurans* tinea corporis in a rehabilitation hospital. Infect Control Hosp Epidemiol 1997;18:322–5.
36. Mossovitch M, Mossovitch B, Alkan M. Nosocomial dermatophytosis caused by *Microsporum canis* in a newborn department. Infect Control 1986;7:593–5.
37. Al Aboud AM, Crane JS. Tinea capitis. [Updated 2022 Aug 8]. In: StatPearls [Internet]. Treasure Island (FL): StatPearls Publishing; 2022 Jan.
38. Dhurat R, Shukla D, Agarwal S, Chitalia J, Ghate S, Jage M. Tinea capitis presenting as diffuse hair loss and significance of trichoscopy: Four case reports. Skin Appendage Disord 2021;7:286–91.

39. Bristow IR, Spruce MC. Fungal foot infection, cellulitis and diabetes: a review. Diabet Med 2009;26(5):548–51.
40. Vinay K, Mahajan R, Sawatkar GU, Kanwar AJ, Kumar M. An unusual presentation of tinea cruris with bullous lesions. J Cutan Med Surg 2013;17(4):224–5.
41. Morrone A, Aldo M, Calcaterra R, Roberta C, Valenzano M, Mariacarla V, et al. Erythema nodosum induced by kerion celsi of the scalp in a woman. Mycoses 2011;54 (4):e237–9.
42. Godse KV, Zawar V. Chronic urticaria associated with tinea infection and success with antifungal therapy—a report of four cases. Int J Infect Dis 2010;14 (Suppl 3):e364–5.
43. Contreras-Barrera ME, Moreno-Coutina G, Torres-Guerrero DE, Aguilar-Donis A, Arenas R. Erythema multiforme secondary to cutaneous *Trichophyton mentagrophytes* infection. Rev Iberoam Micol 2009;26(2):149–51.
44. Young JR, Dewolfe VG. Recurrent lymphangitis of the leg associated with dermatophytosis. Report of 25 consecutive cases. Cleve Clin 1960;27:19–24.
45. Warycha MA, Leger M, Tzu J, Kamino H, Stein J. Deep dermatophytosis caused by *Trichophyton rubrum*. Dermatol Online J 2011;17(10):21.
46. Want R, Huang C, Zhang Y, Li R. Invasive dermatophyte infection: a systematic review. Mycoses 2021;64:340–8.

CHAPTER 4

Laboratory Investigations

• Nayankumar H Patel • Jyothi Jayaraman

INTRODUCTION

In routine clinical practice, scope of laboratory investigation is limited to confirmation of the clinical diagnosis or as a tool to differentiate one from the other similar dermatosis. For epidemiological purpose, investigations help in establishing species of causative fungi causing an outbreak, establishing drug susceptibility to antifungals, and studying the host immune response to fungi.

The uprise of the new species – *T. indotineae* in the country over past few years, and its subsequent worldwide spread, has led to a renewed interest in techniques required for precise molecular characterization of dermatophytes, and in knowing drug susceptibility patterns of the prevalent species to guide clinical management. Further, there is a heightened interest in documenting antifungal resistance mechanisms and virulence mechanisms of this new species to achieve better therapeutic outcomes.

SMEAR EXAMINATION

Taking skin scrapings followed by microscopic examination of potassium hydroxide (KOH) mount is a simple laboratory technique employed in diagnosis of fungal infections of skin, hair and nails. It is of particular importance in dermatophytosis due to ease of testing and faster results as compared to the gold standard fungal culture, and hence it is routinely employed.

KOH is a strong alkaline solution which can soften and disintegrate the keratin debris without affecting the fungal cell wall and thus aids in easy visualization of the fungal elements.

Methodology

Materials

Sterile glass slide, cover slip, KOH solution (10, 20 or 40%), microscope and Bunsen's burner, and equipment for specimen collection (scalpel blade, nail clipper, etc.).

Preparation

Various concentrations of KOH solution are available but commonly used is the 10% concentration. It is prepared by addition of 10 g of KOH crystals to 50 ml of distilled water and stirring until complete dissolution. Glycerol (10 ml) is added to prevent drying and distilled water is added to prepare a solution of 100 ml volume.

Specimen Collection

1. *Dermatophytosis affected skin*: Area selected is first cleaned with alcohol. Blunt edge of a sterile scalpel blade is used to gently scrape the skin from advancing edge or border of the skin lesion. Material collected may be transported in a folded black paper or directly transferred onto the glass slide. In case of blisters, fine scissors/scalpel blade is used to cut open the blister roof which is then used as the specimen.
2. *Tinea capitis*: Infected short stubs of hair or lustreless hair along with the root can be collected gently by using epilation forceps. In black-dot infections, scraping the skin of the scalp along with stumps of infected roots and scales would give a high yield of dermatophytes. Other methods such as rubbing, using moist gauze piece or toothbrush have also been tried.[1–3]
3. *Tinea unguium*: Full thickness nail specimen is ideal. Nail clippings are taken (as proximal as possible) using a nail clipper and nail scrapings are also collected (from under surface of the nail-plate, using flat end of a dental probe, as most infections begin at the hyponychium.[3] In Superficial white onychomycosis cases, superficial scrapings may yield positive results.[4]

Procedure[2]

1. The specimen is placed on a sterile glass slide.
2. Appropriate strength of KOH solution is added. For routine use 10–20% concentration is sufficient. In case of thick or hyperkeratotic lesions, and nail specimens, 20–40% solution is preferred.
3. Cover slip is placed and then gently pressed to prevent formation of air bubbles.
4. Excess solution may be removed using blotting paper.
5. Skin specimens usually need around 10–15 minutes for the clearing action of KOH, while nail specimens may require up to 24 hours; hence cutting into small pieces is useful to shorten the time required.
6. Slide may be gently preheated to hasten the keratin digestion, prior to the microscopic examination.
7. Low power examination (10×) is then performed under low lighting conditions by lowering the condenser. Lighting is of paramount importance as over illumination may render the fungal elements invisible.
8. High power magnification (40×) under good illumination is further performed to study the morphology of fungi.

Results

Septate hyphal elements which are long, branching, with or without arthroconidiospores, are characteristic of dermatophytes **(Fig. 4.1)**. These appear refractile on lower magnification. Use of high power helps to appreciate the morphological characteristics. Some artefacts such as polygonal shaped cholesterol forming deposits around epithelial cell margins known as "**Mosaic fungus**", cloth or cotton fibers and air bubbles may be mistaken for the fungal elements. Hence, prior cleansing of the area of specimen collection with alcohol to avoid contaminants and use of a clean glass slide is important.[3] Epithelial cell margins become less apparent on change of fine magnification, as compared to the dermatophyte hyphal elements **(Fig. 4.2)**.

In case of tinea capitis, arthrospores are seen either penetrating the hair shaft (endothrix) or lie outside the hair shaft (ectothrix) **(Fig. 4.3)**.

In case of onychomycosis, KOH mount is useful in differentiating dermatophytes from non-dermatophytes showing hyphae versus pseudohyphae with blastoconidia.[2]

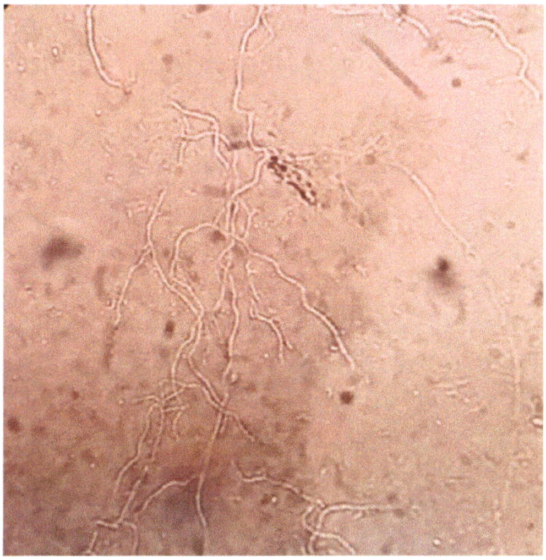

FIGURE 4.1: Long, branched, septate hyphae of dermatophytes on KOH mount

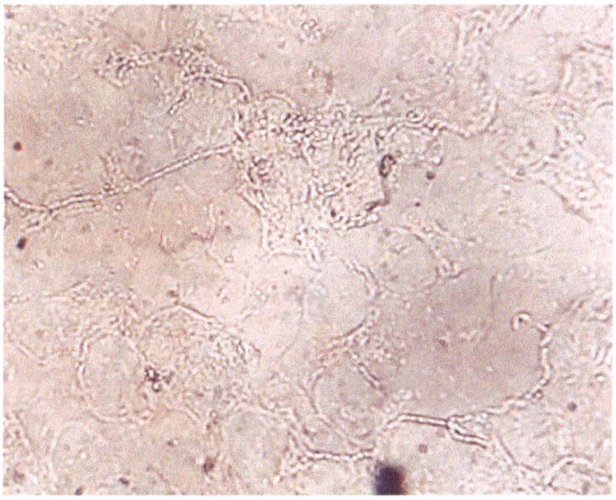

FIGURE 4.2: Well demarcated hyphae in contrast with less apparent epithelial cell margins on changing fine magnification

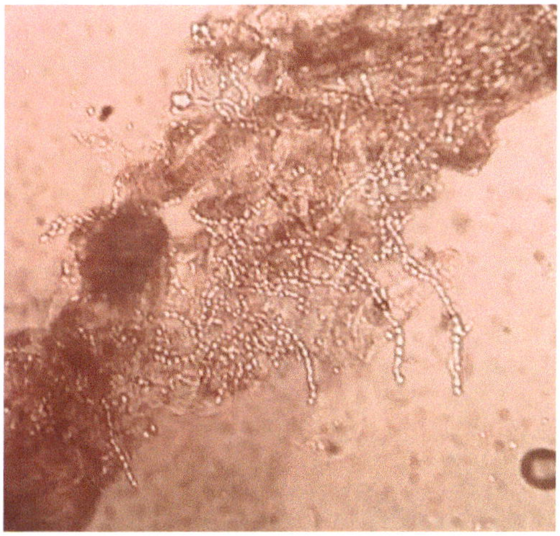

FIGURE 4.3: KOH mount of hair showing hyphae and arthroconidia penetrating the hair shaft

Modifications

1. Use of 40% Dimethyl sulphoxide (DMSO) for a rapid keratolysis, along with 10% KOH solution can significantly reduce the resting time from 15 minutes to 5 minutes in skin specimens. Similar benefits are noted with nail specimens where it considerably shortens the waiting period. Added advantages are prevention of drying of specimens and that it precludes the need for pre-warming.

   Addition of contrast stains such as Parker blue stain (fungal elements stain blue-violet), 1% Chicago sky blue (fungal elements stain blue), fluorescent stains, e.g. Calcofluor white (fungal elements show apple green fluorescence in UV light) can increase the sensitivity of KOH mount testing.[1] Calcofluor white (CFW) is a fluorescent blue dye commonly used in microbiology laboratories for fungal identification. It binds to the chitin in the fungal cell wall and brightly fluoresces on exposure to ultraviolet (UV) light (**Fig. 4.4**). Although considered a superior method for dermatophyte detection, bedside use of this technique is limited by the increased cost and complexity associated with fluorescence microscopes. A modification used CFW and an inexpensive and easily available handheld 395-nm light-emitting diode flashlight (TaoTronics model TT-FL001, TaoTronics, Sunvalley Group, Shenzhen, China) as an effective means of detection.
2. *Cellophane tape method*: In this technique, a cellophane tape is pressed over skin lesion and then it is applied on a sterile glass slide containing 1–2 drops of KOH solution. It is useful when sparse scales are seen and in children who are apprehensive with use of scalpel blade; and is a faster technique as compared to the traditional method. It may also be used for collecting specimen towards fungal culture by transferring the material directly into the culture plates.[1,3]

Advantages of KOH Mount[1]

1. Over all sensitivity is up to 60–70%, depending on expertise of examiner.
2. Simple technique.
3. Reliable outpatient technique and requires very few material.
4. Economical and with faster results as compared to fungal culture which may take up to 2–3 weeks to yield results.
5. Easy to perform and interpret with minimal training.

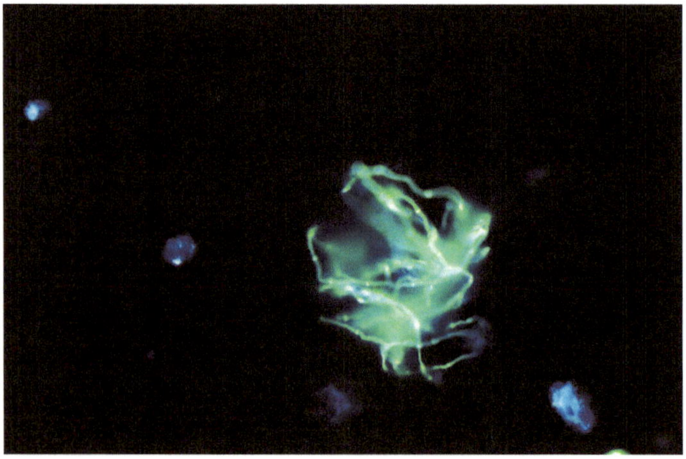

FIGURE 4.4: Fluorescence of fungus under UV light using the Calcofluor white dye

6. Useful screening test in doubtful cases of dermatophytosis.
7. In onychomycosis, it helps to differentiate dermatophytes from non-dermatophytes, and thus to choose an appropriate treatment.

Future Directions

Utility of KOH mount as a prognostic tool is a hitherto less explored field. A change in morphology of hyphae from long, branching hyphae (which may extend beyond the viewing field on microscopy) to short stumpy hyphal elements that have lost branching has been reported following a good treatment response **(Fig. 4.5)**. Reduction in branching may indicate reduced spark cell proliferation action of ergosterol and fragmentation indicates break in structural integrity of dermatophytes. Hence, continuing treatment till complete clearance of these hyphae has been reported to present with fewer relapses.[5, 6] Another study has suggested a semi-quantitative grading termed as "Hyphal index", akin to Bacteriological index (BI) used in Hansen's disease, to study the fungal load and test its utility as a prognostic marker, and to compare the effectiveness of two different antifungals.[7] Further research may be necessary for the standardization and validity of these tools.

DERMOSCOPY

Dermatoscopy or epiluminescence microscopy is an effective, non-invasive technique used in diagnosis of the cutaneous disorders. It employs the use of a hand-held device known as dermatoscope or dermoscope that functionally resembles a magnifying lens and has an inbuilt system for illumination. This technique helps the visualization of subtle features of cutaneous lesions on the surface as well as in depth study till the level of reticular dermis.[8] In this chapter, we review the utility of dermoscopy in dermatophytosis affecting the skin, hair, nails.

Principle

Transillumination of the skin lesion to study the details by using higher magnification is employed in a dermoscope. Advanced dermoscopes are equipped with image capture technology and analytical capacity by using an inbuilt software.

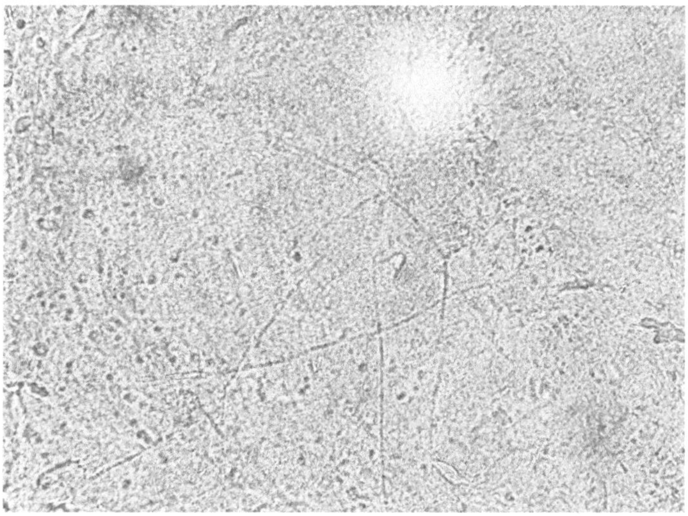

FIGURE 4.5: Short hyphae with loss of branching signifying good treatment response

Technique

There are two techniques which can be employed, namely—contact and non-contact. In the contact technique, there is a contact plate on the dermoscope that is applied on a skin lesion in the presence of a linkage fluid in between the two surfaces and it has a limitation of lower magnification, i.e. only up to 20×. The non-contact technique employs the use of a cross-polarized lens and is not in direct contact with the skin which is especially useful in infectious disorders and can magnify the lesion up to 200×. However, it has disadvantages such as lower illumination and resolution.[9]

Utility of Dermoscopy in Dermatophytosis

Skin Lesions

Various aspects to be noted during dermoscopic evaluation of dermatophytosis on skin are globules, scales, background color, follicular area, color of terminal and vellus hair. Reddish brown colored globules due to acute inflammatory changes, minimal scaling, pale or bright red background are commonly seen in the new lesions. In older lesions, due to melanin deposition as a part of post-inflammatory stage, dark brown to black colored globules and abundant scales may be seen over a greyish background.[10] Halo around brown globule has been reported in a case report by Knopfel et al.[11]

Scales in follicular and perifollicular areas and skin creases have been reported. Of particular interest is the presence of fine scales along the palmar creases in tinea manuum. This finding may help in differentiating it from close clinical mimics such as psoriasis and hand eczema.[10, 12]

Dilution of the pigment in terminal and vellus hairs leading to hypopigmented hairs and interrupted medulla of terminal hairs is suggestive of invasion of the hair shaft by dermatophytes. It however, does not correlate with the duration of the infection. Vellus hair infection has been noted as an indicator for need to start oral antifungals, and in treated cases, it may be suggestive of need for prolonged therapy.[10, 11]

Other findings that have been reported are red dots or tips of microvasculature, micropustules (due to epidermal neutrophilic abscesses) seen around the hair follicles and are suggestive of inflammation.[10]

Tinea capitis

Dermoscopy has been found to be particularly useful in diagnosis of hair and scalp disorders and is denoted by the term "trichoscopy".

Infiltration of hair shaft by hyphae can affect the integrity of the hair shaft leading to comma shaped, zig-zag and cork screw hairs. Further breakage can lead to broken, dystrophic hair and black dots.[13] **Comma hairs** are produced by twisting of hair shaft filled with fungal hyphae and are of uniform thickness and pigmentation. Although it is characteristically seen in tinea capitis, it has been reported in alopecia areata and trichotillomania as well.

Zig-zag shaped hairs have been noted in ectothrix type of tinea capitis. Hairs are bent at sharp angles due to transverse shaft fracture.[14]

Cork screw hairs were described by Hughes et al. as a dermoscopic indicator of endothrix tinea capitis in the black children.[15] These have been more commonly reported in *Trichophyton* tinea capitis as compared to *Microsporum* tinea capitis. This finding may be useful to differentiate between these infections at an early stage and enable us to choose appropriate antifungal therapy.[16]

Morse code appearance, characterized by appearance of multiple transverse white bands in the hair shaft, are due to collection of spores around the hair shaft and often associated with ectothrix infection.[14] It suggests a heavy load of infection. Presence of diffuse scaling, morse code and bent hairs may suggest tinea capitis by *Microsporum* species. Woods lamp examination to look for yellow-green fluorescence is of added value in such cases.[14, 16]

Other findings such as bent hairs, "i" hairs and presence of white sheath have also been noted in tinea capitis.

Tinea incognito

Tinea incognito can manifest with varying morphology and atypical presentation, making the diagnosis a challenge especially when side laboratory facilities are not readily available for a KOH mount or fungal culture. Erythematous, concentric areas, presence of follicular micropustules and halo around black-colored dots have been described. In hair bearing sites, comma hairs, morse code hairs and cork screw hairs have been noted.[14, 17]

Onychomycosis

Dermoscopy is a quick, non-invasive alternative to KOH examination or fungal culture which often yield negative results and are time consuming. The procedure of examining the nails with a dermoscope is known as 'onychoscopy'.

In distal subungual onychomycosis, presence of longitudinal streaks of white, brown, yellow color along with onycholysis has been described. In a study by Kaya IZG et al. longitudinal striations were associated with *T. tonsurans* infections.[18]

Aurora pattern which is the irregular streaks of color noted in the onycholytic nail plate resembling the northern lights or 'Aurora borealis' may be noted in some cases **(Fig. 4.6)**.[14]

White longitudinal indentations facing proximally in areas of onychomycosis with jagged edges termed as "spikes" is yet another characteristic finding.[14, 16] These findings can help to differentiate onychomycosis from traumatic onycholysis **(Figs 4.6 and 4.7)**.

Subungual hyperkeratosis with a "ruin like" appearance is also known to be associated with total dystrophic onychomycosis.[14, 18]

Transverse striate pattern and homogeneous leukonychia has been associated with white superficial onychomycosis.[18]

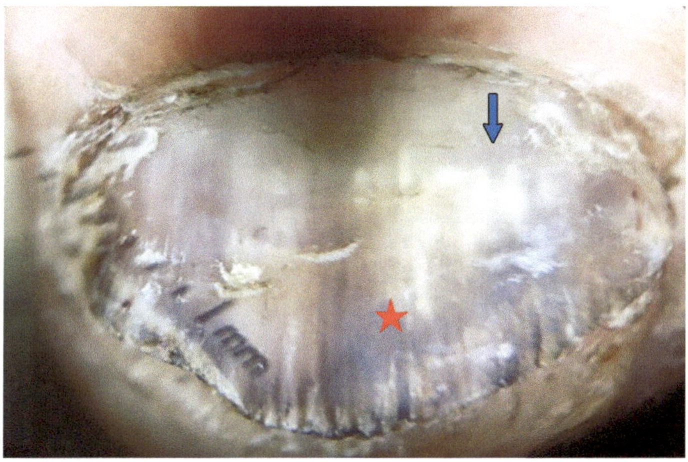

FIGURE 4.6: Aurora borealis pattern (arrow) and longitudinal striations (star) facing proximally, called as spikes, seen on dermatoscopy in onychomycosis

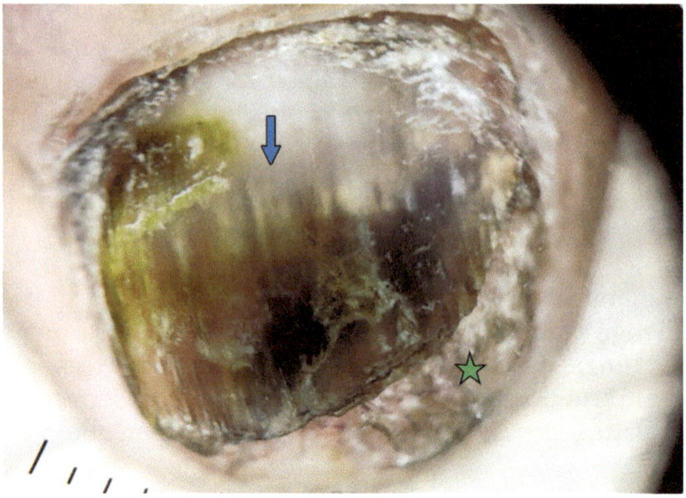

FIGURE 4.7: White longitudinal indentations with jagged edges (arrow) with subungual hyperkeratosis (star) in dermatoscopy of onychomycosis

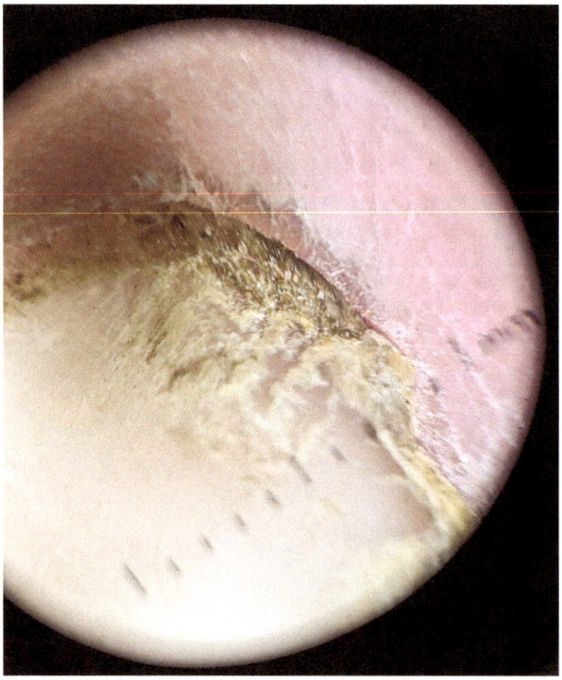

FIGURE 4.8: Filamentous yellow lines, yellow clods and structures representing fungal colonies on dermatoscopy of nail

Melanonychia is another finding which may be seen, and unlike true melanonychia of melanoma, it does not arise from melanocytes. Appearance may be of brown-black discoloration of the nail plate which is not longitudinal or homogeneous. In addition, a reverse triangular pattern of yellow brown color has also been described.[16]

Presence of filamentous yellow lines and yellow clods and structures represent fungal colonies on dermoscopic examination **(Fig. 4.8)**.[20]

White fluffy cotton wool like shadows which are better visualized using a polarizing dermoscope and lamellar micro-splitting in the nail plate are some of the newer findings described in a study by Kayarkatte MN et al.[19]

In the past decade, with the epidemic of recalcitrant dermatophytosis and need for faster diagnostic techniques, dermoscope has evolved as a user friendly, noninvasive tool in the hands of a trained dermatologist.

BIOPSY

Histopathological examination (HE) is usually not performed in case of dermatophytosis, as other noninvasive methods like direct KOH smear examination and culture study along with clinical correlation is sufficient for establishing diagnosis. Biopsy is usually advised in cases with atypical morphology or cases mimicking other dermatosis clinically, especially in dermatophytosis involving non-glabrous skin and scalp. For onychomycosis, sensitivity of HE of nail clipping exceeds that of KOH examination and culture, as a standalone test.[21] Biopsy from active margin of lesion is recommended for evaluation of fungi and inflammatory epidermal and dermal reaction. One has to remember that no single pattern on HE is diagnostic of dermatophyte infection. All the reaction patterns seen in cases of dermatophytosis overlap with other common inflammatory disorders like psoriasis and eczema **(Figs 4.9 and 4.10)**. Careful search for fungal elements in stratum corneum and follicular epithelium is a must before possibility of dermatophytosis is ruled out. Stratum corneum may show parakeratosis, compact orthokeratosis or normal basket wave cornification. Orthokeratosis underlying mounds of parakeratosis, also known as 'sandwich sign', may not be present in all cases **(Fig. 4.11)**.[22] Collection of neutrophils in stratum corneum is not unusual **(Fig. 4.12)**. Epidermis may show variable reaction pattern like acanthosis with or without spongiosis. Dermal changes include variably degree of perivascular infiltrates, mostly lymphocytes with or without neutrophils. Perifollicular inflammation may also be sometimes present. Identification of septate or non-septate hyphae is usually possible even on hematoxylin and eosin (H&E) stained sections. Periodic acid-Schiff (PAS) stain can improve the detection rate in some cases **(Fig. 4.13)**. In a study by Patil DP et al., highest detection rate for surface as well as hair follicle fungus was observed with Grocott-Gomori's methenamine silver (GMS) stain.[23]

For onychomycosis caused by dermatophyte, biopsy of nail plate obtained through nail avulsion or punch biopsy technique can demonstrate hyphae. Jeelani S et al., have

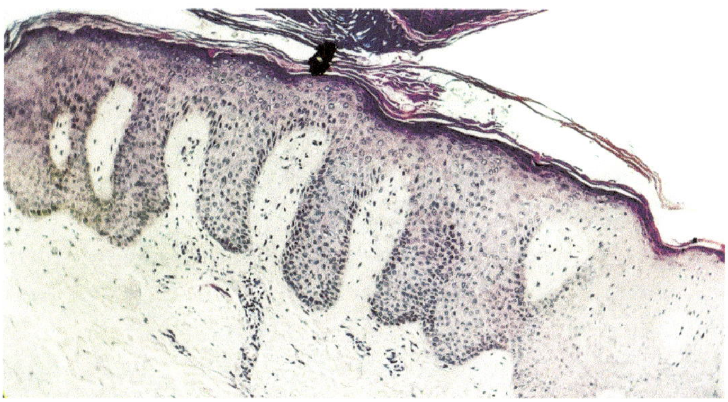

FIGURE 4.9: Psoriasis like picture showing papillomatosis and acanthosis in dermatophytosis. Note the presence of fungal elements in stratum corneum

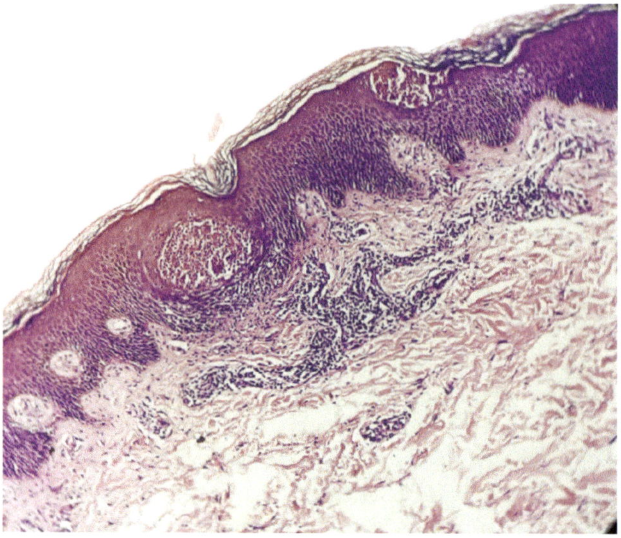

FIGURE 4.10: Acute spongiotic dermatitis like pattern in dermatophytosis

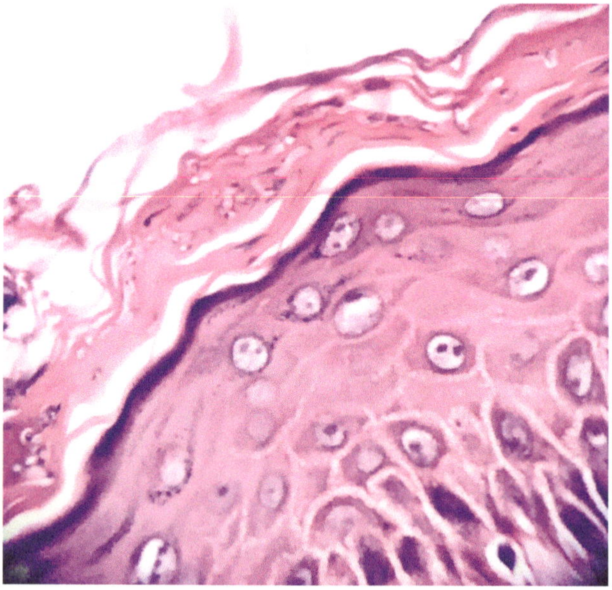

FIGURE 4.11: Orthokeratosis underlying parakeratosis, the sandwich sign

demonstrated simple HE examination of nail clipping is more sensitive in detecting fungal hyphae compared to direct examination and culture study.[1] Fungal hyphae can be visualized in upper layer or under surface of nail plate, depending upon clinical pattern of onychomycosis. Nail bed biopsy (usually not required) in cases of onychomycosis shows variable patterns like psoriasiform hyperplasia or spongiosis.

In cases of tinea capitis, biopsy from the lesion will demonstrate fungal hyphae in surface as well as follicular epithelium. Fungus invading hair cortex in cases of endothrix and presence over hair cuticle in cases of ectothrix can be evident using special stains like Periodic Acid Schiff (PAS) and Gomori Methanamine Silver (GMS).

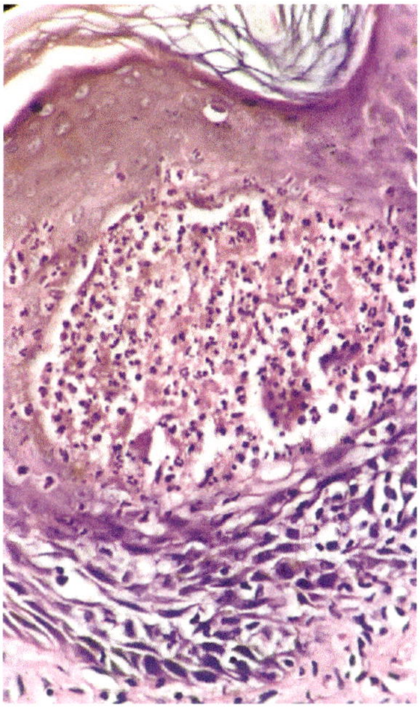

FIGURE 4.12: Neutrophilic collection in stratum corneum in dermatophytosis

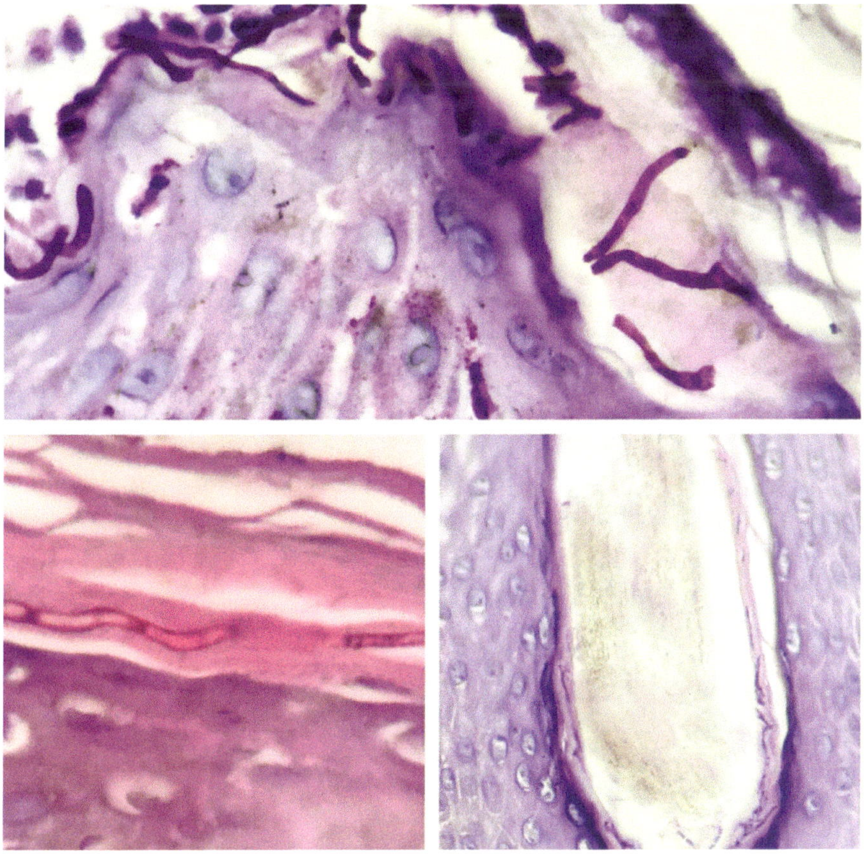

FIGURE 4.13: Fungal hyphae seen clearly using the PAS stain

FUNGAL CULTURE

Isolation and Identification of Dermatophytes in Culture

For definitive identification of species of dermatophyte fungal culture is conventionally used. Culture also helps in establishing the viability of fungi observed in direct examination (KOH). Fungal culture is also the first step for obtaining sufficient growth of dermatophyte for further antifungal sensitivity testing, molecular identification and whole genome sequencing. Low detection rate ranging from 20% to 35% remains major challenge with this conventional and relatively cheaper technique.

Media and Inoculation Method for Culture Study

To obtain the growth of the dermatophyte on culture Sabouraud dextrose agar (SDA) is conventionally used. Culture media should support the growth of dermatophyte at the same time inhibit growth of other bacteria and non-dermatophyte fungi. For this, Cycloheximide (to inhibit non-dermatophytes) and antibacterial like gentamicin (0.0025%) and/or chloramphenicol (0.005%) are added into SDA. Dermatophyte test medium (DTM) and dermatophyte identification medium (DIM) allows more selective growth of the dermatophyte over other non-dermatophyte fungi and bacteria. Specimen should be inoculated on two different media, one selective against non-dermatophytic molds and bacteria, second being non-selective which allows growth of non-dermatophytic molds and bacteria. This is important particularly in sample from nail, palm and sole where non-dermatophytic molds or fungi can be possible etiological agent (*Scytalidium* species).[24] **Table 4.1** shows characteristic of various media used for growth of dermatophytes.

TABLE 4.1: Various media used for growth of dermatophyte

Media	Ingredients	Characteristics
Sabouraud dextrose agar (SDA)	Dextrose, peptone, agar, and distilled water	Allows growth of dermatophyte and non-dermatophyte fungi
Sabouraud peptone-glucose agar (Emmons' modification)	Added cycloheximide and chloramphenicol	Semi-selective as inhibits growth of non-dermatophytic fungi
Dermatophyte test medium	Phenol red	Color changes to red in presence of dermatophyte growth due to phenol red Some nonpathogenic dermatophytes can give red color too. Some isolates may give false negative results *Disadvantage:* Observation of reverse of colony not possible
Cycloheximide-free Sabouraud glucose agar	Sabouraud glucose agar with gentamicin and chloramphenicol	Allows growth of non-dermatophytic fungi
Littman oxgall agar	Peptic digest of animal tissue, dextrose, oxgall, crystal violet agar, final pH (at 25°C)	Reduces the colony diameters of fast-growing contaminants, thus allowing outgrowth of slower-growing fungi
Casamino acids-erythritol-albumin medium	Cycloheximide, antibacterial agents, and suspended egg albumin	Highly selective medium for isolating dermatophytes from lesions heavily contaminated by bacteria or by the cycloheximide-tolerant *C. albicans*

Species Identification

Once the growth of dermatophyte is obtained on SDA, next step is to identify the exact species of dermatophyte causing infection. This is conventionally achieved by observing the developing colony on culture plate. Both top and reverse surface of growth need to be examined to observe colony characteristics and color change related to specific species of dermatophytes (**Table 4.2**).

Second step is direct microscopic examination using lactophenol cotton blue tease mounts. Microscopic characteristics of macro and microconidia helps in identifying the species of dermatophytes (**Table 4.2**).

Hair perforation test where the hair are inoculated with isolated fungus and examined at the interval of 4 weeks for microscopic wedge shaped indentations, helps in differentiating *T. mentagrophytes* from *T. rubrum* and *M. canis* from *M. equinum*. Urease test which is performed by inoculating isolated fungus in Christensen's medium, which turns deep red due to the production of urease, helps in differentiating *T. mentagrophytes* (positive) from *T. rubrum* (negative). Some of the strains of *T. indotineae* also shows positive urease test.

Colony characteristics of *T. indotineae*

Study by Tang C et al., showed all three *Trichophyton indotineae*, *T. mentagrophytes* and *T. interdigitale* produce expanding, cottony to powdery colonies. The reverse of *T. interdigitale* strains was mostly brown ochre, that of *T. mentagrophytes* mostly brown ochre to pale brown,

TABLE 4.2: Shows colony and microscopic characteristic of important dermatophyte species

Species	Top of colony	Reverse of colony	Microscopic morphology
M. audouinii	White to tan silky growth like mouse fur	Salmon pink to tan	Thick walled chlamydospores, conidia are rare and irregular
M. canis	White, thinning towards the edge, cottony with buff center	Yellow or orange	Abundant thick walled spindled shape macroconidia
M. gypseum	Cinnamon or brown powdery surface	Yellow buff to brown	Abundant thin walled macroconidia
T. concentricum	Compact heap folded colonies, with gray tan or brown surface	Tan brown or reddish tone	Conidia absent, hyphae may be swollen and distorted
T. mentagrophytes	Intensely granular surface with white or cream center. Edge of the colonies may be spikey	Yellow tan red to brown (**Fig. 4.14**)	Clusters of microconidia and cigar shaped macroconidia with terminal rat tail filaments
T. interdigitale	Rapidly growing white powdery colonies with cream or pinkish surface	Tan or reddish brown with paler edges	Spherical microconidia arranged in bunches
T. rubrum	White downy or cottony and domed surface (**Fig. 4.15**)	Dark brown center with pale cream border	Tear drop microconidia and pencil shaped macroconidia
T. indotineae[25–27]	Fast-growing, cottony or powdery, colonies (**Fig. 4.16**)	Pale brown to yellow orange	Round microconidia, cigar-shaped macroconidia, chlamydospores

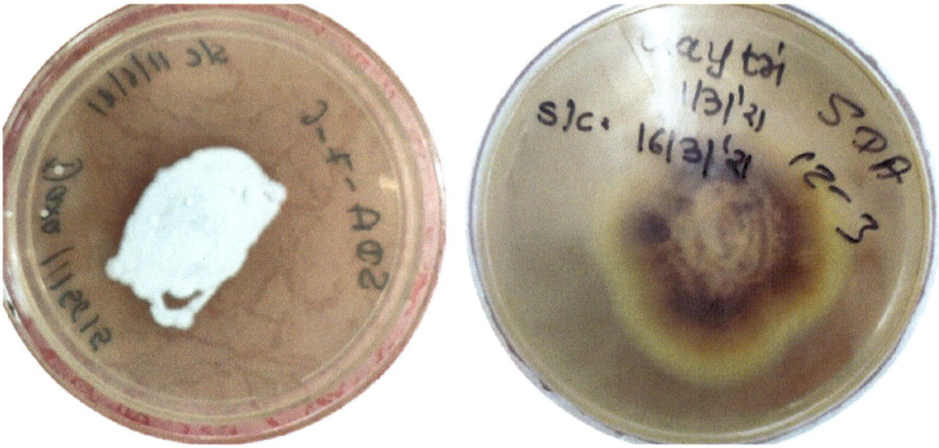

FIGURE 4.14: *Trichophyton mentagrophyte* showing white granular surface on the top and brown colony on the reverse side on SDA

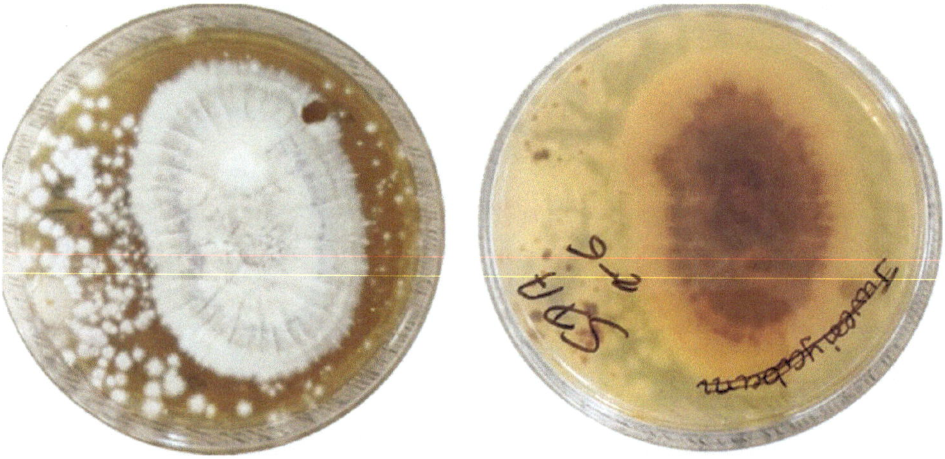

FIGURE 4.15: *Trichophyton rubrum* colony growth showing white cottony and domed surface on top and brown center with cream borders on reverse side on SDA

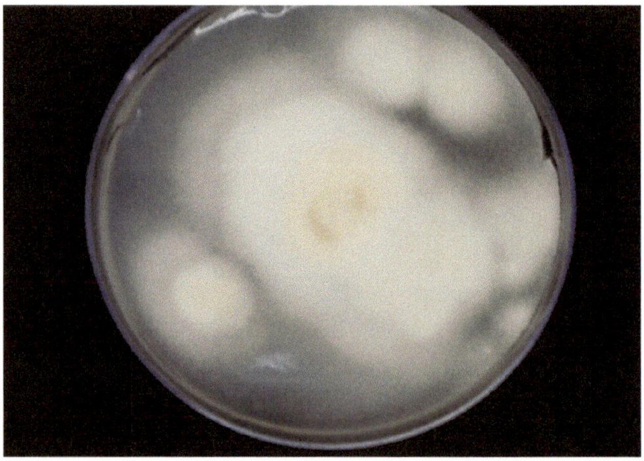

FIGURE 4.16: *Trichophyton indotineae* showing white powdery colonies on SDA

and of *T. indotineae* mostly pale brown to yellow-orange. Positive hair perforation test was observed in 27.8% strains of *T. indotineae*. Keratin azure test, performed to test the production of keratinase was found to be positive in 85.1% strains of *T. indotineae* whereas 27.1% strains showed positive urease test.[26]

NEWER TECHNIQUES FOR IDENTIFICATION OF DERMATOPHYTES

Matrix Assisted Laser Desorption Ionization-time of Flight Mass Spectrometry (MALDI-ToF)

In this spectrometry technique, isolate of fungus are coated with matrix. Sample within the matrix is further ionized using LASER beam. Desorption and ionization of sample produce singly protonated ions. Protonated ions are then accelerated with fix charge which differ in their time of flight (ToF).[28] So different species of dermatophyte will have different ToF. Limitation of this technique is it requires a good database for comparison of results. *T. interdigitale* and *T. mentagrophytes* may not be reliably differentiated with this technique.[29] Recently, online web application developed by Sorbonne University (Paris, France) and the Belgian collection of microorganisms (BCCM-IHEM, Brussels, Belgium) known as mass spectrometry identification (MSI-2) has improved detection rate for *T. indotineae* to 96% with sensitivity of 99.6%.[30]

Molecular Techniques for Identification of Dermatophyte Species

Conventional culture technique has limitation in term of low sensitivity and long incubation period before culture growth can be observed (7–10 days). In addition, species identification may not be always possible if good growth conidia are not obtained. Since the last decade molecular techniques are rapidly taking over conventional method for identification of dermatophyte species.[31]

Species Identification from Culture Growth

Conventional polymerase chain reaction (PCR) using available target genes (box). Internal transcribed spacer (ITS) rDNA region is most commonly used target gene. Results are compared with available online database for species identification. Study by Brillowska-Dabrowska et al. showed higher sensitivity of PCR compared to conventional techniques in identifying the dermatophytes.[32] In view of acceptance of genome-based classification of dermatophytes, molecular technique should be employed whenever it is possible.

Dermatophyte Identification Directly from Clinical Samples

Identification of dermatophytes directly from clinical sample (skin scrapping, nail, hair, etc.) using real time PCR technique is being extensively explored in last few years in research settings. Majority of studies have documented that sensitivity of PCR based assays surpass that of other methods in detecting the dermatophytes from clinical samples, ranging from 88.9% for in-house assays and 65.4% for commercially available kits.[33–35] What detail this assay can provide-in term of "just presence of dermatophyte" to exact species detected, depends on primer used during assay (pan dermatophyte *vs* species specific). Identification of multiple species of dermatophytes and few non-dermatophytes (e.g. Candida) is being made possible with commercially available kits, yet identification of all species may not be possible. Melting curve characteristics (temperature at which amplified DNA material denature) may add to specificity of species identification but require further validation.[2]

Role of Whole Genome Sequencing in Dermatophytes

Whole genome sequencing has limited role in routine laboratory identification of dermatophytes but is a useful research tool. It is used for identification and classification of (new) causative fungi during new outbreaks or epidemics. It also helps in identifying single amino acid polymorphisms in various genes which in turn provides further insight into phylogenetic classification of organism.[36]

ANTIFUNGAL SUSCEPTIBILITY TESTING

Uses of Antifungal Susceptibility Testing

Utility of antifungal susceptibility testing (AFST) for measurement of minimum inhibitory concentration (MIC) is limited in day-to-day management of dermatophytosis. The reason for this is that AFST is a technically demanding procedure, it is difficult for laboratories to standardize this procedure and, it required time for obtaining primary growth of fungi from clinical specimens. In addition to above mentioned procedural difficulties, discordance in clinical response and MIC values is not uncommon. Nevertheless, establishment of epidemiological cut-off values, based on AFST of large number of clinical isolates, for various antifungal drugs can guide management of infections caused by the particular species in that geographical area. At present, AFST is neither being utilized nor is recommended in all cases of dermatophytosis, but it can be employed in particular patients having recalcitrant infection.

Methods for AFST

Various methods for AFST have been explored by scientists in recent time each having its own advantages and disadvantages (**Table 4.3**).

Antifungal sensitivity testing is extremely labor intensive and involves multiple steps which can be affected by technician's expertise and observer's difference. For example, media used, inoculum size, incubation temperature and observation by microbiologist in term of presence or absence of growth at particular concentration of antifungal drug.

TABLE 4.3: Various methods used for antifungal sensitivity testing of dermatophytes

Method	Advantages	Disadvantages
Broth microdilution	• Gold standard for AFST, recommended by CLSI, EUCAST and BSAC. Plates can be made in house by laboratory • Most accurate and reproducible	• Subjective evaluation in CLSI guidelines (EUCAST recommends spectrometry) • Making plates is time consuming
Disk diffusion	• Disc can be made in laboratory, relatively inexpensive • Good for resource limited laboratories	• Not include in standard guidelines for dermatophytes • Interpretation is subjective • Disc diameter is only categorical, does not co-relate with MIC values
Agar dilution	Inexpensive	Not recommended for dermatophytes
Gradient diffusion[35]	• Inexpensive compared to broth microdilution • Can be used for both yeasts and filamentous fungi • Good for resource-limited settings	• Interpretation is somewhat subjective • Must be purchased commercially

Detail discussion of steps of AFST is beyond scope of this book but interested readers can go through CLSI (Clinical Laboratory Standards Institute)–USA reference method for broth dilution (https://clsi.org/) and reference EUCAST method (https://www.eucast.org/). Both methods recommend chemically defined RPMI medium over chemically non-defined Sabouraud dextrose agar. Inoculation size of 10^3 conidia/ml is considered optimum for testing. Incubation temperature of 35°C is recommended. Results are read at the end of 72 to 96 hours. Dimethyl sulfoxide is recommended solvent to prepare solution of antifungal compound.

Minimum Inhibitory Concentration (MIC)

Broth dilution method for AFST provides a value of lowest concentration of drug at which growth of isolated fungus is completely inhibited, which is interpreted as MIC of that drug, for that isolate. MIC50 and MIC90 denotes the concentration of drug at which growth of 50% or 90% isolates of a particular strain (respectively) is inhibited. MIC50 and MIC90 values can be determined only after testing large number of isolates of particular species, for a particular antifungal. *Epidemiological cut-off value* (ECV) is defined as a MIC value at which wild type (without resistance) strain is separated from one with known mutation or acquired resistance. ECV values do not take into consideration clinical outcome of patient treated with particular antifungal, because of which it can give only epidemiological indication of susceptibility of particular strain to antifungals in specific geographical area. *Clinical break points* (CBP), on the other hand is the concentration of antifungal beyond which particular strain of fungus is resistant to antifungal. To determine CBP combination of MIC values, pharmacokinetic and pharmacodynamics data (serum level of drug) and clinical outcome data (cured or not) are taken into consideration.

Newer Techniques in Detection of Resistance

Whole genome sequencing (WGS) provides excellent tool for identifying antifungal resistant genes and site of mutation. However, being a high cost and time-consuming procedure with availability only in few referral labs, limit its extensive use in clinical practice. Other more targeted sequencing techniques like amplified refractory mutation system–polymerase chain reaction (ARMS–PCR), Tetra-primer-amplification refractory mutation system-PCR (T-ARMS-PCR), restriction site mutation (RSM) and high-resolution melt (HRM) analysis are useful in detecting single nucleotide polymorphism in resistance imparting genes (like squalene epoxidase, Erg11, etc.).[37,38] These use a set of allele-specific PCR primers that allows amplification of alleles carrying mutation and do not amplify the wild type allele.

Advanced techniques including proteomic and genomic analysis on isolates from therapeutically recalcitrant case with isolation of gene mutations and enzymatic abnormalities have been also done and have found mutations in SQLE, ERG4, ERG11, MDR1, MFS genes, and a novel ERG3 mutation. Proteomic analysis established the aberrant expression of acetyl Co-A transferase in the resistant strain and upregulation of thioredoxin reductase and peroxiredoxin.[39] There is a need to use advanced techniques in therapy resistant cases and such cutting edge research can help us understand clinical failures.

CONCLUSION

The diagnosis of dermatophyte infections, including those affecting the skin, hair, and nails, benefits from a variety of diagnostic tools, each with its strengths and limitations. The KOH mount remains a simple and effective method for visualizing dermatophytes, with the ability to identify characteristic refractile hyphae and arthrospores. Dermoscopy provides a non-invasive, rapid approach to diagnose dermatophytosis, particularly in tinea capitis, by identifying specific hair and skin features. While histopathological examination is not the first-line test for dermatophyte diagnosis, it is valuable for distinguishing dermatophytosis from other skin conditions. The culture study continues to be the gold standard for fungal identification, despite its limitations such as long incubation periods and potential contamination. Furthermore, molecular techniques, such as PCR and whole genome sequencing, offer promising advances in terms of sensitivity, speed, and the ability to explore genetic characteristics, which contribute to a better understanding of fungal pathogenesis, host interactions, and drug resistance. Together, these diagnostic methods, when used appropriately, enable dermatologists to effectively diagnose and manage dermatophyte infections, ensuring better patient outcomes.

Key Points

- KOH mount and dermoscopy are simple, office based, non-invasive, handy, quick, useful techniques in diagnosis of dermatophyte infections of skin, hair, and nails.
- Longitudinal striae, spikes, ruin like appearance and aurora pattern are some of the findings of onychomycosis on dermoscopy.[40]
- No one histological pattern is diagnostic of dermatophytosis on skin biopsy. Spongiotic and psoriasiform pattern are routinely observed in biopsy specimens.
- HP examination of nail clipping, as a standalone test is more sensitive to smear examination and culture study in diagnosis of onychomycosis.
- Whole genome sequencing is important step in identification of species or causative fungi and it helps in identification of single amino acid polymorphism in various gene, which may be responsible for different host preference, infective, immune response and drug resistance.

REFERENCES

1. Gautam M, Bhatia S. Mount the menace! – Potassium hydroxide in superficial fungal infections. Indian J Paediatr Dermatol 2020;21:343–6.
2. Kurade SM, Amladi SA, Miskeen AK. Skin scraping and a potassium hydroxide mount. Indian J Dermatol Venereol Leprol 2006;72:238–41.
3. Hay RJ, Ashbee HR. Mycology. Superficial mycoses. In: Griffiths CEM, Barker J, Bleiker T, Chalmers R, Creamer D, editors. Rook's Textbook of dermatology, 9th ed. Oxford: Wiley Blackwell 2016. pp. 32.7–32.8.
4. Grover C, Khurana A. Onychomycosis: Newer insights in pathogenesis and diagnosis. Indian J Dermatol Venereol Leprol 2012;78:263–70.
5. Khurana A, Agarwal A, Agrawal D, Sethia K. Re-emerging role of KOH smear examination in the era of recalcirant dermatophytoses. Dermatol Ther. 2021;34(2):e14891.
6. Singh S, Beena P M. Comparative study of different microscopic techniques and culture media for the isolation of dermatophytes. Indian J Med Microbiol 2003;21:21–4.
7. Chandramohan A, Srinivas CR. Hyphal index following a potassium hydroxide mount in dermatophytosis. Cureus. 2021;13(12):e20576.
8. Sonthalia S, Yumeen S, Kaliyadan F. Dermoscopy overview and extradiagnostic applications. [Updated 2022 Aug 8]. In: StatPearls [Internet].
9. Nischal K C, Khopkar U. Dermoscope. Indian J Dermatol Venereol Leprol 2005;71:300–3.
10. Ankad BS, Mukherjee SS, Nikam BP, Reshme AS, Sakhare PS, Mural PH. Dermoscopic characterization of dermatophytosis: A preliminary observation. Indian Dermatol Online J 2020;11:202–7.
11. Knöpfel N, del Pozo LJ, Escudero Mdel M, Martín-Santiago A. Dermoscopic visualization of vellus hair involvement in tinea corporis: A criterion for systemic antifungal therapy? Pediatr Dermatol 2015;32:e226–7.

12. Errichetti E, Stinco G. Dermoscopy in General Dermatology: A Practical Overview. Dermatol Ther (Heidelb). 2016;6(4):471–507.
13. Elghblawi E. Idiosyncratic findings in trichoscopy of tinea capitis: Comma, zigzag hairs, corkscrew and morse code-like hair. Int J Trichol 2016;8:180v3.
14. Bakos RM, Leite LL, Reinehr C, Escobar GF. Dermoscopy of skin infestations and infections (entomodermoscopy) – Part II: viral, fungal and other infections. An Bras Dermatol 2021;96:746–58.
15. Hughes R, Chiaverini C, Bahadoran P, Lacour J-P. Corkscrew hair: A new dermoscopic sign for diagnosis of tinea capitis in black children. Arch Dermatol 2011;147:355–6.
16. Lim SS, Shin K, Mun JH. Dermoscopy for cutaneous fungal infections: A brief review. Health Sci Rep 2022;5(1):e464.
17. Piccolo V, Corneli P, Russo T, Zalaudek I, Alfano R, Argenziano G. Dermoscopy as a useful tool in diagnosis of tinea incognito. Int J Dermatol 2019;58(2):e32–e34.
18. Kaya Islamoglu ZG, Demirbas A, Unal M, Findik D. Nail digital dermoscopy in onychomycosis: A correlation with clinical type, gender, and culture examination. Erciyes Med J 2019;41(3):288–94.
19. Kayarkatte MN, Singal A, Pandhi D, Das S, Sharma S. Nail dermoscopy (onychoscopy) findings in the diagnosis of primary onychomycosis: A cross-sectional study. Indian J Dermatol Venereol Leprol 2020;86:341–9.
20. Ankad BS, Gupta A, Alekhya R, Saipriya M. Dermoscopy of onycholysis due to nail psoriasis, onychomycosis and trauma: a cross sectional study in skin of color. Indian Dermatology Online Journal 2020;11(5):777.
21. Jeelani S, Ahmed QM, Lanker AM, Hassan I, Jeelani N, Fazili T. Histopathological examination of nail clippings using PAS staining (HPE-PAS): Gold standard in diagnosis of onychomycosis. Mycoses 2015;58(1):27–32.
22. Murali M, Tirumalae R. Histopathologic patterns in dermatophyte infections: Clues to diagnosis. Indian Journal of Dermatopathology and Diagnostic Dermatology 2021;8(2):38.
23. Patil PD, Pande S, Mahore S, Borkar M. Histopathology of hair follicle epithelium in patients of recurrent and recalcitrant dermatophytosis:A diagnostic cross-sectional study. International Journal of Trichology. 2019;11(4):159.
24. Weitzman I, Summerbell RC. The dermatophytes. Clinical microbiology reviews. 1995;8(2):240–59.
25. Nenoff P, Uhrlaß S, Verma SB, Panda S. *Trichophyton mentagrophytes* ITS genotype VIII and *Trichophyton indotineae*: A terminological maze, or is it? Indian J Dermatol Venereol Leprol 2022;88:586–9.
26. Ngo TM, Nu PA, Le CC, Ha TN, Do TB, Thi GT. First detection of *Trichophyton indotineae* causing tinea corporis in Central Vietnam. Medical Mycology Case Reports. 2022.
27. Tang C, Kong X, Ahmed SA, Thakur R, Chowdhary A, Nenoff P, et al. Taxonomy of the *Trichophyton mentagrophytes/T. interdigitale* species complex harboring the highly virulent, multiresistant genotype *T. indotineae*. Mycopathologia 2021;186:315–26.
28. Singhal N, Kumar M, Kanaujia PK, Virdi JS. MALDI-TOF mass spectrometry: an emerging technology for microbial identification and diagnosis. Frontiers in microbiology. 2015;6:791.
29. Kidd SE, Weldhagen GF. Diagnosis of dermatophytes: from microscopy to direct PCR. Microbiology Australia 2022;43(1):9–13.
30. Normand AC, Moreno-Sabater A, Jabet A, Hamane S, Cremer G, Foulet F, et al. MALDI-ToF mass spectrometry online identification of *Trichophyton indotineae* using the MSI-2 application. Journal of Fungi 2022;8(10):1103.
31. Rudramurthy SM, Shaw D. Overview and update on the laboratory diagnosis of dermatophytosis. Clinical Dermatology Review 2017;1(3):3.
32. Brillowska-DaaBrowska A, Swierkowska A, Lindhardt Saunte DM, Arendrup MC. Diagnostic PCR tests for *Microsporum audouinii, M. canis* and *Trichophyton infections*. Medical Mycology 2010;48(3):486–90.
33. Ross IL, Weldhagen GF, Kidd SE. Detection and identification of dermatophyte fungi in clinical samples using a commercial multiplex tandem PCR assay. Pathology. 2020;52(4):473–7.
34. Kabtani J, Diongue K, Dione JN, Delmas A, L'ollivier C, Amoureux MC, et al. Real-time PCR assay for the detection of dermatophytes: Comparison between an in-house method and a commercial kit for the diagnosis of dermatophytoses in patients from Dakar, Senegal. Journal of Fungi. 2021;7(11):949.

35. Ndiaye M, Sacheli R, Diongue K, Adjetey C, Darfouf R, Seck MC, et al. Evaluation of the multiplex real-time PCR DermaGenius® assay for the detection of dermatophytes in hair samples from senegal. J Fungi (Basel). 2021;8(1):11. doi: 10.3390/jof8010011.
36. Kumar P, Das S, Tigga R, Pandey R, Bhattacharya SN, Taneja B. Whole genome sequences of two *Trichophyton indotineae* clinical isolates from India emerging as threats during therapeutic treatment of dermatophytosis. 3 Biotech 2021;11(9):1–0.
37. Berkow EL, Lockhart SR, Ostrosky-Zeichner L. Antifungal susceptibility testing: Current approaches. Clinical Microbiology Reviews. 2020;33(3):e00069–19.
38. Norris HA, Elewski BE, Ghannoum MA. Optimal growth conditions for the determination of the antifungal susceptibility of three species of dermatophytes with the use of a microdilution method. Journal of the American Academy of Dermatology 1999;40(6):S9–13.
39. Bhattacharyya A, Sadhasivam S, Sinha M, Gupta S, Saini S, Singh H, Khurana A, Sachdeva S, Sardana K, Ghosh S. Treatment recalcitrant cases of tinea corporis/cruris caused by *T. mentagrophytes - interdigitale* complex with mutations in ERG11 ERG 3, ERG4, MDR1 MFS genes & SQLE and their potential implications. Int J Dermatol. 2023 May;62(5):637–648. doi: 10.1111/ijd.16622. Epub 2023 Mar 17. PMID: 36929499.
40. Grover C, Rathod D. Onychoscopy. IADVL Atlas of Dermoscopy, 1st Edn., Jaypee Brothers Medical Publishers Ltd. ISBN 9789390595648, DOI 10.5005/jp/books/18665, 2022.

CHAPTER 5

Differential Diagnosis of Dermatophytoses

• *Shital Poojary* • *Prachisingh Rajpoot*

INTRODUCTION

Dermatophytosis can masquerade as several common dermatological diseases. In the ongoing epidemic of chronic and recurrent dermatophytosis, atypical clinical patterns have become the rule rather than an exception. Apart from host factors and changes in the causative organism, the abuse of topical steroids further alters the clinical pattern. This chapter covers the differential diagnosis of all site-specific dermatophytosis.[1]

Some of the atypical clinical morphological patterns of dermatophytosis which have been reported include the following:[2]

- Psoriasiform
- Seborrheic dermatitis like
- Erythema multiforme like
- Lupus erythematosus like
- Erythroderma
- Tinea pseudoimbricata

TINEA CORPORIS

Tinea corporis commonly presents as annular scaly plaques with central clearing and papules/ pustules along the border of the lesions. There may occasionally be bullous or nodular lesions.

Differential diagnosis of tinea corporis include the following:

Seborrheic dermatitis: Ill-defined plaques of tinea corporis (especially tinea incognito) on the chest or mid back may resemble seborrheic dermatitis. However involvement of typical seborrheic areas such as nasolabial fold and scalp and presence of greasy scales help to differentiate this condition from tinea corporis.

Psoriasis: It is an important differential diagnosis of tinea corporis when the distribution of lesions is atypical and extensor aspects of extremities are involved. Especially, annular lesions of psoriasis need to be differentiated from tinea corporis. Presence of typical erythematous plaques with silvery white scales on the knees, elbows and scalp, and associated changes in the nails, (irregular pits, onycholysis), are helpful in differentiating psoriasis from plaques of tinea corporis which typically have fine scales on the border of the plaque. Rarely atypical psoriasiform tinea corporis may occur (**Fig. 5.1a to c**). In such cases, a potassium hydroxide (KOH) mount would be needed to confirm the diagnosis.

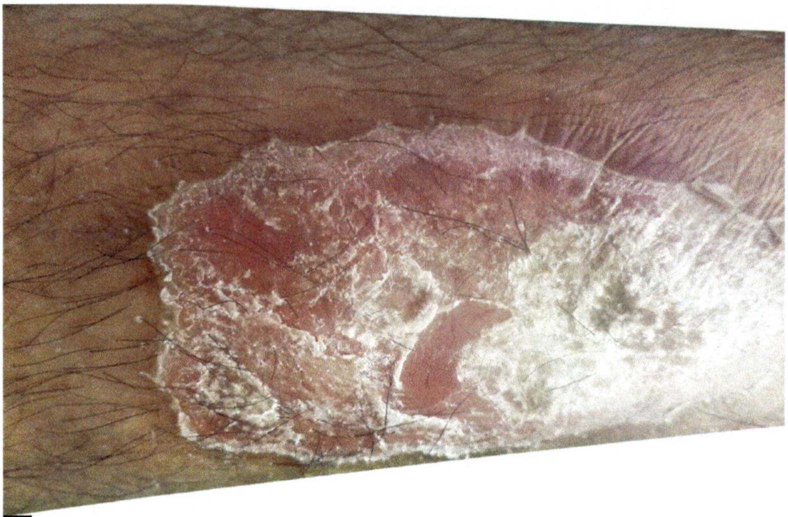

a

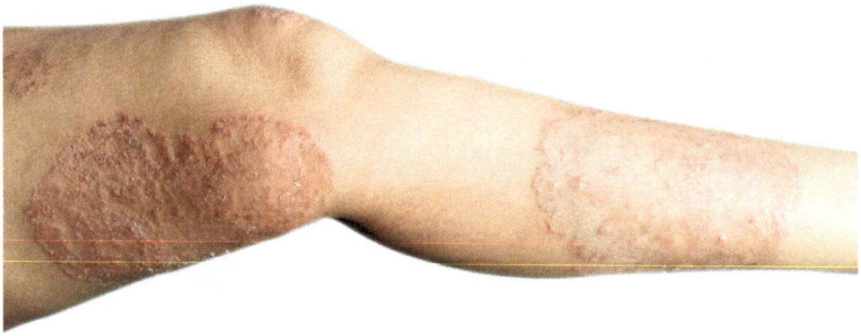

b

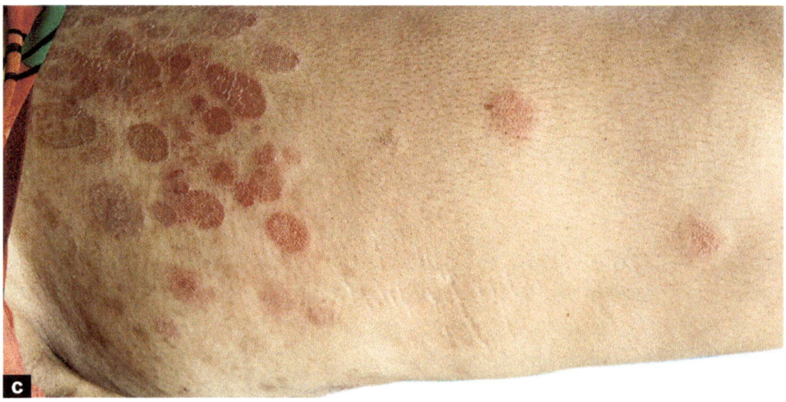

c

FIGURE 5.1a to c: (a) Classical psoriasis plaque which is pink to salmon colored with whitish silvery scales; (b) Tinea plaque with fine scaling at border; (c) Psoriasiform tinea plaque which is well-defined with uniform scaling

Impetigo: Circinate variant of dermatophytosis can be confused with patches of impetigo. However, the typical honey colored crusts distinguish impetigo from tinea corporis **(Fig. 5.2a and b)**.

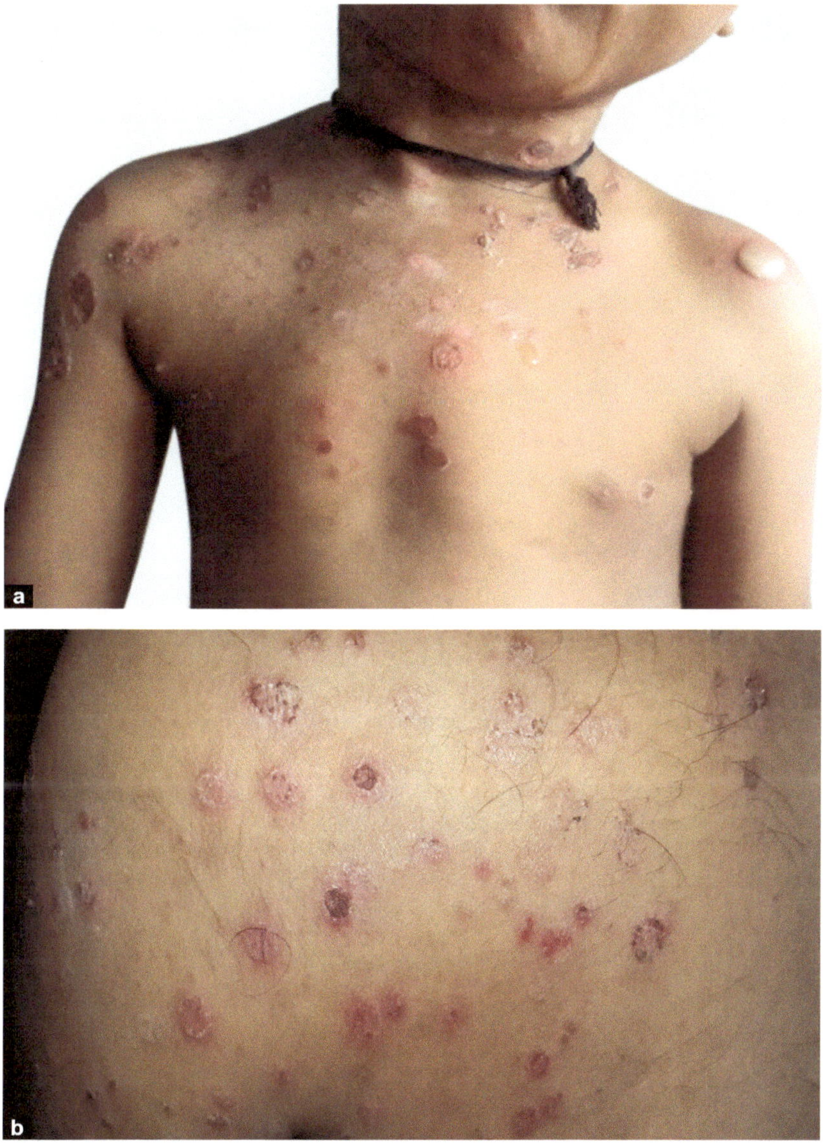

FIGURE 5.2a and b: (a) Impetigo: Circular plaques with central crusting and few plaques with vesicles/ vesicopustules on border resembling tinea; (b) Inflammatory tinea corporis: Plaques with pustules on the peripheral border and few plaques with secondary impetiginization

Lichen simplex chronicus: In chronic cases of dermatophytosis, lichenification can occur due to persistent rubbing/scratching **(Fig. 5.3)**. Such plaques can mimic lichen simplex chronicus. However, involvement of typical sites of lichen simplex chronicus such as ankles, shins point to the diagnosis, and in addition its, longer duration and intense pruritus are clues to diagnosis.

Pityriasis rosea: The annular plaques seen in pityriasis rosea, both the herald plaque and secondary lesions are a close differential diagnosis of tinea corporis. However, the presence of hanging curtain sign, classical Christmas tree distribution of the lesions help in differentiating the annular plaques of pityriasis rosea from tinea corporis **(Fig. 5.4)**.

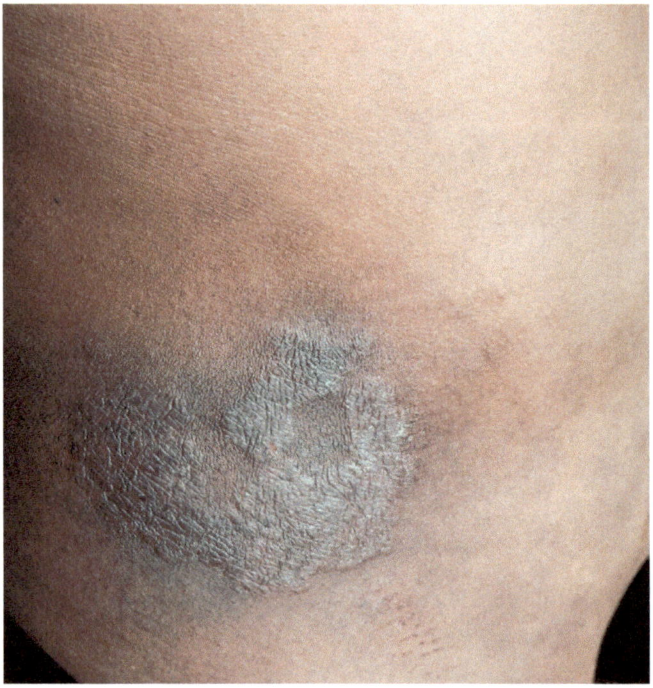

FIGURE 5.3: Lichenified tinea corporis

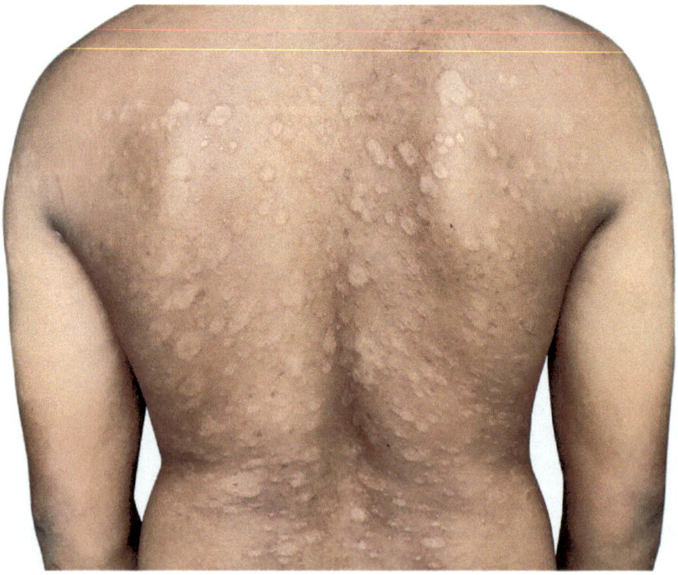

FIGURE 5.4: Annular erythematous plaques with collarette scales and characteristic distribution along cleavage line giving configuration of "Christmas tree" in pityriasis rosea

Figurate erythemas: Erythema annular centrifugum (EAC) closely resemble plaques of tinea corporis with annular lesions, flat advancing border and trailing scale at the inner border of the lesions **(Fig. 5.5a and b)**. However lesions of EAC mostly have incomplete polycyclic lesions. Histopathology is required for confirmation of diagnosis of EAC.

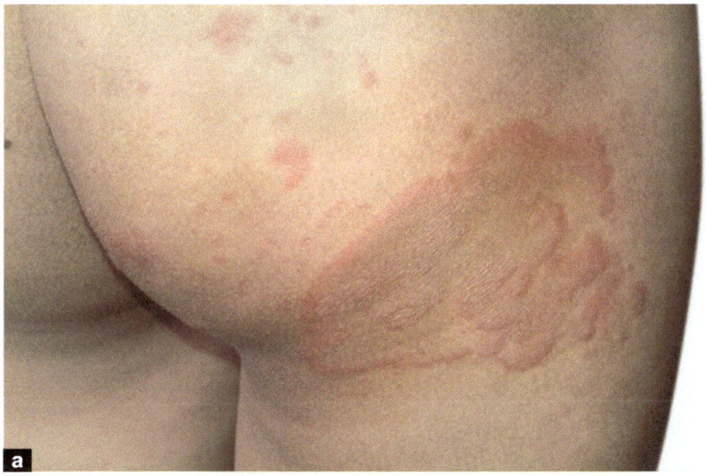

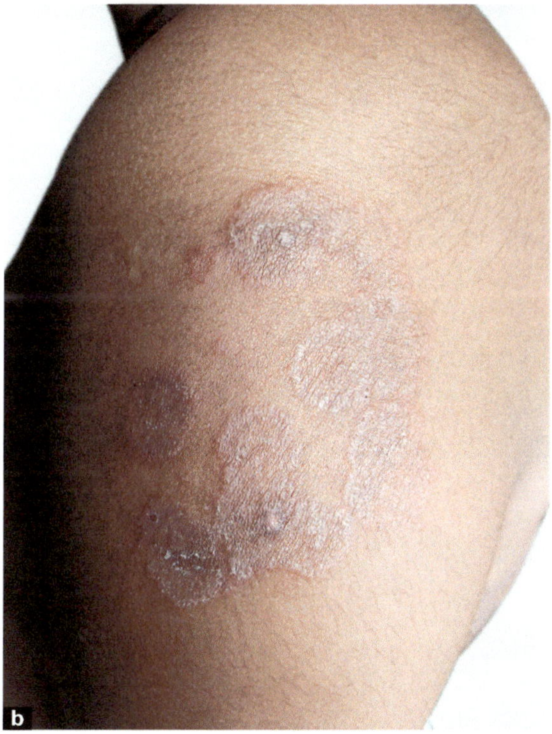

FIGURE 5.5a and b: (a) Classical annular erythematous plaque of tinea corporis with scaling at advancing edge; (b) Tinea resembling erythema annulare centrifugum

TINEA CAPITIS

Tinea capitis clinically presents as inflammatory and non-inflammatory types. The non-inflammatory types (gray patch and black dot type) presents predominantly as non-cicatricial patches of alopecia with scaling and broken hair stubs. Inflammatory type of tinea capitis (Kerion, favus) presents as alopecia with boggy swelling/pustules.

All entities resulting in patchy alopecia with inflammatory changes of scalp should be considered in differential diagnosis of tinea capitis **(Fig. 5.6a to c)**.[1]

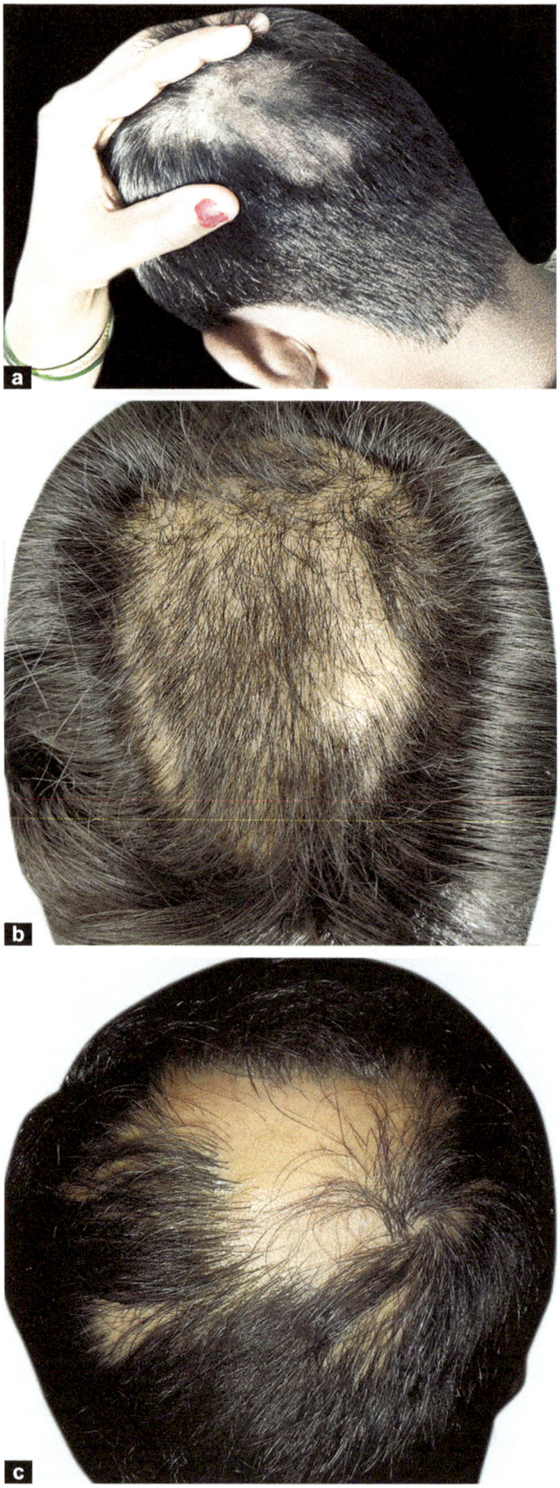

FIGURE 5.6a to c: (a) Multiple alopecia patches with broken hairs and scaling in tinea capitis; (b) Smooth patch of alopecia in alopecia areata; (c) Irregular patch of hair loss with varying lengths of broken hair, Friar tuck pattern of trichotillomania

Alopecia areata: It present with patches of alopecia without any scaling. The classical feature of alopecia areata, exclamation hairs, need to be carefully differentiated from broken hairs of tinea capitis. Other trichoscopic features of alopecia areata such as presence of black dots, yellow dots, coudability sign, pigtail hairs also help to differentiate. In cases where diagnosis is in doubt, a biopsy can help in confirming diagnosis of alopecia areata.

Trichotillomania: Trichotillomania presents with irregular patches of non-cicatricial alopecia and needs to be differentiated from non-inflammatory variant of tinea capitis. Trichoscopic features like broken hair shafts of varying length, flame sign, perifollicular hemorrhage easily differentiates this entity from tinea capitis.

Seborrheic dermatitis: It is usually diffuse compared to localized and patchy involvement in tinea capitis. The scales are yellowish, greasy, while dry scales and broken hairs are a hallmark of tinea capitis. Involvement of other seborrheic areas such as nasolabial fold, medial end of eyebrows, anterior chest, mid back corroborate the diagnosis. Trichoscopy shows thin arborizing vessels, yellowish scales and structureless areas in seborrheic dermatitis.

Psoriasis: Psoriasis is characterized by plaques with whitish to silvery scales without any broken hairs. Hair loss when present is not very prominent. Presence of corona psoriatica can be a clincher for diagnosis.

Pediculosis capitis: Secondary infection of the scalp especially in extensive pediculosis capitis leading to matting and crusting can be mistaken for inflammatory variant of tinea capitis, i.e. kerion.[1]

Furunculosis: Furunculosis presents as inflammatory nodules and needs to be differentiated from inflammatory variant of tinea capitis. Examination of the pus for bacteria and a KOH mount can help in confirming the diagnosis.

Discoid lupus erythematosus: Discoid lupus erythematosus (DLE) presents as patches of cicatricial alopecia with dyspigmentation, scales and follicular plugging. As it is cicatricial type, it is mostly easily distinguished from non-inflammatory type of tinea capitis. Late stages of inflammatory tinea capitis in which occasionally scarring can occur may need to be differentiated from DLE.

TINEA BARBAE

Bacterial folliculitis: Folliculitis presents as *painful* papules topped with pustules and can closely resemble tinea barbae. There is however absence of easy pluckability of hairs and alopecia. A smear from the purulent discharge and KOH mount helps in easy differentiation.

Sycosis barbae: It is characterized by pustules and nodules with scarring (cut fig like appearance). The disease is often recurrent and scarring characterizes the disease.

Acne: Severe variant of acne with papules, pustules, nodules and cyst in the beard area needs to be differentiated from tinea barbae occasionally. Involvement of other areas of face and other polymorphic lesions such as comedones helps in clinching the diagnosis.

TINEA FACIEI

Tinea faciei needs to be differentiated especially from photosensitive disorders as lesions of tinea faciei itself may have some degree of *photosensitivity* with intense erythema.

Seborrheic dermatitis: It is distinguished by greasy yellowish scales and involvement of seborrheic areas. A subtle but distinct border of the annular plaque of tinea faciei also helps in diagnosis (**Fig. 5.7**).

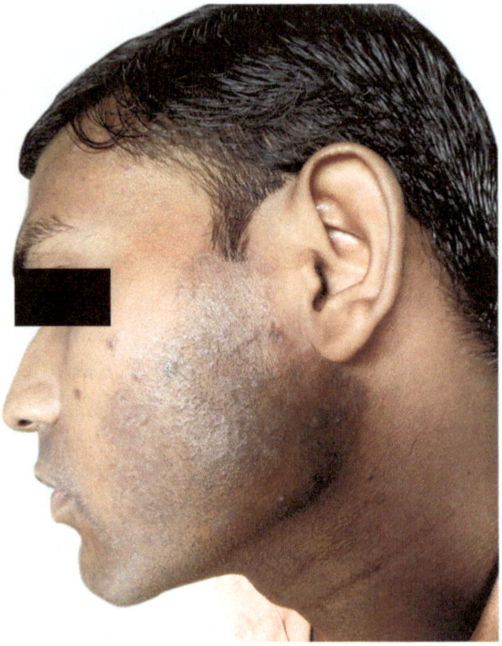

FIGURE 5.7: Tinea faciei involving seborrheic areas of face, predominantly beard area

Lupus erythematosus: Annular plaques of DLE need to be differentiated from tinea faciei. Depigmentation in central part with surrounding hyperpigmentation (dyspigmentation) and associated atrophy, carpet tack scales distinguish these lesions from tinea faciei **(Fig. 5.8a)**. Rarely, tinea faciei with secondary photosensitivity may resemble malar rash of SLE **(Fig. 5.8b and c)**.

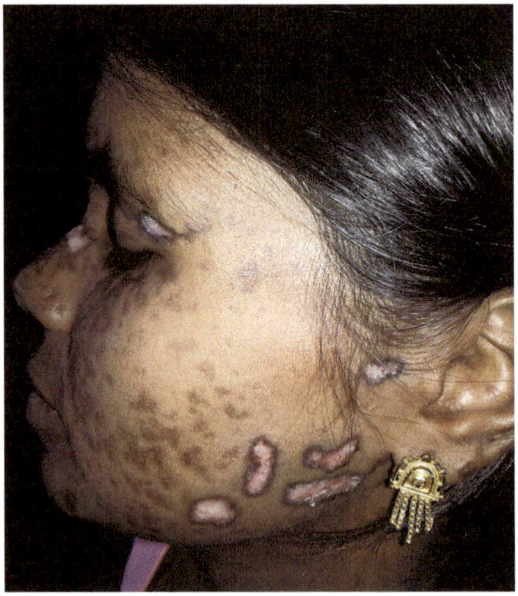

FIGURE 5.8a: Atrophic annular plaques with central depigmentaion and surrounding hyperpigmented border in discoid lupus erythematosus

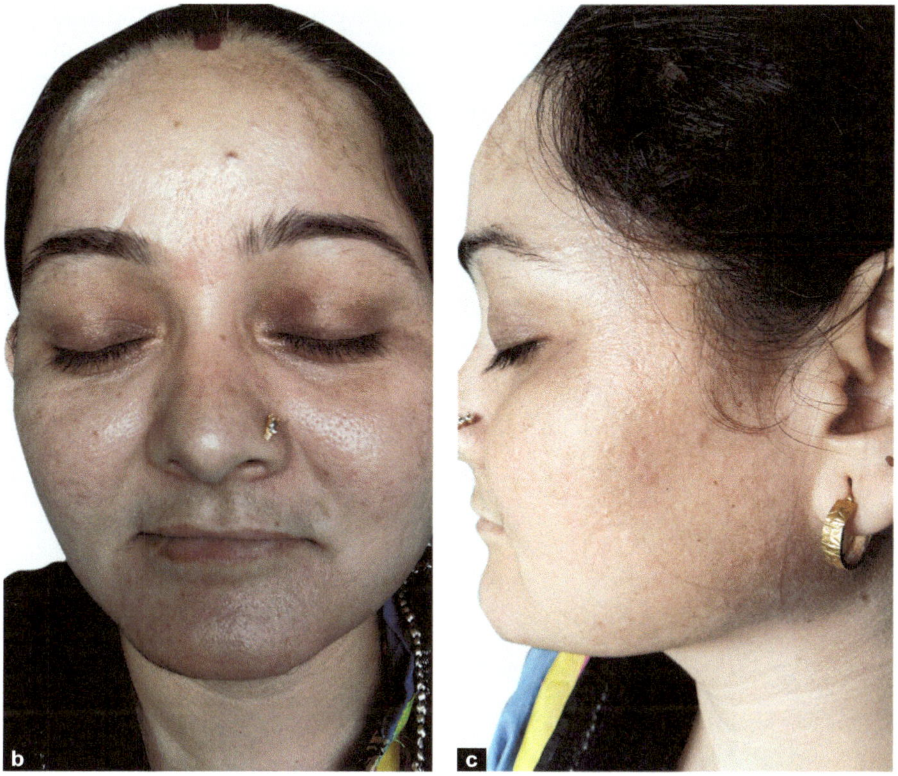

FIGURE 5.8b and c: Tinea faciei resembling malar rash of SLE but with a distinct classical border at mandibular margin

Polymorphous light eruption: Polymorphous light eruption (PMLE) presents as erythematous to lichenoid plaques on photo exposed areas. Lesions respond to strict photoprotection. Usually, there is absence of scaling **(Fig. 5.9)**.

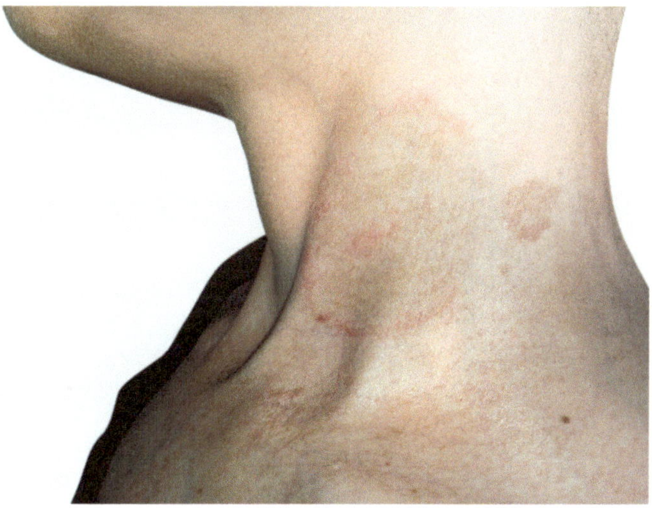

FIGURE 5.9: Annular to circular plaques of tinea on photoexposed areas resembling polymorphous light eruption

Impetigo: Impetigo may coexist with tinea faciei or may need to be distinguished from tinea faciei. Staphylcocci in culture does not rule out dermatophytes. Dermoscopy may be helpful which shows dotted vessels, reddish brown dots and globules and superficial white scales.[3]

Rosacea: Papulopustules, telangiectasias pose diagnostic challenges in cases of topical steroid induced modified tinea faciei. Careful examination of scrapings in KOH is helpful (**Fig. 5.10a and b**).

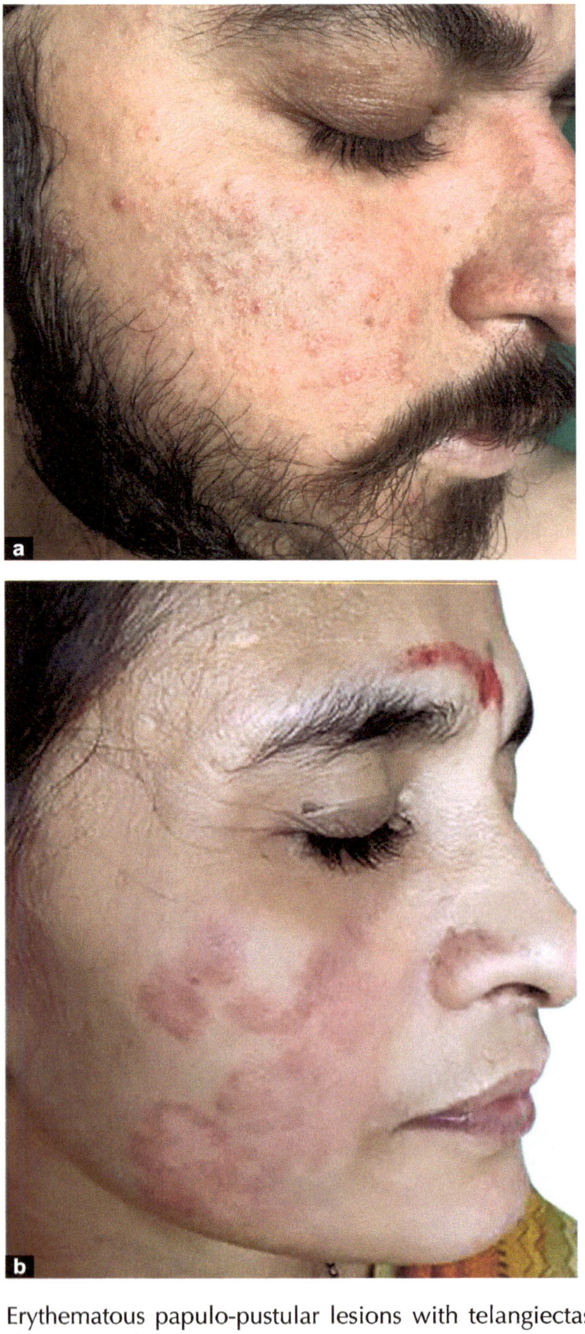

FIGURE 5.10a and b: (a) Erythematous papulo-pustular lesions with telangiectasias in Rosacea; (b) Tinea faciei after topical steroids abuse resembling Rosacea

TINEA PEDIS

Morphological variants of tinea pedis include non-inflammatory (Papulosquamous, moccasin, intertriginous type) and inflammatory type (vesicobullous type).

Candidiasis: Intertriginous tinea pedis needs to be differentiated from candidiasis and is suspected when predominantly web spaces are involved. Whitish macerated skin favours the diagnosis of Candida intertrigo. KOH mount will aid in confirmation of diagnosis.

Bacterial infections: Intertrigo due to staphylococci, streptococci and gram negative bacteria like *Acinetobacter* can resemble inflammatory variant of tinea pedis and there is often associated odor. KOH mount helps in distinguishing the lesions.

Juvenile planter dermatosis in young children may mimic tinea pedis. The lesions are predominant on the forefoot and bilateral while tinea pedis is likely to be unilateral in distribution. The lesions have a glazed appearance as against scaly plaques of tinea pedis. Scrapings are useful in such cases.

Plantar psoriasis: Plantar psoriasis presents as scaly plaques on the instep, soles and can be a close differential diagnosis of papulosquamous type of tinea pedis. The lesions are likely to be present bilaterally. Associated classical psoriatic nail involvement in form of pits, onycholysis can be corroborative in diagnosis of psoriasis.

Contact dermatitis: Acute and cumulative contact dermatitis both have to be differentiated from Tinea pedis. Common allergens arise from contact with detergents, rubber and plastic footwear. A thorough history and distribution of lesions in pattern of contact is helpful in the diagnosis (**Fig. 5.11**). Scrapings are useful to confirm diagnosis in such cases.

TINEA MANNUM

Irritant contact dermatitis and chronic hand eczema: As with tinea pedis, contact dermatitis has to be considered in differential diagnosis of tinea mannum. The allergens however are different and include detergents, cement, etc. Although asymmetric and unilateral involvement favours diagnosis of tinea mannum, scrapings and dermoscopy are useful in such cases. Presence of yellow scales, brown-orange dots or globules (corresponding to tiny spongiotic vesicles)

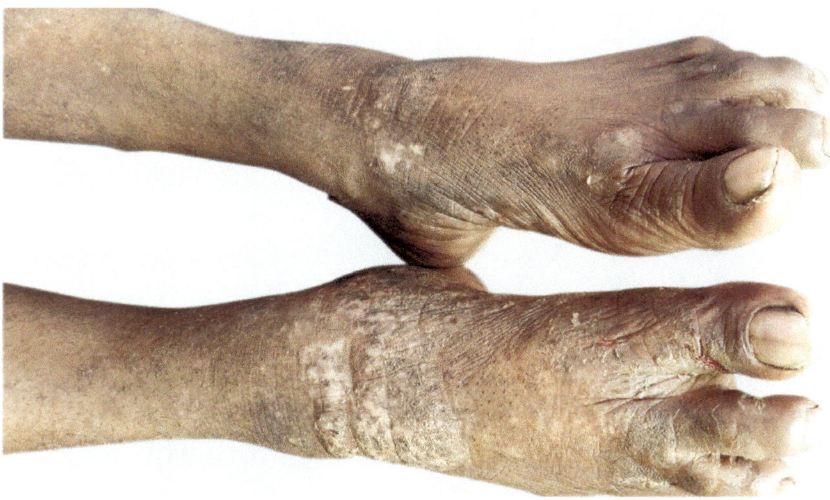

FIGURE 5.11: Foot eczema due to contact dermatitis to footwear with bilateral patterned involvement

and yellow-orange crusts are characteristic of chronic hand eczema, while dermoscopy of tinea mannum shows a peculiar finding of whitish scaling mainly located in the creases.[4] In most cases of tinea mannum, nails are also involved.

Palmar psoriasis: Scaly plaques of psoriasis need to be distinguished from tinea mannum. Presence of psoriatic plaques at other classical sites like extensors, scalp, nails can be corroborative in diagnosis of psoriasis. Dermoscopy is helpful in such cases as with tinea pedis.

Pityriasis rubra pilaris: Palms show diffuse and thick hyperkeratosis. Dermoscopy reveals structureless orange areas or relatively large amber scales over a white-to-pink background.[5] Involvement of other areas with distinctive follicular papules is likely to be present and helps in diagnosis.

TINEA CRURIS

Tinea cruris needs to be differentiated from other infective and non-infective conditions as below:

Candidiasis: Maceration is more likely to occur, often without distinct raised margins. Satellite pustules are characteristic, and when they rupture, they leave a collarette of scales at the edges. Occasionally, maceration may also be observed in tinea cruris; however, the presence of distinct margins and the absence of satellite pustules aid in its diagnosis **(Fig. 5.12)**.

Pityriasis versicolor: Lesions are usually non-inflammatory and asymptomatic and present as perifollicular hypopigmented to hyperpigmented macules. The characteristic furfuraceous scaling, positive scratch sign and golden yellow fluorescence seen on Wood's lamp help to differentiate.

Erythrasma: Characteristic erythematous, usually asymptomatic patches without any scaling with coral-red fluorescence under Wood's lamp aids in the diagnosis.

Psoriasis: Flexural psoriasis can be a close mimicker as the characteristic scaling is often not evident in the intertriginous areas. Pink to salmon colour of plaques and regular dotted vessels on dermoscopy are key features in differentiating from tinea cruris.

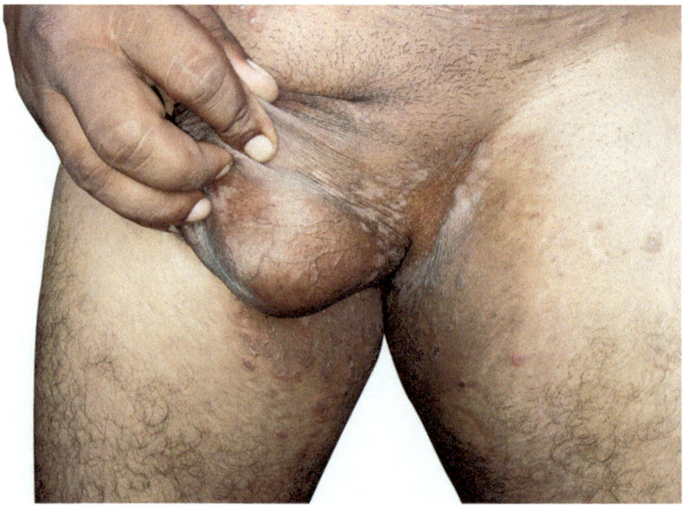

FIGURE 5.12: Erythematous plaques of tinea cruris with maceration in groin folds resembling candidiasis

TINEA UNGUIUM

Nail psoriasis: Destructive changes of nail bed and nail plate produced by dermatophytes is sometimes difficult to differentiate from nail psoriasis **(Fig. 5.13a and b)**. Scrapings and culture using nail clippings are helpful in such cases. Dermoscopy in onychomycosis shows jagged edge of proximal margin of onycholysis with sharp structures directed to proximal nail fold whereas it is regular onycholysis in psoriasis along with other findings like coarse pitting on nail plate, oil drop sign, dilated globose vessels, splinter hemorrhages. Other classical patterns such as 'aurora borealis' pattern is also useful in diagnosis of tinea unguium.

Candidiasis: Nail plate is affected proximally with sparing of free edges. Swelling of proximal and lateral nail fold is also associated, which is rare in dermatophytes.

Lichen planus: The nail plate is mostly thinned in lichen planus with characteristic features being pup tent sign and pterygium. In absence of classical features and only dystrophic changes, KOH and culture of nail clippings and sometimes nail biopsy may be required.

It is also important to remember that damaged nails such as those due to psoriasis or lichen planus are sometimes prone to dermatophyte infection and hence changes of both diseases may be present.

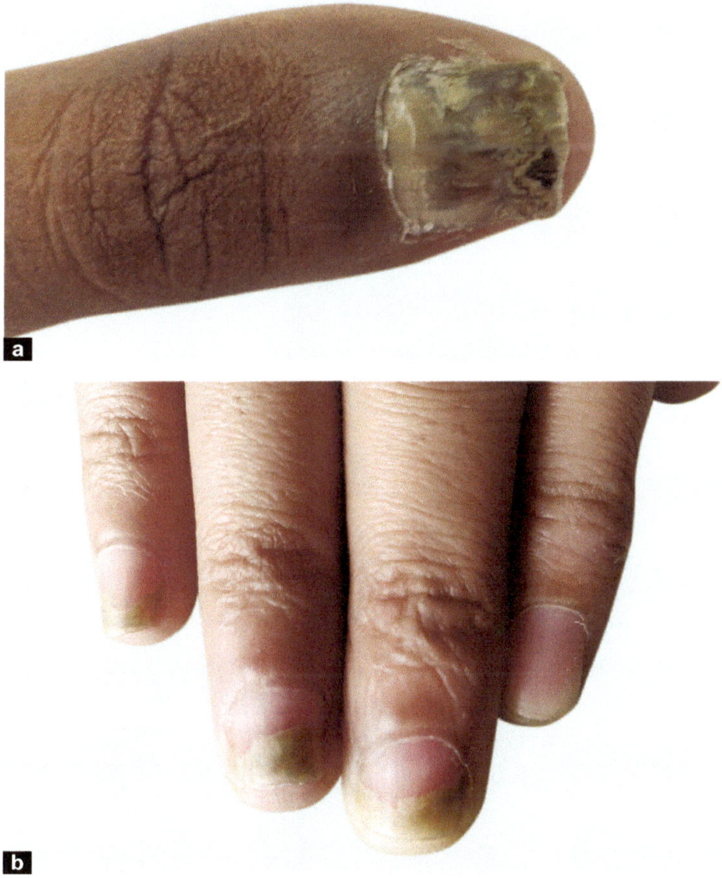

FIGURE 5.13a and b: (a) Onycholysis with jagged edges at proximal margins in tinea unguium; (b) Regular onycholysis with erythema at the proximal end in nail psoriasis

ERYTHRODERMIC TINEA

Tinea corporis can cause erythroderma with extensive involvement and diffuse scaling. A high degree of suspicion is required, and a simple KOH mount is sufficient for diagnosis. An underlying immunocompromised state or prolonged usage of topical steroids are contributory factors **(Fig. 5.14a and b)**.

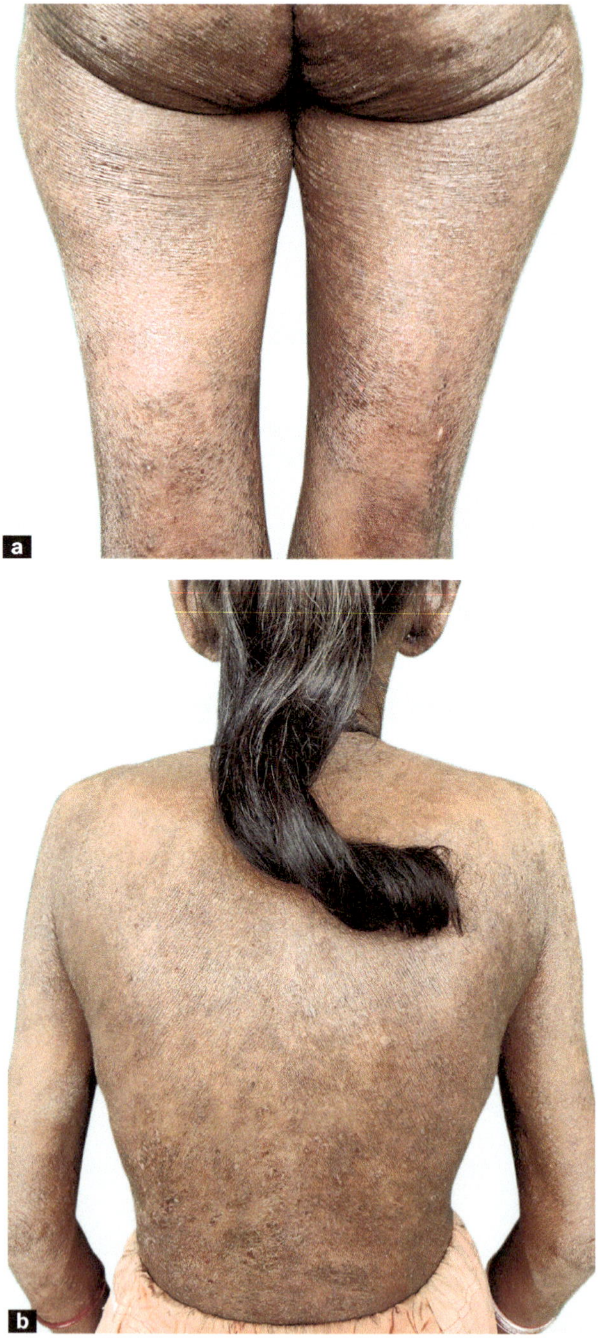

FIGURE 5.14a and b: Erythroderma in a patient of extensive tinea

CONCLUSION

Classical patterns of dermatophytosis are easy to diagnose clinically. Atypical patterns and associated factors such as topical steroid abuse may make diagnosis difficult. Changing clinical patterns have been observed in pediatric population as well.[6] There are increasing reports of resistance with rise in MICs to terbinafine and itraconazole along with squalene epoxidase mutations.[7,8] Dermoscopy and a simple KOH mount are often sufficient to confirm diagnosis.

Key Points

- Chronic and recurrent dermatophytosis often presents with atypical patterns, including psoriasiform, seborrheic dermatitis-like, erythroderma, and lupus erythematosus-like features.
- Common conditions that mimic tinea corporis include psoriasis (with silvery scales), impetigo (honey-colored crusts), pityriasis rosea (Christmas tree distribution), and lichen simplex chronicus (lichenification due to scratching).
- Conditions such as alopecia areata, trichotillomania, seborrheic dermatitis, and discoid lupus erythematosus can resemble tinea capitis and require careful differentiation through clinical features and diagnostic tools like KOH mounts.
- Tinea cruris may be confused with conditions like candidiasis (with satellite pustules) or erythrasma (coral-red fluorescence)
- Tinea unguium often needs differentiation from nail psoriasis and lichen planus through dermoscopy and fungal cultures.
- Diagnosis of dermatophytosis in challenging cases often relies on KOH mounts, dermoscopy, and sometimes histopathology, particularly in cases altered by steroid misuse or immunosuppression.

REFERENCES

1. Hay RJ, Ashbee HR. Fungal infections. In: Griffith C, Barker J, Bleiker Tanya, Chalmers R, Creamer D, (eds). Rook's Textbook of Dermatology, 9th edn. Wiley Blackwell, UK. 2016;1:32.6–32.96.
2. Dogra S, Narang T. Emerging atypical and unusual presentations of dermatophytosis in India. Clinical Dermatology Review 2017;1(Suppl 1): S12–S18.
3. Ankad BS, Mukherjee SS, Nikam BP, Reshme AS, Sakhare PS, Mural PH. Dermoscopic characterization of dermatophytosis: A preliminary observation. Indian Dermatol Online J 2020;11(2):202–7.
4. Errichetti E, Stinco G. Dermoscopy in tinea manuum. An Bras Dermatol 2018;93(3):447–8.
5. Errichetti E, Stinco G. Dermoscopy as a supportive instrument in the differentiation of the main types of acquired keratoderma due to dermatological disorders. J Eur Acad Dermatol Venereol 2016;30:e229–e231.
6. Poojary S, Jaiswal S, Bhalala K, Bagadia J, Shah K, Arora S, et al. A cross sectional observational study of pediatric dermatophytosis: Changing clinico mycological patterns in western India. Indian Journal of Paediatric Dermatology 22(3):p 236–40.
7. Poojary S, Miskeen A, Bagadia J, Jaiswal S, Uppuluri P. A Study of *in vitro* antifungal susceptibility patterns of dermatophytic fungi at a tertiary care center in western India. Indian J Dermatol. 2019;64(4):277–84.
8. Ebert A, Monod M, Salamin K, Burmester A, Uhrlaß S, Wiegand C, et al. Alarming India-wide phenomenon of antifungal resistance in dermatophytes: A multicentre study. Mycoses. 2020;63(7):717–28.

CHAPTER 6

Old and New Topical Antifungal Agents

• *Meghana Phiske*

INTRODUCTION

Topical antifungal medication is cream, solution, lotion, powder, gel, spray or lacquer applied to skin to treat fungal infection. They are considered first-line therapy, due to high efficacy and low potential for systemic adverse effects and are important adjuvants for uncomplicated, superficial dermatophytosis, being also preferred in pregnancy and for infants.[1,2]

They are compounded into various types of vehicles to facilitate penetration and efficacy depending on site of involvement. They readily penetrate stratum corneum, killing fungi or inhibiting their growth, achieving clinical and mycologic eradication.[3]

Advantages and disadvantages of topical antifungals are mentioned in **Table 6.1**.

CLASSIFICATION OF TOPICAL ANTIFUNGALS

They are classified as polyenes, azoles and allylamines/benzylamines. Other antifungals include ciclopirox olamine, oxaborole, tavaborole and selenium sulfide.[1]

Polyenes

These drugs were the first agents with specific antifungal properties. They contain macrolide ring of carbon atoms with several conjugated double bonds, hence named polyenes. Clinically significant and readily available polyenes are nystatin and amphotericin B **(Table 6.2)**.[1]

Azoles

New class of compounds with broader spectrum of activity including action against dermatophytes not susceptible to polyenes.[1] They have excellent capacity for stratum corneum penetration. Systemic absorption is prevented, even when applied on inflamed skin due to their strong keratinophilic property. Subgroups include imidazoles, triazoles and thiazoles.[4] Azoles interfere with cytochrome P-450-dependent enzyme, lanosterol 14α-demethylase, which catalyzes conversion of lanosterol to ergosterol. Decreased availability of ergosterol and accumulation of intracellular 14α-methylsterols results in increased membrane rigidity, membrane permeability changes, alterations in critical membrane bound enzymes, inhibition of growth and ultimately cell death.[1] Tioconazole (imidazole group), may be useful for onychomycosis in nail formulation.[4] Details of azoles is mentioned in **Table 6.3a to c**.

TABLE 6.1: Advantages and disadvantages of topical antifungals[2]	
Advantages	**Disadvantages**
Lack of systemic side effects and complications due to limited systemic absorption	Difficult to use in extensive dermatophytic infections
Very low incidence of drug interactions	Application of inadequate amount results in poor response
Ease of use	Inability to apply in difficult-to-reach areas (e.g. natal cleft) may leave residual foci of infection
Comparatively low cost of therapy	Low effectiveness in onychomycosis due to inadequate penetration
Additional benefit of anti-inflammatory activity of several topical antifungals (azoles and allylamines)	Rarely contact dermatitis

TABLE 6.2: Details of polyene antifungals[1, 4]		
Polyenes class of topical antifungal	**Nystatin**	**Amphotericin B**
	First specific antimycotic to become available for human use	• Mostly available in systemic form • Topical liposomal gel is under investigation
Source	Produced by *Streptomyces noursei* and *Streptomyces albidus*	
Structure	• Tetraene antibiotic with both conjugated diene and conjugated tetraene moiety in the molecule • It also contains a sugar moiety, mycosamine, as part of its composition	
Mechanism of action	• Both fungistatic (at low concentrations) and fungicidal activity (at high concentrations) *in vitro* • Acts by binding irreversibly to membrane sterols of susceptible species of *Candida*, resulting in a change in membrane permeability and the subsequent leakage of essential intracellular components • Essentially insoluble in water and not absorbed from intact skin, gastrointestinal tract, or vagina	
Indication	• Clinically and mycologically effective for cutaneous and mucocutaneous mycotic infections caused by *Candida albicans* and other susceptible species • Clinically ineffective for dermatophyte infections	
Formulation and dosing	• Available in cream, ointment, lotion and powder formulations for twice-daily cutaneous application • Also available in suspension and slowly dissolving pastille formulations for the treatment of oral candidiasis	
Adverse effects	• Burning, pruritus, rash, eczema, and pain on application • Very rare occurrences of hypersensitivity reactions	

TABLE 6.3a: Details of azole topical antifungals[1, 4]

Azole class of topical antifungal	Miconazole	Clotrimazole	Ketoconazole	Oxiconazole
Structure	• Synthetic β-substituted 1-phenethylimidazole derivative • Penetrates stratum corneum well, and can be detected there for 4 days after a single application	• A 1-[(2-chlorophenyl) (diphenyl) methyl]-1H imidazole • Broad-spectrum imidazole antifungal agent	• Water-soluble imidazole derivative synthetic antimycotic	• Acetophenone-oxime derivative of basic imidazole structural unit • Penetrates stratum corneum rapidly to reach fungicidal concentrations • Remains in epidermis for up to 7 days
Indication	• Active *in vitro* against *Trichophyton rubrum, Trichophyton mentagrophytes*, and *Epidermophyton floccosum* • Effective for tinea pedis, tinea corporis, tinea cruris • Activity against some Gram-positive bacteria, modestly effective in erythrasma, impetigo, and ecthyma	• Active against *Trichophyton rubrum, T. mentagrophytes*, and *Epidermophyton floccosum* • Effective in the treatment of tinea pedis, corporis, cruris • Activity against some Gram-positive bacteria	• Effective for tinea pedis, tinea cruris, and tinea corporis • Broad spectrum of activity against dermatophytes • Anti-inflammatory action	• First topical antifungal approved for once daily application • *In vitro* highly effective against *T. rubrum, T. mentagrophytes, Trichophyton tonsurans*, and *E. floccosum* • Effective for tinea pedis, including hyperkeratotic plantar and interdigital subtypes
Formulation and dosing	Available as a cream with twice-daily application	Available in cream, lotion, and solution formulations for twice-daily application.	Available as a cream and shampoo	• Available as 1% cream and 1% lotion, latter useful for large or hairy areas (trunk and back) • Used once or twice daily
Adverse effects	Well tolerated, rare side effects include burning, irritation, maceration, and allergic dermatitis at application site	Well tolerated, with isolated reports of erythema, burning, irritation, stinging, peeling, blistering, edema, pruritus, and urticaria at site of application	Irritation, pruritus, stinging and rarely contact dermatitis	Well tolerated, with isolated reports of pruritus, erythema, burning, irritation, maceration and fissuring

TABLE 6.3b: Details of azole topical antifungals[1, 3, 4]

Azole class of topical antifungal	Econazole	Sulconazole	Sertaconazole	Luliconazole (see Fig. 6.1)
Structure	• Deschloro derivative of miconazole • Absolute concentrations in stratum corneum after local application far exceeds minimal inhibitory concentration (MIC) for dermatophytes • Inhibitory concentrations are detected up to mid-dermis • Faster onset of action	• Has sulfide (thiol) bond between constituent rings • Inhibits lanosterol 14α-demethylase • Has modest antibacterial activity against Gram-positive bacteria • Remains in stratum corneum up to 4 days • Percutaneous absorption (higher than other azoles) is clinically insignificant	• Contains benzothiophene ring which uniquely distinguishes it from other imidazole antifungals • Relatively lipophilic compared with other azoles, leading to a greater reservoir effect in stratum corneum • Can be either fungistatic or fungicidal depending on concentration of drug and specific organisms involved • Anti-inflammatory and antipruritic effects causing increased compliance	• Is R-enantiomer of lanoconazole, is an imidazole antifungal • Has a unique chemical structure which is augmented by introduction of an imidazole moiety into ketene dithioacetate structure • This modification allows an unusually high potency against filamentous fungi while maintaining broad spectrum
Indication	• Effective for tinea pedis, corporis, cruris • Activity against some Gram-positive and Gram-negative bacterial organisms	Effective for dermatophytosis caused by common organisms	• Antifungal spectrum includes: *E. floccosum*, *T. mentagrophytes*, *T. rubrum*, and *C. albicans* • Has modest activity against Gram-positive bacteria	• MIC is 1–4 times lower than lanoconazole and terbinafine for *T. rubrum* and *T. mentagrophytes* • Effective for tinea corporis, tinea pedis and tinea cruris caused by *T. rubrum* and *E. flocossum* • Has excellent penetration capability through nail layer proving useful for onychomycosis
Formulation and dosing		Available as 1% cream and 1% solution, to be applied 1–2 times daily until clinical resolution (2 to 4 weeks)	Available as 1% cream, gel, powder, and solution, to be used twice daily	Available as 1% topical cream to be applied once daily
Adverse effects	Isolated reports of pruritus, erythema, burning and stinging	Well tolerated, with isolated reports of allergic contact dermatitis	Excellent safety profile, with rare reports of allergic contact dermatitis	Well tolerated, with rare reports of allergic contact dermatitis and cellulitis

TABLE 6.3c: Details of azole topical antifungals[1–5]

Azole class of topical antifungal	Efinaconazole	Eberconazole	Lanoconazole	Bifonazole
Structure and chemical properties	• First topical triazole approved for toenail onychomycosis • Has potent broad spectrum antifungal activity against dermatophytes • Drug reaches infection site by transungual delivery and spreads through subungual space • Keratin binding is not strong, so low keratin affinity is thought to result in increased availability of free drug to nail infection site • Methylene-piperidine group at C-4 position of efinaconazole molecule may be responsible for its relatively low keratin binding. • Has low surface tension which also leads to increased penetration and spreading	Imidazole azole with broad antimicrobial activity	Racemic imidazole antifungal agent	Substituted imidazole antifungal agent
Indication	• Indicated for fungal infections of nail in mild-to-moderate tinea unguium without lunula involvement attributed to *T. rubrum* and *T. mentagrophytes* in immunocompetent • Because of its low- risk of AE, quick treatment duration, and broad-spectrum activity, it may be useful for pediatric and geriatric patients • Is fungistatic, not fungicidal, hence it may induce resistance in dermatophytes	• Good efficacy against dermatophytes • Possesses antibacterial property against Gram-positive bacteria • Has anti-inflammatory activity similar to aspirin and ketoprofen, and this effect is due to inhibition of 5-lipo-oxygenase and cyclo-oxygenase-2	• Widely used in Japan for tinea pedis, tinea corporis • Has anti-inflammatory activity due to inhibition of IL-8.	Has broad spectrum of activity *in vitro* against dermatophytes, molds, yeasts, dimorphic fungi and Gram-positive bacteria
Formulation and dosing	Available as 10% topical solution, is to be applied once daily for 48 weeks with brush applicator to affected toenail and its undersurface, nail folds, nail bed and hyponychium	Available as 1% cream		• Efficacious and safe as once daily application for dermatophytosis • Available as 1% cream, gel, solution and powder forms
Adverse effects	None reported	Mild-to-moderate application site reactions		

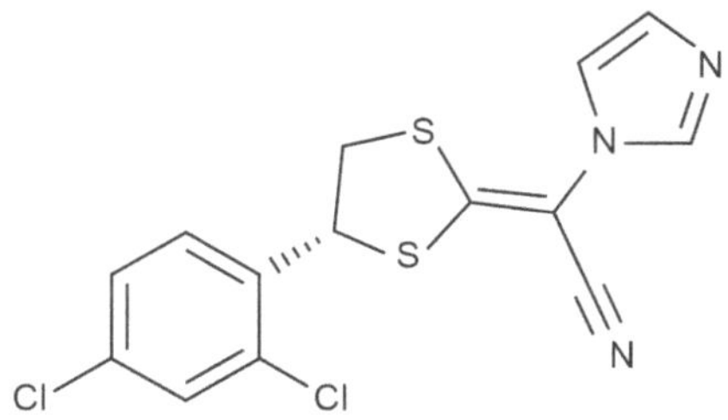

FIGURE 6.1: Luliconazole chemical structure

Allylamines and Benzylamines

Allylamines are a new class of broad-spectrum antifungals, with fungistatic and fungicidal activity, and include Naftifine and terbinafine. Butenafine is first and only representative of benzylamine class.[1] Details of Allylamines and Benzylamines are mentioned in **Table 6.4**.

Other Antifungals

Details of other topical antifungals is mentioned in **Table 6.5**.

NEWER TOPICAL ANTIFUNGALS

ME-1111

Novel antifungal with fungicidal activity. Ideal antifungal for onychomycosis as it has potent anti-dermatophyte activity, low molecular weight leading to increased penetration, maintaining good inhibitory activity even in presence of keratin and low propensity to develop resistance in dermatophytes. It selectively inhibits fungal succinate dehydrogenase, an important enzyme involved in mitochondrial respiratory electron transfer leading to ATP production blockade.[2, 3] This is probably an indication of extensive structural damage to hyphae due to its fungicidal activity **(Fig. 6.4)**.[2] With regards to penetration and attainment of high concentrations in deeper nail layers, 10% ME-1111 topical formulation is superior to 8% Ciclopirox nail lacquer.[5]

Pramiconazole

Newer triazole under development, with good *in vitro* and clinical activity against dermatophytes. Topical Pramiconazole have shown superior efficacy compared to Itraconazole and Terbinafine against *Microsporum canis* in guinea pigs.[3]

Arasertaconazole

Novel 14α-lanosterol demethylase inhibitor, under development.[3]

BB-2603

Newer squalene epoxidase inhibitor in spray formulation currently ongoing trials for onychomycosis and tinea pedis.[3]

Oxaboroles

New class of drug with broad-spectrum antifungal activity against *T. rubrum* and *T. mentagrophytes*. It acts by blocking protein synthesis via inhibition of leucyl aminoacyl transfer RNA synthetase. Premature termination of protein synthesis leads to growth inhibition and fungal death.[3]

TABLE 6.4: Details of Allylamines and Benzylamines[1, 3, 4]

Allylamines and Benzylamines	Naftifine	Terbinafine (*see* Fig. 6.2)	Butenafine	Amorolfine
Structure and chemical properties	Synthetic allylamine antifungal, with highly lipophilic nature which allows for efficient penetration and high concentrations in stratum corneum and hair follicles	• Broad-spectrum synthetic antimycotic agent of allylamine chemical family, with both fungistatic and fungicidal properties • Highly lipophilic, resulting in high concentration in and efficient binding to stratum corneum, sebum, and hair follicles, thereby reducing the probability of reinfection • 10 to 100 times more potent *in vitro* • Key structural modifications to allylamine group include: benzene ring, with an additional triple bond (the acetylene group), and addition of branched side chain leading to significantly increased antifungal activity *in vitro* and *in vivo*	• Structurally similar to various allylamines with butyl benzyl group in place of allylamine group • Fungicidal concentrations in stratum corneum, for at least 72 hours after application as a result of interaction with or fixation to cutaneous lipids, leading to a depot effect	Morpholine antifungal drug
Mechanism of action	• Both fungicidal and fungistatic • Through squalene epoxidase inhibition, it leads to decreased ergosterol synthesis, increased accumulation of sterol precursor squalene, and subsequent disruption of fungal cell membrane • Has anti-inflammatory activity by targeting prostaglandin pathway	Through squalene epoxidase inhibition, it leads to decreased ergosterol synthesis, increased accumulation of sterol precursor squalene, and subsequent disruption of fungal cell membrane	• Acts by squalene epoxidase inhibition, leading to decreased ergosterol synthesis, increased accumulation of sterol precursor squalene, and subsequent disruption of fungal cell membrane • Has anti-inflammatory activity	Inhibits D14 reductase and D7–D8 isomerase which depletes ergosterol

(*Contd.*)

TABLE 6.4: Details of Allylamines and Benzylamines[1, 3, 4] *(Contd.)*

Allylamines and Benzylamines	Naftifine	Terbinafine (see Fig. 6.2)	Butenafine	Amorolfine
Indication	• Effective in tinea pedis, tinea cruris, tinea corporis • Effective monotherapy for moccasin tinea pedis • Has strong activity against *T. mentagrophytes*	FDA approved for interdigital-type tinea pedis (athlete's foot), tinea cruris (jock itch), and tinea corporis (ringworm)	• Effective for short-term therapy for interdigital tinea pedis, tinea corporis, and tinea cruris • Continued mycologic and clinical improvement after completion of therapy, suggesting a continued benefit after dose completion related to strong keratin binding	Used for onychomycosis in lacquer formulation, which reduces propensity to form antifungal-resistant spores and limits risk of reinfection
Formulation and dosing	Available as cream and gel formulations, applied once to twice daily	Available as a 1% cream and lotion, to be applied once daily	Available as cream for once daily application	Available as cream for once-twice daily application and nail lacquer
Adverse effects	Well tolerated, with isolated reports of pruritus, erythema, mild burning and irritation and rarely, allergic reactions	Well tolerated, with few adverse effects like irritation, burning/tingling sensation, pruritus, and dryness at application site	Burning, pruritus and redness at application site	Allergic contact dermatitis

TABLE 6.5: Details of other topical antifungals[1, 3–5]

Other topical antifungals	Ciclopirox olamine	Selenium sulfide	Tavaborole (see Fig. 6.3)	Tolnaftate	Undecylenic acid
Structure and chemical properties	• Hydroxypyridone antifungal with a unique structure and a mode of action unrelated to other available antifungals • Does not affect sterol biosynthesis.	Liquid antiseborrheic, antifungal for topical application only	• First FDA approved oxaborole antifungal for onychomycosis caused by *T. rubrum* or *T. mentagrophyte* • Low molecular weight (152 kDa) and highly specific fungal protein synthesis inhibitor that forms boron-based bond at enzyme-editing site to prevent catalytic turnover of leucyl-tRNA synthetase and block fungal protein synthesis resulting in suppression of fungal cell activity • Has 1000-fold greater selectivity for fungal leucyl-tRNA synthase compared to mammalian leucyl-tRNA synthetase • Low molecular weight enables its good penetration through thick nail plate • Has low propensity to develop resistance	Synthetic thiocarbamate used as an antifungal agent	Organic unsaturated fatty acid derived from castor oil with natural fungicidal property

(Contd.)

TABLE 6.5: Details of other topical antifungals[1, 3–5] *(Contd.)*

Other topical antifungals	Ciclopirox olamine	Selenium sulfide	Tavaborole (see Fig. 6.3)	Tolnaftate	Undecylenic acid
Mechanism of action	• Acts by interfering with active membrane transport of essential macromolecular precursors, disrupting cell membrane integrity and inhibiting enzymes essential for respiratory processes • High affinity for trivalent cations, and subsequent blockade of enzymatic cofactors is main mode of action. • Also has inherent anti-inflammatory activity. • Has exhibited strong activity in vitro and in vivo against Gram-positive and Gram-negative bacteria. • Inhibits prostaglandin and leukotriene synthesis in human polymorphonuclear (PMN) leukocytes. • Due to unique and multilevel mechanism of action resistance is rarely reported	Has cytostatic effect on cells of epidermis and follicular epithelium, which allows for shedding of fungi in stratum corneum via reduction in corneocyte adhesion	• Functions by inhibiting fungal protein synthesis through leucyl-transfer ribonucleic acid (tRNA) synthetase (LeuRS • This aminoacyl-tRNA synthetase warrants accurate translation of genetic code by catalyzing attachment of an amino acid to its corresponding tRNA • LeuRS is inhibited when boron atom within oxaborole ring of tavaborole binds to oxygen atoms of tRNALeu terminal adenosine which in turns blocks *tRNA Leu* active site, thereby preventing translation of *tRNA* by *Leu*RS • Not likely to induce resistance	Inhibition of squalene epoxidase	Disrupts the structural and functional stability of the fungal cell membrane

(Contd.)

TABLE 6.5: Details of other topical antifungals[1, 3–5] *(Contd.)*

Other topical antifungals	Ciclopirox olamine	Selenium sulfide	Tavaborole (see Fig. 6.3)	Tolnaftate	Undecylenic acid
Indication	• *In vitro*, exhibits high inhibitory activity against dermatophytes • Its antimicrobial profile includes: clinically relevant dermatophytes, yeasts and is therefore broader than that of most other drugs • Approved for treatment of tinea pedis, corporis	Effective adjuvant with griseofulvin for tinea capitis	• Should be applied to affected area of onychomycosis once daily for 48 weeks and over entire surface of toenail and underneath tip of the toenail • Mycologic cure rate is lower than oral antifungal agents (30–36% *vs* 50–76%, respectively), however, it might provide an important alternative or adjuvant to available antifungal therapies • Good substitute for oral antifungals in patients with associated comorbidities	Dermatophytosis on glabrous skin	Effective for dermatophytosis on glabrous skin relieving itching, burning and irritation
Formulation and dosing	• Available as a cream, gel, or suspension (0.77%) and nail lacquer (1.0%) • Suspension formulation is suited for extensive skin surface, e.g. widespread tinea corporis		Available as solution 5%	Available in cream, powder, spray, and liquid aerosol forms	In 3% concentration, it is active ingredient in medications for skin infections
Adverse effects	Well tolerated, with few adverse effects reported like burning, pruritus, and rarely allergic hypersensitivity		Well tolerated, commonly application site related or ingrown toenail		

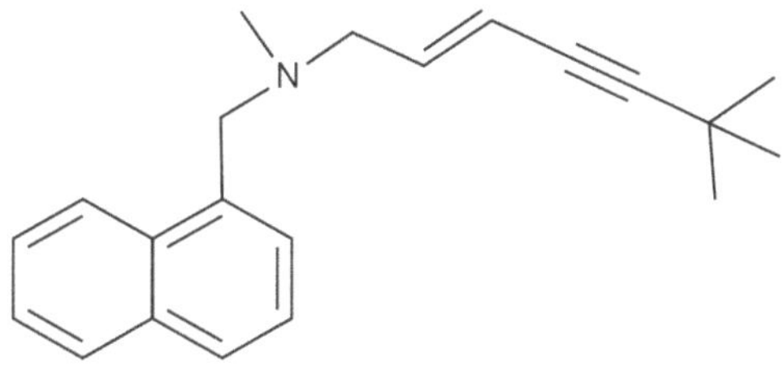

FIGURE 6.2: Chemical structure of Terbinafine

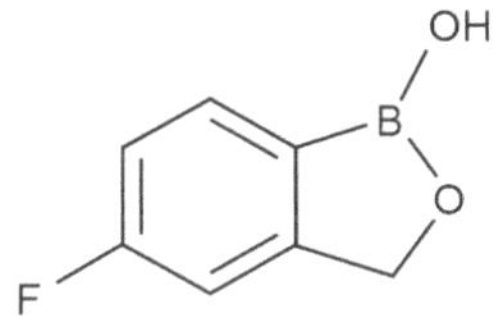

FIGURE 6.3: Chemical structure of Tavaborole

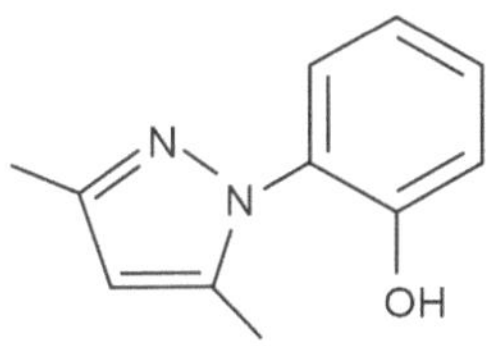

FIGURE 6.4: Chemical structure of ME-1111

Hydroxypyridones

Weak acids with broad-spectrum antimicrobial activity and low incidence of resistance. Prototype is Ciclopirox, others include Rilopirox and Octopirox. They act by chelating trivalent metal cations causing inhibition of metal-dependent enzymes leading to less degradation of cytoplasmic peroxides, increased sensitivity of cells to oxidative stress and decreased levels of iron permeases or transporters.[3]

AR12

Acetyl-CoA synthase inhibitor, effective for onychomycosis.[3]

NP213

New topical synthetic peptide, under investigation for treating onychomycosis. Designed and developed based on host defense peptide structure and pattern of action, it acts by novel mechanism. Positively charged peptide rapidly penetrates negatively charged nail and circumvents proteolytic activity of dermatophyte peptidases and proteases due to its all-arginine composition and cyclic structure **(Fig. 6.5)**. It causes lysis of cytoplasmic membranes without affecting cell wall integrity. As it has high efficacy and biostability that establishes disease-free microenvironment within nail apparatus, it can become useful therapeutic tool in future.[5]

Quinoline Derivatives

Have selective and potent anti-dermatophytic activity. Compound 5 has safe toxicological profile at topical level, suggesting its indication as strong candidate for development of new effective compound against dermatophytosis.[6]

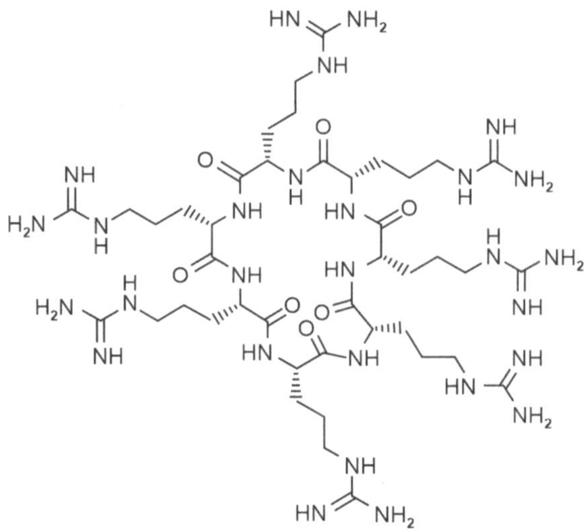

FIGURE 6.5: Chemical structure of NP-213

NEWER FORMULATIONS OF TOPICAL ANTIFUNGALS (Table 6.6)[2, 3]

Anhydrous Gel Formulations

Higher solubility of drug in anhydrous vehicle may result in higher thermodynamic activity allowing greater partitioning and increased bioavailability of antifungal into skin, e.g. sertaconazole anhydrous gel.[2]

Transfersomes

Flexible and ultra-deformable drug carriers composed of complex lipid vesicles used for noninvasive drug delivery through skin/nail. Nail acts as hydrophilic gel network through which transfersome carrier can easily traverse, increasing drug concentration in nail bed. TDT-067 (terbinafine 15 mg/ml in transfersome) can deliver high concentrations of Terbinafine to infection site in nail bed.[2] Used as carriers for griseofulvin and amphotericin B in dermatophytosis with better efficacy.[3]

Microemulsion Gel

Microemulsions are clear, stable, isotropic mixtures of oil, water surfactant, and co-surfactant. Enhanced drug solubility, good thermodynamic stability and higher transdermal permeability are its advantages. Clotrimazole microemulsion formulations have significantly higher skin retention compared to clotrimazole creams.[2]

Liposomes/Ethosomes

Ethosomes are soft malleable vesicles constituting phospholipids, ethanol and water. They act as noninvasive delivery carriers for targeting antifungal drugs to deep skin layers for long time, e.g. terbinafine HCl ethosomes.[2] Transferosomes have been used as carriers for griseofulvin and amphotericin B for dermatophytosis with better efficacy.[3]

Poloxamer 407-based Formulations

Permeation coefficient from these formulations was higher in comparison to nail lacquer.[2]

TABLE 6.6: Newer formulation for old topical antifungals[2, 3]

Name of old topical antifungal	Newer formulation	Advantages
Amphotericin B	Microemulsion and nanoemulsion	Increased skin retention of the drug leading to better *in vitro* antifungal activity
Amphotericin B	Lipid-based gel formulation	Good safety profile
Amphotericin B	Amphotericin B nanoliposomes Nanotechnology may provide an increase in potency without affecting drug activity	Liposomal Amphotericin B formulation has displayed lower MIC compared to Amphotericin or liposomes without evidence of resistance Nanoliposomes could be an effective way to deliver drug transungually by using appropriate particle size and encapsulation
Amphotericin B	Topical amphotericin formulation (ABL01) for onychomycosis has been recently studied	
Econazole	Aqueous micellar solutions	13-fold higher deposition of drug compared to conventional preparation
Clotrimazole, miconazole, ketoconazole, fluconazole, terbinafine, and griseofulvin	Solid lipid nanoparticles and nanostructured lipid carriers	Increase occlusion, better penetration, less degradation of active drug, and sustained release over longer duration leading to increased efficacy
Griseofulvin and amphotericin B	Ultra-deformable or flexible liposomes	Better efficacy
Terbinafine	• MOB015B is Terbinafine 10% solution • MOB015B formula contains urea, lactic acid, and propylene glycol as enhancers of penetration • P-3058 is a Terbinafine reformulation that contains the novel excipient hydroxypropyl chitosan as a film-forming agent • BB2603 is another topical Terbinafine-based agent under investigation. It uses polyhexamethylene biguanide (PHMB) as an excipient and is administered as low-velocity spray	Higher concentrations in the nail plate (median value 1610 μg/g) and nailbed (median value 45 μg/g) than oral Terbinafine (up to 1000-fold and 40-fold, respectively)

(Contd.)

TABLE 6.6: Newer formulation for old topical antifungals[2, 3] *(Contd.)*

Name of old topical antifungal	Newer formulation	Advantages
Terbinafine	Terbinafine-based formulation using poly(pseudo) rotaxanes (PPR) technology	
Terbinafine	Terbinafine-based PPRs are water-soluble preparations consisting of micelles, α-cyclodextrin, and Terbinafine	Small amphiphilic surfactants solubilize Terbinafine and form 2% (w/v) gels PPRs exhibit viscoelastic properties that favor high concentrations in deep layers and prolong drug presence at application site
Terbinafine	Subungual insert (HTS-519) has been evaluated in completed open-label phase II trial	
Terbinafine	Subungual gel	
Ciclopirox	Ciclopirox, dissolved in lipid diffusion enhancers, hydrosoluble preparations, formulation containing isopropyl alcohol, potassium hydroxide, and urea	Have led to excellent efficacy and permeation for onychomycosis
Luliconazole	Luliconazole 10% solution (recently approved) is administered on nail as 5% w/w solution.	• Drug concentration increases in dose-dependent manner, as it is positively associated with duration of application • It penetrates nail plate and rapidly achieves fungicidal levels in nail unit independent of nail plate thickness

Nail Penetration Enhancer Containing Nanovesicles

Newer formulations of sertaconazole, i.e. anhydrous gel, microsponge, microemulsion, nanovesicles, loaded hydrogel, bioadhesive gel, transdermal and nail patches, are under development to enhance dermal delivery and skin retention of drug.[3]

Film-forming Solution

Film-forming Terbinafine solution, forms thin film allowing fungicidal effect to be maintained for 13 days following single application.[2]

Nail Solution

Luliconazole, 10% nail solution, has shown high penetration in nails at 7 days after 29-day application for onychomycosis.[2]

Ethyl Cellulose Microsponges

Ethyl cellulose microsponges as topical carriers of eberconazole causes four-fold retention in stratum corneum allowing increased drug efficacy.[3]

Colloidal Nanocarriers

Colloidal nanocarriers containing drug, leads to increased penetration in stratum corneum.[3]

Solid Lipid Nanoparticles and Nanostructured Lipid Carriers

They increase occlusion, cause better penetration, less degradation of active drug, and sustained release over longer duration leading to increased efficacy. They have been used for clotrimazole, miconazole, ketoconazole, fluconazole, terbinafine, and griseofulvin. Solid lipid nanoparticles of clotrimazole and miconazole have shown sustained and 10-fold better retention than hydrogels.[2,3]

Newer formulation for old topical antifungals is mentioned in **Table 6.6.**[2,3]

CONCLUSION

There is need for newer antifungals due to growing epidemic of recurrent/chronic dermatophytosis.[3] Due to widely increasing resistance, older drugs in newer formulations are being studied and are likely to be added to existing list to achieve maximum cure.

Key Points

- Topical antifungals offer advantages such as lack of systemic adverse effects, low incidence of drug interactions, ease of use, lower cost of therapy and additional anti-inflammatory effects (in case of azoles and allylamines).
- Topical antifungals are classified as polyenes, azoles, allylamines/benzylamines and others (cyclopirox olamine, undecylenic acid, selenium sulfide, etc.).
- Newer antifungals such as oxaboroles and ME-1111 target enzymes different from the conventional antifungal agents.
- Conventional antifungal agents have been incorporated in novel formulations using nanotechnology, to enhance penetration and bioavailability in the skin.

REFERENCES

1. Aditya G, Rachel M, Kelly F. Comprehensive dermatologic drug therapy, 4th edn. Stephen Wolverton; 2021.pp.481–92.
2. Shital P. Topical antifungals: A review and their role in current management of dermatophytosis. Clin Dermatol Rev 2017;1(1):24–9.
3. Kanika S, Sanjay S, Sunil D. Newer topical treatments in skin and nail dermatophyte infections. Indian Dermatol Online J 2018;9(3):149–58.
4. Arijit C, Sujata S. IADVL textbook of dermatology, 4th edn. In: Sacchidanand S; 2015. Chapter 59,Topical Therapy in Dermatology; 2015.pp.2243–2313.
5. Stamatios G, Maria K, Aikaterini T, Dimitrios R. Novel and investigational treatments for onychomycosis. J Fungi 2022;8(10):1079.
6. Gabriella M, Denise D, Thaís R, Aline Z, Mário T, Luís O, et al. Quinolines derivatives as promising new antifungal candidates for the treatment of candidiasis and dermatophytosis. Braz J Microbiol 2020;51(4):1691–1701.

CHAPTER 7

Old and New Systemic Agents and Major Drug Interactions

• Preethi B Nayak • Vivek M Pai

INTRODUCTION

Antifungal drugs which are used in treatment of dermatophytosis typically fall into the following structural families: (1) Triazoles–Itraconazole, Fluconazole, Voriconazole, Posaconazole and Ravuconazole, (2) Imidazoles–Ketoconazole, and (3) Allylamines–Terbinafine, Naftifine. Griseofulvin belongs to Caspofungin group of antifungals. This chapter focuses on Terbinafine, Itraconazole and Fluconazole, as the traditional agents, Griseofulvin and Ketoconazole, now have limited use in the management of onychomycosis and other dermatomycoses. Newer generation of systemic antifungal agents are Voriconazole, Posaconazole, and Ravuconazole.

The salient drugs act by inhibiting the ergosterol synthesis pathway while others act via inhibition of the cell wall. The main drugs that are prescribed by clinicians focus on the cytoplasmic membrane synthesis (**Fig. 7.1**).

Indications for systemic antifungal therapy are extensive tinea corporis, multiple site involvement, tinea pedis/tinea manuum, chronic/recurrent dermatophytosis, tinea capitis, onychomycosis, tinea incognito and special forms–Majocchi granuloma, tinea imbricata.[1-4]

IMIDAZOLES AND TRIAZOLES

The mechanism of action of Imidazoles (Ketoconazole) and Triazoles (Fluconazole and Itraconazole) is the same. They inhibit the fungal cytochrome P450 enzyme 'lanosterol 14-α-demethylase' and thus impair ergosterol synthesis leading to a cascade of membrane abnormalities in the fungus (**Fig. 7.1**). The lower host toxicity of Triazoles compared to Imidazoles has correlated with their lower affinity for mammalian CYP450 enzymes and lesser propensity to inhibit mammalian sterol synthesis.[2,3]

Fluconazole

It is a water-soluble triazole. It is a fungistatic drug. It was initially approved for use in humans in France and the United Kingdom in 1988. Fluconazole is well absorbed orally, and its dermatological uses include dermatophyte infections (tinea).

Pharmacokinetics

Formulation: Tablet, oral suspension, IV

Half-life: 30 hours

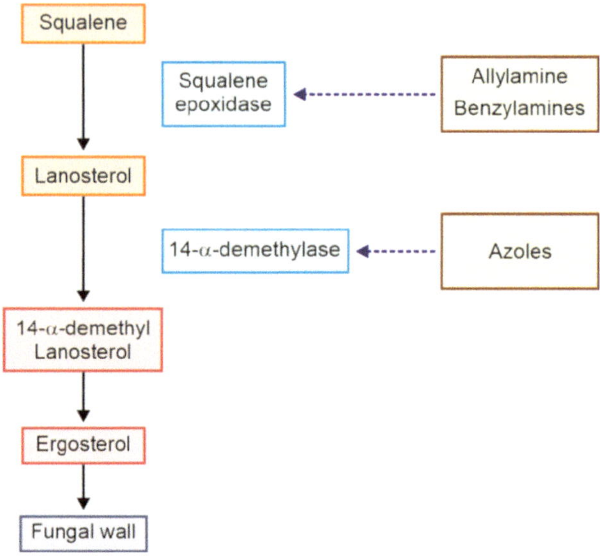

FIGURE 7.1: Site of action of the main class of oral antifungals used for dermatophytosis

Bio-availability: 90%, not affected by food intake
Metabolism: Little first pass hepatic metabolism
Excretion: Renal
Dosage: 50, 100, 150, 200, 300, 400 mg tablets, IV 2 mg/ml, oral suspension 50 mg/5 ml and 200 mg/5 ml.

Fluconazole is 94% absorbed. Fungicidal concentrations are achieved in nails, vagina and saliva; penetration into brain and CSF is good. Dose reduction is needed in renal impairment. It is a potent CYP2C9 inhibitor, moderate CYP3A4 inhibitor. When Fluconazole 50–400 mg is given once daily, steady-state concentrations are achieved within 5–10 days, but may be attained more rapidly by doubling the dose on the first day. When two doses of Fluconazole (150 mg once weekly) are administered, the drug accumulates in the stratum corneum through sweat and by direct diffusion through the dermis and epidermis.

Indication

1. Genital candidiasis and oropharyngeal candidiasis.
2. Systemic candidiasis, including candidemia and disseminated candidiasis.
3. Superficial mycoses: Tinea pedis, tinea corporis, tinea cruris, pityriasis versicolor and cutaneous candidiasis.

Other uses include:
- Tinea capitis in children (off-label).
- Recalcitrant toenail onychomycosis (off-label).
- Prophylaxis or treatment of systemic mycoses such as cryptococcosis and candidosis in HIV infection, treatment of histoplasmosis and coccidioidomycosis and prevention of fungal infections in immunocompromised patients.

Recommended dose and duration: (Dermatophytoses)

- Tinea corporis—Pulse dose of 150 mg once weekly.
- Tinea pedis—50 mg daily for 2–4 weeks up to 6 weeks.

- Onychomycosis—300 mg once weekly till abnormal looking nail has grown out. This may take 3–6 months and 9–12 months for fingernail and toenail onychomycosis, respectively.
- Tinea capitis–6 mg/kg/day (continuous dose) for 3 weeks, 8 mg/kg once weekly (pulsed dose) for 4–8 weeks.

Side Effects

Gastrointestinal: Nausea, vomiting, and abdominal pain.

Skin: Rash, fixed drug eruption, Stevens-Johnson syndrome (SJS), increased sweating, alopecia.

Hepatic: Elevated liver enzymes.

Miscellaneous: Headache, fatigue, anaphylaxis, and oliguria.

Not recommended in pregnancy (Category C) and lactation (secreted in breast milk).[2–6] Important drug interactions of Fluconazole are summarized in **Table 7.1**.

Special Situations

Pregnancy: Contraindicated in pregnancy, as it has been associated with birth defects in the children born to mothers taking high-dose long-term treatment.

Lactation: Fluconazole is excreted in breast milk at similar levels to plasma and should not be used during lactation.

Children: Fluconazole is licensed for use in children, including neonates, in the treatment of mucosal candidiasis, invasive Candida infections and cryptococcal infections, but not for superficial skin infection. Clearance is faster than in adults, so higher doses are needed (up to 12 mg/kg/d for severe infection).

Conclusion

Relevant to tinea corporis/cruris, Fluconazole may achieve high levels in the skin but the MIC is high and consistent results are rarely achieved in the present epidemic.

Itraconazole

It is a Triazole that was synthesized in 1980. It was first approved for invasive fungal infections in 1987. It is fungistatic, but effective in immunocompromised patients. Steroid hormone synthesis inhibition is absent in Itraconazole, and serious hepatotoxicity is rare.

Pharmacokinetics

Formulation: Capsule, tablet, oral suspension, IV

Half-life: 21 hours

Bio-availability: 55%, highest levels with full meal or with cold beverage

Metabolism: Extensive hepatic metabolism

Excretion: Renal

Dosage: 100 mg capsule, 200 mg tablet, IV, oral suspension 10 mg/ml.

In patients with liver cirrhosis, careful monitoring is suggested. Itraconazole is delivered to the skin mainly as a result of passive diffusion from the plasma to the keratinocytes,

TABLE 7.1: Drug interactions–Itraconazole and Fluconazole

Interactive drug group	Itraconazole (CYP3A4 inhibitor)	Fluconazole (Potent CYP2C9 and moderate CYP3A4 inhibitor)
Contraindications		
Antiarrhythmic agents	Quinidine, Dofetilide	Quinidine
Antipsychotics	Pimozide	Pimozide
Non-sedating antihistamines	–	Astemizole
Others	Cisapride, Ergot alkaloids, oral Midazolam, Statins – Lovastatin and Simvastatin	Cisapride
Interactions		
Anticoagulants–Warfarin	Monitoring in drug dosage	Monitoring in drug dosage
Anticonvulsants– Phenytoin, carbamazepine	Lowers antifungal levels	Lowers antifungal levels
Antineoplastics–Vinca alkaloids, Busulfan, Docetaxel	Increases levels of vinca alkaloids, Busulfan, Docetaxel	Increases levels of vinca alkaloids
HMG-CoA reductase–Atorvastatin, Cerivastatin, Fluvastatin and Simvastatin	Increases levels of Atorvastatin, Cerivastatin	Avoid fluconazole along with Atorvastatin, Fluvastatin and Simvastatin
Gastric acid suppressors –H2-receptor antagonist, Omeprazole	Decreases the itraconazole level	–
Immunosuppressants–Cyclosporine, Tacrolimus, Sirolimus	Increases the level of cyclosporine, tacrolimus, sirolimus	Monitoring is required
Macrolide antibiotics–Erythromycin	Increases the level of itraconazole	Avoid use of Fluconazole and Erythromycin together
NSAIDs–Celecoxib, Naproxen, Lornoxicam, Meloxicam, Diclofenac, Ibuprofen	–	Monitor the patient, reduce dose if needed
Antiretroviral–Nevirapine, Ritonavir, Indinavir, Saquinavir	Nevirapine lowers antifungal levels. Ritonavir and Indinavir increases antifungal levels Saquinavir levels get increased with Itraconazole	Monitor the drug dose when Fluconazole and Saquinavir is taken together
Polyenes–Amphotericin B	Amphotericin B (pre-treatment with Itraconazole may reduce activity–use with caution)	–
Azoles–voriconazole	–	Avoid with Voriconazole

with *strong drug adherence to keratin*. Itraconazole becomes detectable in the sweat within 24 hours after the initial intake of drug. There is extensive excretion of itraconazole into sebum. Itraconazole is highly protein bound, has a large volume of distribution (10 L/kg), accumulates in vaginal mucosa, skin and nails, but penetration into CSF is poor. It is largely metabolized in liver by CYP3A4; an active metabolite is produced which is excreted in feces.

Indication

- Dermatophytosis (tinea corporis, tinea pedis, etc.).
- Onychomycosis caused by dermatophytes and/or yeast.
- Pityriasis versicolor.
- Vulvovaginal and oropharyngeal candidiasis.

Itraconazole has a broad spectrum of antifungal action and is also widely used to treat systemic fungal infections (e.g. aspergillosis, candidiasis, cryptococcosis and histoplasmosis), deep mycoses (e.g. sporotrichosis, chromoblastomycosis, paracoccidiodomycosis and histoplasmosis) and for prophylaxis of fungal infection in patients with neutropenia and HIV.

Recommended dose and duration:

- Tinea corporis—Itraconazole 100 mg BD for 3–4 weeks. In the recent times, most often used dose is Itraconazole 200 mg OD for a longer duration up to 6–8 weeks.
- Tinea pedis—Itraconazole 200 mg OD for 4 weeks.
- In continuous dose for tinea capitis, capsules 5 mg/kg/day and oral solution 3 mg/kg/day can be used for 4–8 weeks or 4 weeks respectively and as pulsed dose for tinea capitis 5 mg/kg/day for a week with 3 weeks off for 2–4 pulses.

Onychomycosis–200 mg/day for 3 months. An intermittent pulse regimen of 200 mg BD for 1 week each month for 3 months is equally effective.

Notably the Stands for Super Bioavailability Itraconazole (SUBA ITZ) formulation is being increasingly prescribed that obviates the variable bioavailability of conventional ITZ. There is no superiority and 65 mg and 50 mg SUBA are as good as C ITZ 100 mg. The approvals are for endemic mycosis and while clinicians can use it for tinea, a national authoritative guideline does not suggest that it will be consistently superior to C ITZ.[7]

Side Effects

Gastrointestinal: Nausea, vomiting, diarrhea, and abdominal pain.

Cutaneous: Skin rash, pruritus, Stevens-Johnson syndrome (SJS)/toxic epidermal necrolysis (TEN), exfoliative dermatitis, leukocytoclastic vasculitis, photosensitivity, alopecia.

Neurological: Headache

Hepatic: Raised liver enzymes (reversible); rarely–hepatitis, hepatic failure.

Miscellaneous: Leukopenia, neutropenia, thrombocytopenia, congestive cardiac failure.

It should not be consumed during pregnancy (category C) and breastfeeding (excreted in breast milk).[2–5, 8]

Interactions and Advise

As Itraconazole is mainly metabolized by CYP3A4, potent inhibitors of this enzyme may increase its bioavailability. Examples include: Ritonavir, Indinavir, Clarithromycin and Erythromycin. Enzyme inducers and medications that reduce gastric acidity and absorption of Itraconazole may reduce its bioavailability, such as Rifampicin, Lansoprazole, Omeprazole, Pantoprazole and Ranitidine.

Multiple drugs are contraindicated with Itraconazole, including Mizolastine, Triazolam, oral mid-azolam, Quetiapine, Pimozide, Dofetilide, Dabigatran, Ticagrelor, Quinidine, and statins metabolized by CYP3A4 (Atorvastatin, Lovastatin and Simvastatin) (**Table 7.1**).

Caution is advised with the following drugs:

- Calcium channel blockers, which is due to pharmacological interactions and additive negative inotropic effects which may precipitate cardiac failure.
- Cardiac glycosides (digoxin).
- Ciclosporin, Tacrolimus and Sirolimus metabolism are inhibited. Reduced dosage and monitoring of drug levels may be required.
- Colchicine is contraindicated in those with renal or hepatic impairment.
- Coumarin anticoagulants' and non-vitamin K oral anticoagulants' (NOACs) effect may be enhanced.
- Inhaled corticosteroids, because metabolism may be impaired with long-term itraconazole, leading to iatrogenic Cushing syndrome.
- HIV protease inhibitors such as Ritonavir, Indinavir and Saquinavir.

Special Situations

Pregnancy and pre-conception—Itraconazole is embryotoxic and teratogenic in animals, so it is contraindicated in pregnancy except for life-threatening infections. Effective contraception must be used during treatment and until the next menstrual period following treatment cessation. It may cause menstrual irregularities.

Lactation: Small amounts of Itraconazole are excreted in human breast milk, so it should not be taken during lactation.

Children: Itraconazole is unlicensed in children under the age of 12 years, but it has been proven to be safe, effective and well-tolerated. It is commonly prescribed for tinea capitis due to *Trichophyton* species.

Elderly: Care should be taken in those at risk of cardiac failure and those taking drugs which may interact with Itraconazole. The prevalence of onychomycosis in older people is high, but generally morbidity is low; therefore, the risks/benefits of treating onychomycosis with any oral antifungal should be carefully considered before embarking on potentially lengthy courses of treatment.

Conclusion

The therapeutic effect in the skin is achieved by passive diffusion into basal keratinocytes, a high rate of excretion in sebum and, to a lesser degree, excretion in sweat. Extensive tissue (protein) binding in skin and hair has been demonstrated, so the active drug persists for several weeks after stopping therapy.

Ketoconazole

It is the first orally effective broad-spectrum antifungal drug, useful in both dermatophytosis and deep mycosis. It is an Imidazole fungistatic antifungal. It is no longer approved by the FDA for use in superficial fungal infections due to the idiosyncratic hepatic toxicity.

Pharmacokinetics

Formulation: Tablet and oral suspension

Half-life: 2 hours in the first 10 hours and 8 hours thereafter

Bio-availability: It is well absorbed in acid milieu.

Metabolism: Extensive hepatic metabolism.

Excretion: Major by bile into intestinal tract, 13% renal, and 4% feces (unchanged).

Dosage: 200 mg tablet, oral suspension 100 mg/5 ml.

Ketoconazole is known for its time-dependent pharmacokinetics and sustained post-treatment antifungal effect.

Indication

FDA in 2013 warned against the use of Ketoconazole tablets to treat skin and nail fungal infections and stated that it could be used to treat serious fungal infections when no other antifungal therapies are available.

Recommended dose: 200 mg OD or BD tablet, higher doses are sometimes required.
A recent case study used the drug in case of multidrug resistance in a dose of 200 mg BD × 28 days.[9]

Side Effects

Gastrointestinal: Nausea and vomiting

Cutaneous: Urticaria

Hepatic: Severe hepatitis [Although the estimated incidence of severe hepatotoxicity was less than 1 in 10,000, in view of this serious hazard and availability of safer drugs, the European Medical Agency (EMA) advised that its use was no longer justified.]

Endocrinological: Adrenal insufficiency, gynecomastia, impotence, alopecia. Ketoconazole is pregnancy category C.[1–4, 8]

ALLYLAMINE

Terbinafine

It is an allylamine that was developed in 1974. Oral terbinafine was first approved for use in the United Kingdom in February 1991. The first allylamine to be approved for use in humans was Naftifine; however, it is only available as a topical treatment.

Mechanism of Action

It acts as a non-competitive inhibitor of 'squalene epoxidase', an early step enzyme in ergosterol biosynthesis by fungi. Accumulation of squalene within fungal cells appears to be responsible for the fungicidal action.

Pharmacokinetics

Formulation: Tablet and oral granules

Half-life: 36 hours

Bio-availability: 40–65%, tablets not affected by food

Metabolism: Significant first pass hepatic metabolism

Excretion: Renal 70%

Dosage: 250 mg tablet, oral granules 125 mg or 187.5 mg.

Terbinafine is a broad-spectrum antifungal drug with keratinophilic and lipophilic properties. Terbinafine is delivered by passive diffusion through sebum and basal keratinocytes to the stratum corneum. It is well distributed in the adipose tissue, skin and nails.

Indication

Terbinafine is FDA approved for the treatment of tinea unguium and tinea capitis. It is used off-label in the treatment of onychomycosis caused by Candida and non-dermatophyte molds, tinea corporis/cruris, tinea pedis, Majocchi's granuloma and tinea imbricata.

Recommended dose and duration:

- Tinea corporis: Terbinafine 250 mg OD for 4–6 weeks.
- Tinea pedis: Terbinafine 250 mg OD for 6–8 weeks.

At present, Terbinafine doses required are 250 mg BD for prolonged durations. Though with increasing resistance a review of the effects should be assessed at about 14 days, as it is delivered to the stratum corneum primarily by sebum and to a lesser extent by diffusion through the dermo-epidermis and in the first 2 weeks of therapy, concentrations within the stratum corneum increase to 75 times greater than plasma concentrations.

In tinea capitis the dose is dependent on the body weight of the child; 10–20 kg: 62.5 mg/day, 21–30 kg: 125 mg/day, 31–40 kg: 125 mg/day, 41–50 kg: 250 mg/day, >50 kg: 250 mg/day.

Side Effects

Terbinafine has the least side effects among all the antifungal drugs.

Gastrointestinal: Diarrhea, dyspepsia, abdominal pain, nausea.

Cutaneous: Skin rash, pruritus, drug rash, alopecia, flare of psoriasis and lupus.

Neurological: Headache.

Hepatic: Raised liver enzymes. Occasional cases of hepatotoxicity have been seen and are related to the HLA typing.

Terbinafine is safer in later pregnancy with category B and it is excreted in breast milk.[2–4,6,8]

Interactions (Table 7.2)

- CYP450 enzyme inducers (e.g. Rifampicin) and inhibitors (e.g. Cimetidine) may accelerate or reduce Terbinafine metabolism, respectively, and its dosage may need adjustment.
- CYP2D6-mediated drug metabolism is inhibited by Terbinafine. Patients taking drugs metabolized by this enzyme (H1-antihistamines, SSRIs, MAOIs type B) may require closer monitoring.
- Oral contraceptive metabolism is not usually affected, but there have been sporadic reports of menstrual disturbances/breakthrough bleeding.
- Warfarin efficacy may be reduced, so closer monitoring is indicated.

Special Situations

Pregnancy and pre-conception: Although there is no evidence of harm, the use of Terbinafine is not recommended in pregnancy unless potential benefit outweighs risk.

Lactation: Avoid as Terbinafine is excreted in milk with a high ratio of drug in milk: plasma of 7:1 after oral administration.

TABLE 7.2: Drug interaction–Terbinafine and Griseofulvin

Interactive drug group	Terbinafine (CYP2D6 inhibitor)	Griseofulvin
Contraindications	No specific drug contraindications	No specific contraindications
Drugs metabolized by CYP2D6 • Tricyclic antidepressants (e.g. Desipramine) • Antiarrhythmics (e.g. Propafenone) • Beta-blockers • Selective serotonin reuptake inhibitors	Careful monitoring May require dose reduction	–
Anticoagulants–warfarin	Increase in prothrombin time	Decreases levels of Warfarin
Oral contraceptives	Ethinyl estradiol–no inhibition by terbinafine	Decreases levels of estrogen containing oral contraceptives
Immunosuppressants–cyclosporine	Increases Terbinafine, Terbinafine increases Cyclosporine clearance	Decreases levels of Cyclosporine
Alcohol	–	Increases action of alcohol, leading to Disulfiram-like reaction
Caffeine	Decreases clearance of Caffeine	–
Rifampicin	Increases Terbinafine clearance by 100%	–
Barbiturates	–	Barbiturate decreases Griseofulvin level
Salicylates	–	Decreases levels of Salicylates

SPIROBENZOFURAN

Griseofulvin

Griseofulvin was isolated from the mold *Penicillium griseofulvum* by Oxford et al. in 1939. In the late 1950s, Griseofulvin was found to be effective in the treatment of superficial fungal infections in humans. Although the use of Griseofulvin has declined over the years, it is still widely used for the treatment of tinea capitis in children.

Mechanism of Action

Griseofulvin interferes with mitosis—multinucleated and stunted fungal hyphae result from its action. It also causes abnormal metaphase configurations. However, it does not cause metaphase arrest; rather the daughter nuclei fail to move apart or move only a short distance. It does not inhibit polymerization of tubulin (microtubular protein which pulls the chromosomes apart), but binds to polymerized microtubules and somehow disorients them.

Pharmacokinetics

Formulation: Tablet and oral suspension

Half-life: 9.5–22 hours

Bioavailability: Fatty meal increases absorption

Metabolism: Hepatic

Excretion: Renal 50%, 36% in feces

Dosage: 50, 200 mg tablet, IV 200 mg/vial, oral suspension 200 mg/5 ml.

Indication

Griseofulvin is best absorbed after a fatty meal and in micronized and ultra-micronized formulations. It is tightly bound to the keratin during cell differentiation and persists in the keratin. Griseofulvin is United States Food and Drug Administration (US FDA) approved for the treatment of tinea corporis, tinea cruris, tinea pedis, tinea capitis and tinea unguium.

Recommended dose and duration:

Tinea corporis: 250 mg twice daily after a fatty meal for 6–8 weeks/until cure.

Tinea pedis: 250 mg twice daily after a fatty meal for 8–10 weeks/until cure.

Tablet strength of ultramicronized form is 330/375 mg.

In the present epidemic the results of this drug are variable and it does not seem to be effective in majority of the cases.

Side Effects

Gastrointestinal: Vomiting, diarrhea, heartburn.

Hematological: Deranged blood values and punctate basophilia, which disappear despite continuation of therapy.

Hepatic: Hepatotoxicity

Skin: Photosensitivity, Erythema multiformae (EMF)-like rash, morbilliform eruption

Renal: Albuminuria

It is pregnancy category C.[2, 5, 6, 8, 10]

Drug interactions of Griseofulvin are presented in **Table 7.2**.

NEWER ANTIFUNGAL DRUGS

Voriconazole

It is a second generation triazole antifungal drug. It is introduced lately to treat difficult to treat fungal infections like invasive aspergillosis, disseminated infections caused by fluconazole resistant *Candida*, *Fusarium* infections, and febrile neutropenia not responding to antibacterial therapy.

Pharmacokinetics

Formulation: Tablet, IV and oral suspension

Half-life: 1–2 hours

Metabolism: CYP2C19, 2C9, 3A4, majorly CYP2C19

Excretion: Renal 80%

Dosage: 50, 200 mg tablet IV 200 mg/vial, oral suspension 200 mg/5 ml.

Indication

Voriconazole is indicated for the following:

Invasive aspergillosis; esophageal candidiasis; candidemia in non-neutropenic patients, disseminated *Candida* infections in skin, serious fungal infections caused by *Scedosporium apiospermum* and *Fusarium* spp. in patients intolerant to other therapy. It is also used in cases of recalcitrant, refractory, extensive superficial fungal infection.

Voriconazole is used is resistant superficial fungal infection, not responding to traditional antifungals.

Dose: If less than 40 kg, then 100 mg every 12 hours; and if greater than 40 kg, 200–300 mg every 12 hours (or 3–4 mg/kg every 12 hours). For severe infections, the dose can be increased to 400 mg every 12 hours.

IV initially: 6 mg/kg every 12 hours for 2 doses, then maintenance with 4 mg/kg every 12 hours.

A study from Bangladesh has used it in a dose of 200 mg BD for 4 weeks (Ali M),[11] but in India itraconazole is still a effective drug and use of voriconazole should be restricted.

Side Effects

Gastrointestinal: Diarrhea, dyspepsia, abdominal pain, and nausea

Skin: Rash, exfoliative dermatitis, and photosensitivity

Neurological: Headache, and dizziness

Liver: Deranged liver enzymes

Miscellaneous: Visual disturbances, rhinitis, upper respiratory tract infection (URTI), fever, QTc prolongation and an acute reaction on IV injection. Voriconazole is a pregnancy category D drug.[2, 10, 12] Drug interactions of Voriconazole are summarized in (**Table 7.3**).

Posaconazole

It is a second generation Triazole antifungal. It is approved for the treatment and prophylaxis of invasive fungal infections.

Pharmacokinetics

Formulation: Tablet and oral suspension

Half-life: 35 hours

Bio-availability: Increased with fat rich food

Metabolism: UDP glucuronidation and p-glycoprotein substrate

Excretion: Fecal 71% renal 13%

Dosage: 40 mg/ml oral suspension

Indication

Posaconazole is FDA indicated for the following: Prophylaxis of invasive Aspergillus and Candida infections in patients 13 years or older who are at high-risk of developing, such infections owing to being severely immunocompromised; treatment of oropharyngeal candidiasis, including oropharyngeal candidiasis refractory to Itraconazole and/or fluconazole.

Side Effects

Gastrointestinal: Diarrhea, nausea, and vomiting

Skin: Rash, and increased sweating

TABLE 7.3: Drug interactions–Newer antifungals–Voriconazole and Posaconazole

Interactive drug group	Voriconazole (Metabolized by CYP2C19, CYP2C9, CYP3A4)	Posaconazole (Strong CYP3A4 inhibitor)
Contraindications		
Antiarrhythmic agents	Quinidine	Quinidine
Antipsychotics	Pimozide	Pimozide
Non-sedating antihistamines	Astemizole, Terfenadine	Astemizole, Terfenadine
Others	Ritonavir (higher dose), Cisapride, Ergot alkaloids, Carbamazepine, Rifabutin, Rifampicin, Sirolimus, long acting Barbiturates	Cisapride, ergot alkaloids
Interactions		
Anticoagulants–Warfarin	Monitoring of drug dosing	–
Anticonvulsants–Phenytoin, Carbamazepine	Voriconazole levels will reduce with phenytoin, needing dose adjustment	Avoid phenytoin and Posaconazole together
Antimycobacterials		Avoid along with Rifabutin
Antineoplastics – Vinca alkaloids, Busulfan, Docetaxel	Increases levels of vinca alkaloids	Increases levels of vinca alkaloids
HMG-CoA reductase – Atorvastatin, Cerivastatin, Fluvastatin, Simvastatin	Monitor when given with Lovastatin	Monitor when given with Lovastatin
Gastric acid suppressors – H2 receptor antagonists, Omeprazole	Monitor when given with Omeprazole	Cimetidine lowers the Posaconazole levels, hence, to be avoided together
Immunosuppressants – cyclosporine, Tacrolimus, Sirolimus	Reduce dosage of Cyclosporine, Tacrolimus, Sirolimus	Monitoring is required
NSAIDs–Celecoxib, Naproxen, Lornoxicam, Meloxicam, Diclofenac, Ibuprofen	Monitor the patient, reduce dose if needed	–
Antiretroviral – Nevirapine, Ritonavir, Indinavir, Saquinavir	Adjust dose of Efavirenz/ voriconazole. Nevirapine increases antifungal levels	No clinical significance
Azoles – Fluconazole	Avoid with Fluconazole	–

Neurological: Headache

Liver: Enzyme derangement

Miscellaneous: Fever, anorexia, insomnia, and fatigue.

Posaconazole is pregnancy category C and excreted in breast milk.[2, 10, 13, 14]
Drug interactions of Posaconazole are summarized in **Table 7.3**.

Ravuconazole

It is a second generation Triazole derivative. Its spectrum is similar to Voriconazole. It was discontinued in the year 2007.[2, 13, 15]

Isavuconazole

It is a second generation Triazole. Isavuconazole sulphate is rapidly hydrolyzed in blood to Isavuconazole. It has a spectrum of activity against *Aspergillus flavus, A. niger, A. fumigatus,* Mucorales-Rhizopus and Mucormycetes.

Pharmacokinetics

Formulation: Oral capsule and IV

Half-life: 130 hours

Bio-availability: 98%, can be taken with or without food

Excretion: Less than 1% in urine

Dosage: 100 mg tablet.

Indication

It is approved for the treatment of invasive aspergillosis and invasive mucormycosis. It is also used in candidemia and invasive candidiasis and also in conditions where other antifungals are not effective.

Recommended dose and duration: 200 mg OD oral or IV, loading dose of 200 mg for 6 doses every 8 hourly.

Side Effects

Nausea, vomiting, diarrhea, headache, hypokalemia and elevated transaminases. It causes QTc shortening in contrast to prolongation which is seen with other triazoles.[2, 16–18]

CONCLUSION

Systemic antifungals play a crucial role in managing superficial fungal infections when topical treatments are insufficient or the infection is widespread. Medications like Terbinafine, Itraconazole, and Fluconazole are effective and well-tolerated options, offering high cure rates for conditions such as onychomycosis and tinea capitis. A tailored approach, guided by the type of infection and patient needs, ensures optimal outcomes while minimizing side effects.

Key Points

- Common systemic antifungal drug classes include Triazoles (e.g. Itraconazole, Fluconazole), Imidazoles (e.g. Ketoconazole), Allylamines (e.g. Terbinafine), and others like Griseofulvin.
- Most antifungals inhibit the fungal ergosterol synthesis pathway, disrupting the fungal cell membrane's integrity.
- Systemic antifungal therapy is prescribed for conditions like extensive tinea corporis, chronic/recurrent dermatophytosis, onychomycosis, and tinea capitis.
- Antifungal drugs may cause gastrointestinal disturbances, skin reactions, liver enzyme elevations, and rare severe reactions like Stevens-Johnson syndrome.
- Antifungals like Fluconazole and Itraconazole interact with various drugs, including anti-coagulants, statins, and immunosuppressants, necessitating monitoring for adverse effects.

REFERENCES

1. Dismukes WE. Introduction to antifungal drugs. Clinical Infectious Diseases. 2000;30(4):653–7.
2. Wolverton SE, Wu JJ. Comprehensive dermatologic drug therapy. Elsevier Health Sciences; 2019.
3. Sardana K, Khurana A. IADVL manual on management of dermatophytosis, 1st edn. CBS Publishers and Distributors; 2018
4. Griffiths CE, Barker J, Bleiker TO, Chalmers R, Creamer D. Rook's textbook of dermatology. John Wiley & Sons; 2016.
5. Tripathi KD. Essentials of medical pharmacology. Jaypee Brothers Medical Publishers Pvt Ltd; 2013.
6. Bouchara JP, Nenoff P, Gupta AK, Chaturvedi V. Dermatophytes and dermatophytoses. Springer International Publishing; 2021.
7. Patel NH, Sardana K, Shenoy MM, Rengasamy M, Khurana A, et al. IADVL SIG Recalcitrant Dermatophytosis Position Statement on Super Bioavailable Itraconazole. Indian Dermatol Online J. 2023 Dec 1;15(1):1–7. doi: 10.4103/idoj.idoj_668_22. PMID: 38283009; PMCID: PMC10810390.
8. Howard KC, Dennis EK, Watt DS, Garneau-Tsodikova S. A comprehensive overview of the medicinal chemistry of antifungal drugs: Perspectives and promise. Chemical Society Reviews. 2020 Apr 27;49(8):2426–80.
9. Sharath S, Sardana K, Khurana A. Multi-drug failure of tinea corporis to terbinafine, itraconazole and fluconazole; translating extensive Indian microbiological and resistance data to a trial of ketoconazole with remarkable efficacy. Indian J Dermatol Venereol Leprol. 2024 Jul 25:1–3. doi: 10.25259/IJDVL_497_2024. Epub ahead of print. PMID: 39152830.
10. Van Daele R, Spriet I, Wauters J, Maertens J, Mercier T, Van Hecke S, Brüggemann R. Antifungal drugs: What brings the future? Medical Mycology. 2019;57(Suppl3):S328–43.
11. Ali M, Ahmed N, Khan S, Kiran A. Efficacy of oral voriconazole versus oral itraconazole, in the treatment of dermatophyte infections. J Ayub Med Coll Abbottabad. 2024 Apr-Jun;36(2):294–298. doi: 10.55519/JAMC-02-12891. PMID: 39609968.
12. Nicola AM, Albuquerque P, Paes HC, Fernandes L, Costa FF, Kioshima ES, et al. Antifungal drugs: New insights in research and development. Pharmacology and Therapeutics. 2019;195:21–38.
13. Nami S, Aghebati-Maleki A, Morovati H, Aghebati-Maleki L. Current antifungal drugs and immunotherapeutic approaches as promising strategies to treatment of fungal diseases. Biomedicine & Pharmacotherapy. 2019;110:857–68.
14. Mota Fernandes C, Dasilva D, Haranahalli K, McCarthy JB, Mallamo J, Ojima I, Del Poeta M. The future of antifungal drug therapy: Novel compounds and targets. Antimicrobial Agents and Chemotherapy. 2021;65(2):10–128.
15. Vanreppelen G, Wuyts J, Van Dijck P, Vandecruys P. Sources of antifungal drugs. Journal of Fungi. 2023;9(2):171.
16. Wall G, Lopez-Ribot JL. Current antimycotics, new prospects, and future approaches to antifungal therapy. Antibiotics. 2020;9(8):445.
17. Sardana K. Systemic drugs in dermatology. Jaypee Brothers Medical Publishers; 2021.
18. Jampilek J. Novel avenues for identification of new antifungal drugs and current challenges. Expert Opinion on Drug Discovery. 2022;17(9):949–68.

CHAPTER 8

Role and Rationale of Oral and Topical Combination Treatments

• Mohammad Adil

INTRODUCTION

The enormous increase in the cases of recalcitrant dermatophytoses have led clinicians to use antifungal drugs in combination with each other and with other compounds having antifungal activity. This chapter attempts to explore the rationale and scientific evidence of combination therapies used for dermatophytoses.

RATIONALE OF COMBINATION THERAPY

Recalcitrant dermatophytic infections has been ascribed to several factors such as resistance to drugs, changes in epidemiological pattern, abuse of corticosteroids, poor quality medications and poor compliance of patients. The widespread emergence of *Trichophyton indotineae* has led to drug resistance and the need for longer treatment durations to clear infection even with terbinafine and itraconazole.[1] Combination therapy may potentially help reduce relapse rates and treatment duration in such cases, though evidence regarding the same is lacking.

A good combination of antifungals should have a wider spectrum of action, suppress resistant mutants, have enhanced fungicidal action, increase compliance by being less toxic and hence improve cure rates.[2] Potential combination with their rationale have been summarized in **Table 8.1**.

Antifungal drugs can be combined in as sequential therapy or as concurrent therapy **(Table 8.2)**.

TABLE 8.1: Rationale of antifungal drug combinations

Rationale	Example
Drugs act via different mechanisms	Combining Griseofulvin (which inhibits fungal cell mitosis) and Itraconazole (which inhibits Ergosterol biosynthesis)
Drugs target sequential steps in the same pathway	Combination of itraconazole and amorolfine (both act via inhibition of ergosterol synthesis) but itraconazole inhibits 14-alpha demethylase and amorolfine inhibits D-14 reductase and D7-D8 isomerase)
Drugs act via different routes	Combination of oral Itraconazole and topical Ketoconazole
One drug increases bioavailability of another at target site	Caspofungin with human antimicrobial peptides (peptides disrupt membrane permeability)

TABLE 8.2: Combination strategies of antifungal drugs	
Sequential therapy	A topical antifungal is administered alone followed by an oral agent. It is used when patient shows poor response to topical treatment
Concurrent therapy	A topical and an oral agent is used simultaneously. It can be used in patients likely to fail therapy

BASIC CONSIDERATIONS FOR COMBINATION OF ANTIFUNGALS

Many methods and several systems for expressing results have been developed to test for antibiotic synergism since the 1950s. Although clinical microbiologists have shown by many studies and publications their interest in the subject, most clinical laboratories do not perform routine *in vitro* testing for coupling of drugs. The most common is the checkerboard method and killing curve. Results with killing curve and disk diffusion methods are qualitative. A combination is considered to be synergistic when the effect observed with a combination is greater than the sum of the effects observed with the two drugs independently. The checkerboard method may be expressed quantitatively as Fractional Inhibitory Concentration (FIC), Fractional Bactericidal Concentration (FBC) and isobologram **(Fig. 8.1)**.

Combination therapy may have synergistic or antagonistic effects **(Table 8.3)**. An example of antagonistic combination is lipophilic azoles (Itraconazole) with amphotericin B. Azoles deplete ergosterol in the cytoplasmic membrane, leaving fewer binding sites for amphotericin B to act. Thus, drugs showing synergy *in vitro* need to be considered for conducting clinical studies to verify the clinical utility of the said combination.

Combination of antifungals must have sound scientific basis and must pass through the three phases of validation: *in vitro* checkerboard studies, animal studies and clinical trials. Such combinations are based on synergistic checkerboard studies which must ideally be tested on the disease-causing fungus and obtained from diseased site. Further, it must be noted that synergy seen *in vitro* may not necessarily translate to *in vivo* success.[3] The factors considered while testing a drug combination are summarized in **Table 8.4**.

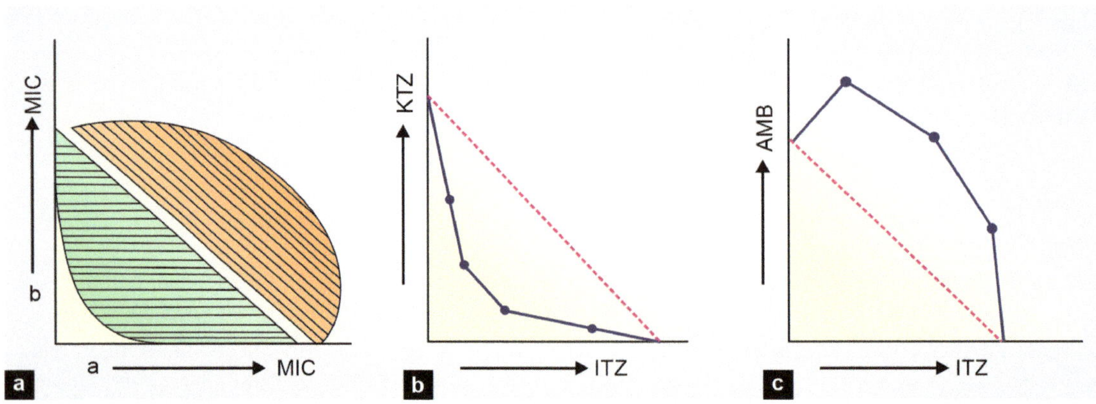

FIGURE 8.1a to c: Checkerboard method. (a) Theoretical isobologram showing synergy zone (green) and antagonism zone (orange); (b) Itraconazole (ITZ) Ketoconazole (KTZ) combination showing syergy (FIC <0.05) in clinical isolates of *Trichophyton mentagrophytes/Trichophyton interdigitale* species complex; (c) Itraconazole (ITZ) Amphotericin B (AMB) combination showing antagonism (FIC>4) in clinical isolates of *Aspergillus fumigatus*

TABLE 8.3: Results of *in vitro* antifungal drug combination studies

Result	Definition	FICI
Synergistic	Antifungal activity greater than the sum of inhibition produced by two antifungals alone	≤0.05
Additive*	Antifungal activity produced by the combination is the sum of the inhibition produced by the two drugs alone	>0.5 but ≤4
Indifferent*	Antifungal activity of the combination is the same as the effect produced by the more active drug when used alone	
Antagonistic	Antifungal activity of the combination is less than that of the less active drug in the combination when used alone	>4

*Additive and indifferent are poorly defined and considered by many experts to be the same

FICI = FIC(A) + FIC(B), where FIC = (MIC combination)/(MIC drug tested alone)

(FICI: Fractional inhibitory concentration index; FIC(A) and FIC(B): Fractional inhibitory concentration of drugs A and B respectively; MIC: Minimum inhibitory concentration)

TABLE 8.4: Factors considered for combination of antifungal drugs

Antifungal drug susceptibility patterns	Susceptibility patterns change over geographic areas
Concentration of the antifungals at the site of action over 24 hours	Concentration in stratum corneum is more important than blood levels
Mechanism of action of the antifungal drugs	Must be complimentary
Duration of exposure of the organism to the drug	Percentage time the drug concentration remains above MIC (%T > MIC)
Total amount of drug exposure	Area under curve in relation to MIC (AUC: MIC)
Maximal drug exposure	Maximum drug concentration at the site in relation to MIC (C_{max}: MIC)
Post-antifungal effect (PAFE)	Suppression of growth of fungus even after drug levels have fallen below MIC levels
Drug toxicity of the combination	Consider if toxic effects are reduced
Likelihood of antifungal resistance to develop	Resistance to antifungal agents must be less likely to develop

TYPES OF COMBINATION THERAPY

Several oral and topical drugs have been tried in different combinations in quest for better therapeutic outcome as discussed below:

1. Combination of Two Antifungals

i. Oral-topical combination: Combining a topical and a systemic antifungal for tinea corporis/cruris is common in clinical practice, although unfortunately not backed by any robust literature as yet. Expert panels have recommended that a combination of oral Itraconazole/Terbinafine with a topical agent be used in cases of tinea pedis and recalcitrant tinea cruris/corporis, despite acknowledging the lack of comparative studies for the same.[4] Checkerboard analysis of isolates from patients with tinea cruris/corporis with *SQLE* gene mutations revealed that combinations of Itraconazole with Luliconazole, Ketoconazole and terbinafine have *in vitro* synergistic effects, implying oral itraconazole plus topical luliconazole or ketoconazole may have synergism in clinical practice, and this could be taken up for therapeutic studies.[5] A systematic review on antifungal combinations in dermatophytosis found six studies using checkerboard analysis which showed synergy with the combinations using amorolfine with terbinafine, itraconazole, fluconazole, griseofulvin, ketoconazole, sertaconazole, sulconazole; cyclopirox with itraconazole, ketoconazole; eficonazole with terbinafine, itraconazole; luliconazole with itraconazole; and tavaborole with itraconazole.[6] However, most included studies in the review were either on laboratory strains, or included dermatophyte and non-dermatophyte fungi together, and those which included clinical isolates were largely from onychomycosis cases. Checkerboard studies on the currently prevalent *T. indotineae* species are limited as yet and urgently needed.[7] Several case reports of combinations of an oral and a topical antifungal agent have been reported in glabrous tinea.[6] However, these reports are not backed with any laboratory evidence to support the use of such combinations.[6] In fact, a recent randomized control trial conducted on 135 patients showed that the patients who received oral itraconazole 200 mg/day with topical luliconazole cream had similar cure rates and relapse rates as those receiving the same dose of itraconazole with a topical bland emollient. The luliconazole group, however, incurred higher medical costs.[8]

For onychomycosis, combination of topical antifungals to oral itraconazole/terbinafine has been shown to achieve improved outcomes compared to oral antifungal used alone. Combination therapy of 5% amorolfine nail lacquer with systemic antifungal agents was found to be superior to oral agents alone in a meta-analysis by Feng et al.[9] The efficacy of griseofulvin is enhanced when used with a topical imidazole. Topical amorolfine lacquer in combination with oral griseofulvin, terbinafine or itraconazole has been shown to be more efficacious in clinical trials.[2, 10] Encouraging results were seen in an open study on onychomycosis patients using 8% ciclopirox nail lacquer with itraconazole.

ii. Oral-oral combination: The use of two oral antifungal agents has not consistently shown significantly better clinical response than monotherapy in any mycosis apart from cryptococcosis.[3] Given the prevalent strain's largely low minimum inhibitory concentration to itraconazole, and high clinical efficacy demonstrated with the drug at all doses,[11] the concurrent use of two oral antifungal agents is not required and is an irrational and unscientific practice. This was demonstrated in a randomized control trial which showed no benefit of a combination of oral itraconazole-terbinafine combination compared to itraconazole alone.[12] The trial showed that a longer duration of monotherapy achieved better cure rates. Though another study showed the oral itraconazole-terbinafine combination to be more efficacious than monotherapy with either drug,[13] but the study had several fundamental flaws such as a small sample size, very short treatment duration, no *in vitro* susceptibility testing and weak scientific and pharmacological rationale.[14] Combination of oral antifungals also predisposes to an increased pill burden, increased risk of drug interactions and other adverse effects (such as hepatotoxicity) and an increased cost of treatment.

2. Combination of Antifungals with Other Chemicals

Whitfield ointment (WO) (6% benzoic acid and 3% salicylic acid) and modified WO (MWO) (5% benzoic acid and salicylic acid each) are keratolytic, accelerate drug penetration and increase shedding of infected stratum corneum. MWO in combination with griseofulvin was found to be effective in difficult to treat tinea corporis/cruris.[15] WO with terbinafine was found to be less effective than WO with clotrimazole.[16] MWO with oral fluconazole 150 mg weekly for 4 weeks was found to be as effective as 1% butenafine cream applied twice daily for tinea of the glabrous skin in a comparative study from Gujarat.[17]

Calcineurin inhibitors (tacrolimus, cyclosporine) and mTOR inhibitor (sirolimus) have intrinsic antifungal activity. *In vitro* studies have shown that tacrolimus has synergistic effect with ergosterol synthesis inhibitors including itraconazole, terbinafine and amorolfine and paves way for studies on its potential clinical application.[18] However, calcineurin inhibitors have immunosuppressive effects and their use has occasionally been associated with unusual deep presentations of dermatophytosis,[19] and hence must be avoided. Newer analogs of FK-506 with lower immunosuppressive activity are under investigation for potential use in fungal infections.

Statins have been found to have synergistic effects in *in vitro* checkerboard studies, when combined with antifungal drugs, particularly terbinafine and azoles.[20] However, azoles are metabolized by the cytochrome P450 pathway and can lead to increased concentration of statins, producing adverse effects such as myositis and rhabdomyolysis.

Isotretinoin was proposed to hasten fungal clearance as it increases epidermal turnover. However, it offers no additional benefit when combined with terbinafine in patients with recurrent tinea cruris/corporis.[21] It decreases sebum secretion, the major route of terbinafine and itraconazole to reach skin. Enhanced epidermal turnover decreases the reservoir effect of these antifungals. Further, isotretinoin is also metabolized by the cytochrome P450 pathway and co-treatment with azoles may lead to decreased blood levels of the latter.[22]

There has been some recent data on use of silver with an *in vitro* study that examined the fungicidal activity of nanocomposites (NCs) based on reduced graphene oxide (rGO) loaded with silver (Ag) nanoparticles (rGO/Ag) against clinical isolates of dermatophytes and *Candida* species.[23] Here, notably, the prevalent species was not studied. Hence, for now, we need more data for this to translate into clinical usage.

LACUNAE IN KNOWLEDGE

While studies on combination of topical and systemic drugs have been conducted in onychomycosis, there are no clinical studies for dermatophytosis at other sites. Further, most studies are based on the rationale of combining drugs based on MIC or mechanism of action alone. Hence, combination therapy in dermatophytosis is fraught with potential adverse effects and medicolegal risks.[5] There is wide variation in the methods employed for *in vitro* study and data analysis for testing of antifungal drug combinations among different laboratories. Multicentric trials have, thus, not been performed due to lack of interlaboratory reproducibility.[24] Further, there is lack of standardized techniques for testing antifungals in animal models as well.

FUTURE DIRECTIONS

There is an urgent need to relook into combination therapy strategies and conduct scientific studies backed by reproducible models which can accurately predict clinical outcomes. Recent *in vitro* studies combining essential oils such as tea tree oil with azoles have shown fungicidal effects.[25] Another potential area of research is the topical use of peptides with oral antifungals, as resistance rarely develops against these compounds, and they act quickly and efficiently. Peptides such as IB-367 and tachyplesin have shown synergy with azoles and allylamines.[26] Other potential compounds that may be combined are antiseptics like chlorhexidine.[27]

CONCLUSION

The surge of recalcitrant cases of dermatophytosis has prompted many clinicians to try various antifungal drug combinations. However, these are not based on scientific evidence.

Use of two oral antifungals is irrational and exposes the patient to various adverse reactions. More scientific studies regarding antifungal combinations are the need of the hour. For now there is just one study from India, which focuses on synergy and suggests that oral itraconazole with topical luliconazole, terbinafine, and ketoconazole would be useful in resistant dermatophyte infections.

Key Points

- Antifungal combination therapy may be used as combination therapy or sequential therapy.
- Use of antifungal combination therapy must have a scientific basis based on *in vitro* studies, animal studies and clinical studies. There are no proper scientific clinical studies on combination of two antifungals in dermatophytosis showing synergy, except in onychomycosis.
- Use of two oral antifungal agents is irrational and such combinations must not be used.
- Antifungals can be potentially used in combination with other compounds such as salicylic acid, Whitfield's ointment, calcineurin inhibitors and other antifungals. However, combination with isotretinoin is not recommended.
- Recent *in vitro* studies indicate use of topical peptides and plant based essential oils may act synergistically with antifungal drugs.

REFERENCES

1. Uhrlaß S, Verma SB, Gräser Y, Rezaei-Matehkolaei A, Hatami M, Schaller M, et al. *Trichophyton indotineae*—an emerging pathogen causing recalcitrant dermatophytoses in India and worldwide – a multidimensional perspective. J Fungi (Basel) 2022; 21;8:757.
2. Baran R, Kaoukhov A. Topical antifungal drugs for the treatment of onychomycosis: an overview of current strategies for monotherapy and combination therapy. J Eur Acad Dermatol 2005;19:21–9.
3. Cuenca-Estrella M. Combinations of antifungal agents in therapy-what value are they? J Antimicrob Chemother 2004;54:854–69.
4. Rengasamy M, Shenoy MM, Dogra S, Asokan N, Khurana A, Poojary S, et al. Indian Association of Dermatologists, Venereologists and Leprologists (IADVL) Task Force against Recalcitrant Tinea (ITART) Consensus on the Management of Glabrous Tinea (INTACT). Indian Dermatol Online J 2020;11:502–19.
5. Sardana K, Gupta A, Sadhasivam S, Gautam RK, Khurana A, Saini S, et al. Checkerboard analysis to evaluate synergistic combinations of existing antifungal drugs and propylene glycol monocaprylate in isolates from recalcitrant tinea corporis and cruris patients harboring squalene epoxidase gene mutation. Antimicrob Agents Chemother 2021;65:e0032121.
6. Brescini L, Fioriti S, Morroni G, Barchiesi F. Antifungal combinations in dermatophytes. J Fungi 2021;7:727.
7. Bidaud AL, Schwarz P, Chowdhary A, Dannaoui E. *In vitro* antifungal combination of terbinafine with itraconazole against isolates of *Trichophyton* species. Antimicrob Agents Chemother 2022;66:e0144921.
8. Rana DK, Shah TS, Rohit MH, Patel NH, Khadela AD, Oza YP, et al. Evaluation of the benefit of the addition of 1% topical luliconazole versus topical bland emollient to the systemic itraconazole therapy for the management of disseminated dermatophytosis: A randomised control trial. Mycoses 2024;67:e13681
9. Feng X, Xiong X, Ran Y. Efficacy and tolerability of amorolfine 5% nail lacquer in combination with systemic antifungal agents for onychomycosis: A meta-analysis and systematic review. Dermatol Ther 2017;30. doi: 10.1111/dth.12457
10. Olafsson JH, Sigurgeirsson B, Baran R. Combination therapy for onychomycosis. Br J Dermatol 2003;149(Suppl 65):15–8.
11. Khurana A, Agarwal A, Agrawal D, Panesar S, Ghadlinge M, Sardana K, et al. Effect of different itraconazole dosing regimens on cure rates, treatment duration, safety, and relapse rates in adult patients with tinea corporis/cruris: A randomized clinical trial. JAMA Dermatol 2022;158:1269–78.

12. Singh SK, Subba N, Tilak R. Efficacy of terbinafine and itraconazole in different doses and in combination in the treatment of tinea infection: A randomized controlled parallel group open labeled trial with clinico-mycological correlation. Indian J Dermatol 2020;65:284–9.
13. Sharma P, Bhalla M, Thami GP, Chander J. Evaluation of efficacy and safety of oral terbinafine and itraconazole combination therapy in the management of dermatophytosis. J Dermatolog Treat 2020;31:749–53.
14. Sardana K, Khurana A, Singh A. Scientific rationale of antifungal drug combination, including oral itraconazole and terbinafine, in recalcitrant dermatophytoses. J Dermatolog Treat 2020;31:43–5.
15. Fonseka S, Bandara DDJ, Wickramaarachchi DC, Narankotuwa NGKHH, Kumarasiri PVR. Treatment of difficult-to-treat dermatophytosis: results of a randomized, double-blind, placebo-controlled study. J Infect Dev Ctries 2021;15:1731–7.
16. Rahangdale V, Deshmukh S, Vaishnavi, Madke B, Singh AL. Effect of salicylic acid 3% + benzoic acid 6% (Whitfield's ointment), clotrimazole 1% cream, and systemic terbinafine on mild-to-moderate tinea corporis: A randomised comparative study. Int J Recent Surg Med Sci 2020;1-4. doi: https://doi.org/10.1055/s-0040-1714163
17. Thaker SJ, Mehta DS, Shah HA, Dave JN, Kikani KM. A comparative study to evaluate efficacy, safety and cost-effectiveness between Whitfield's ointment + oral fluconazole versus topical 1% butenafine in tinea infections of skin. Indian J Pharmacol 2013;45:622–4.
18. Zhang J, Tan J, Yang L, He Y. Tacrolimus, not triamcinolone acetonide, interacts synergistically with itraconazole, terbinafine, bifonazole, and amorolfine against clinical dermatophyte isolates. J Mycol Med 2018;28:612–6.
19. Yamamoto T, Nishioka K. Deep dermatophytosis during topical tacrolimus therapy for psoriasis. Acta Derm Venereol 2003;83,291–2.
20. Nyilasi I, Kocsubé S, Krizsán K, Galgóczy L, Papp T, Pesti M, et al. Susceptibility of clinically important dermatophytes against statins and different statin-antifungal combinations. Med Mycol 2014;52:140–8.
21. Verma KK, Senthilnathan G, Bhatia S, Xess I, Gupta V, Dwivedi SN, et al. Oral isotretinoin combined with oral terbinafine versus oral terbinafine alone to treat recurrent dermatophytosis: An open-label randomised clinical trial. Indian Dermatol Online J 2021;12:820–5.
22. von Bernuth H, Wahn V. Systemic treatment with isotretinoin suppresses itraconazole blood level in chronic granulomatous disease. Pediatr Allergy Immunol 2014;25:405–7.
23. Gottardo B, Zoccal ARM, Maschio-Lima T, Lemes TH, Paziani MH, Von Zeska Kress MR, et al. Antifungal activity of nontoxic nanocomposite based on silver and reduced graphene oxide against dermatophytes and *Candida* spp. ACS Biomater Sci Eng. 2023;9(12):6870–9.
24. Bidaud A-L, Schwarz P, Herbreteau G, Dannaoui E. Techniques for the assessment of *in vitro* and *in vivo* antifungal combinations. J Fungi 2021;7:113.
25. Roana J, Mandras N, Scalas D, Campagna P, Tullio V. Antifungal activity of *Melaleuca alternifolia* essential oil (TTO) and its synergy with itraconazole or ketoconazole against *Trichophyton rubrum*. Molecules 2021;26:461.
26. Simonetti O, Silvestri C, Arzeni D, Cirioni O, Kamysz W, Conte I, et al. *In vitro* activity of the protegrin IB-367 alone and in combination compared with conventional antifungal agents against dermatophytes. Mycoses 2013;57:233–9.
27. Perrins N, Howell SA, Moore M, Bond R. Inhibition of the growth *in vitro* of *Trichophyton mentagrophytes*, *Trichophyton erinacei* and *Microsporum persicolor* by miconazole and chlorhexidine. Veter Dermatol 2005;16:330–3.

CHAPTER 9

Long-term Follow-up after Successful Treatment and Management of Relapses

• Konakanchi Venkata Chalam • Nayankumar H Patel

INTRODUCTION

The prevalence of dermatophytosis ranges between 20% and 25% across the globe. In recent times, dermatophytosis has become a menace in India. Recurrent and persistent infections have become common and appropriate treatment is to be meticulously followed to achieve complete cure. Recalcitrant dermatophytosis is the prevailing clinical scenario currently, and one must delve into complexities to offer appropriate treatment and thus, cure. Once the clinical and mycological cure is achieved, follow-up of the cases is mandatory with necessary counseling about adherence to the general measures, and appropriate treatment is to be offered if there is a relapse, which is not very uncommon. Specifically, we will discuss the importance of long-term follow-up care and how to manage relapses in patients. We will cover various factors contributing to relapse like those related to dermatophyte species, host, environment, drugs, and approach to treatment. Additionally, we will highlight the critical role of regular check-ups and open communication with healthcare providers to ensure the best possible outcomes. The following terminology shall be used in further discussion.[1]

- *Recalcitrant dermatophytosis:* This is a term that encompasses cases of relapse, reinfection, recurrence or persistent infection.
- *Chronic dermatophytosis:* Tinea persisting beyond 6 months to 1 year can be labeled as chronic dermatophytosis.
- *Relapse:* The occurrence of lesions of tinea after 6–8 weeks following clinical cure.

The reported incidence of recurrence in a study conducted in Sikkim in 2015 was 34.3%.[2] Clinical manifestations of recalcitrant dermatophytosis include *Tinea pseudoimbricata, Tinea faciei*, erythroderma, hypopigmented patches mimicking leprosy, due to the irrational use of combination creams containing potent steroids.[3] Lesions may also appear initially at the periphery of already cleared lesions in early relapse. Confirmation of the diagnosis is by KOH mount of skin scrapings and treatment includes systemic antifungals at least for 4 weeks along with topical azoles preferably.[1] A complete cure ideally is achieved once there is a negative mycological report (KOH) following the resolution of lesions and symptoms.[4] A minimum follow-up of twelve weeks is required to identify early relapse.

FACTORS CONTRIBUTING TO RELAPSE

The following are the factors that contribute to relapse:

Dermatophyte Species

The new recently identified dermatophyte species, *Trichophyton indotineae* is responsible for the current scenario in India and is notoriously resistant to terbinafine. Adaptation to humans, high virulence, and extended survival on fomites underscores the need to adhere to general measures strictly. Whether indiscriminate usage of potent topical corticosteroids in combination with antifungals is contributing to this switch in species is speculative.[5,6]

Host Factors

Majority cases that relapse have defective skin barriers due to the indiscriminate use of potent topical corticosteroids. Furthermore, associated skin diseases like atopic dermatitis and ichthyosis lead to xerosis and incessant scratching, which again can lead to relapse and chronicity. The predominance of Th2 immunological response is accountable for this. Virulence of dermatophytosis is directly related to alkaline pH, patients need to be educated not to use soaps aggressively.[7] It is during this phase that liberal use of moisturizers is advised. Many patients continue to use corticosteroid-containing creams apart from the standard prescription and this leads to multiple relapses. This should be ascertained in every visit.

Environment

Geographic areas and climatic conditions determine the prevalence of dermatophytes. The spread of infection can occur directly or indirectly through a contaminated environment. Humans, animals, and soil can be a source of infection. Predisposing factors in case of relapse could be a hot and humid climate, low socio-economic status, overcrowding, poor hygiene, or because of migration or reinfection from other family members.[8]

Drug-related Factors

Bioavailability is an issue with conventional Itraconazole, which can be addressed with the use of super-bioavailable Itraconazole. Super-bioavailable Itraconazole contains Itraconazole in a uniform non-pellet formulation containing a pH-dependent polymeric matrix-hypromellose phthalate. This leads to dissolution and enhanced absorption in the small intestine. Higher bioavailability, consistent serum levels, and low inter-individual variability are advantageous and thus can be useful in cases of relapse. 50 mg, 58 mg, and 65 mg of super- bioavailable Itraconazole is found to be equivalent to 100 mg of conventional Itraconazole.[9] Serum levels of SUBA Itraconazole can go up by 22% if used along with Omeprazole.[10] Co-administered drugs can be the cause of treatment failure due to drug-drug interaction. Drug interactions with Itraconazole are summarized in **Table 9.1**.[11,12]

TABLE 9.1: Drug interactions with Itraconazole leading to failure[11,12]

Drugs leading to decreased absorption of Itraconazole	Drugs leading to an increase in the metabolism of Itraconazole
Antacids, H2-receptor antagonists (Famotidine, Ranitidine), proton pump inhibitors	Rifampicin, Rifabutin, Phenytoin, Phenobarbital, Carbamazepine, Isoniazid
Isotretinoin reduces sebum secretion, and Itraconazole being secreted in sebum does not attain the required skin levels	

Multiple studies across India reported Terbinafine resistance between 18% and 61%. Sardana et al. in a study conducted in a tertiary care center in 2018, opined that *in vitro* resistance (>1 μg/ml) to antifungals may not be a cause of treatment failure.[13] In a multicentric study conducted in 2019 in India, *Trichophyton mentagrophytes* Internal Transcribed Spacer (ITS) type VIII was the predominant species isolated with high Terbinafine resistance.[14] Hence, this has led to increased usage of Itraconazole in India, in cases of recalcitrance.

The checklist of assessment and intervention measures to be followed in a case of relapse is given in **Box 9.1**.

BOX 9.1: Check list in a case of relapse

- Re-assess if there is tinea unguium, tinea pedis, or tinea manuum
- Whether adherent to the general measures-maintaining good hygiene, regular bathing, avoid wearing clothes while the skin is damp
- Ascertain if other family members are affected by a similar problem
- Check out if he or she is continuing to use the steroid-antifungal combination creams or other irritants
- Make certain that the patient is avoiding hot and humid climates
- Whether the patient is atopic-if on moisturizer or not
- Rule-out underlying immunosuppression like diabetes, etc.
- Confirm if he or she is on systemic steroids or other immunosuppressants
- Enquire if there is contact with pets
- Confirm about drug compliance and drug interactions

MANAGEMENT OF RELAPSE IN DERMATOPHYTOSIS

It would be prudent to probe into the above-listed factors responsible to offer appropriate and successful management. Counseling regarding strict adherence to the general measures is the key to a complete cure, more so in a case of relapse.

General Measures

Homemakers, agriculturists, and field workers, working in hot and humid climates should be encouraged to wear loose-fitting cotton clothes.[15] Restructuring of kitchen environment to reduce heat exposure is recommended based on a study showing a positive correlation between chronic tinea and personal history of cooking.[16] Students from hostels have extensive tinea as they wear undergarments on damp skin and share towels and beds. Fomites such as hats and combs must also be treated.[17] They should be counseled regarding this and regular daily bathing. Laundering the linen at 60°C will facilitate the effective clearance of infection, should be reiterated.[18] Additionally, drying the washed clothes inside out in sunlight must be stressed, which will help reduce familial dermatophytosis. At each visit, inquiry about similar complaints in other family members must be practiced.

Investigations

A list of investigations to be done in cases of relapse:

- **Direct microscopy (KOH mount):** It is vital to confirm the presence of fungal elements with 10–20% KOH, as patients would require prolonged treatment. The addition of 1% Chicago sky blue stain allows swift recognition.[19]

- **Fungal culture:** Fungal cultures are conclusive, but 20% can be false-negative despite positive KOH. This may be noticed in treated cases because of a lack of viable fungal elements.[20]
- **Special tests:** These include *in vitro* susceptibility testing and squalene gene mutations.

Pharmacological Interventions

Though Terbinafine was the first-line systemic option, due to the emergence of drug resistance, as high as 32% reported in the Singh et al. study from Delhi, it is no longer the preferred drug. However, updosing to 250 mg BID can still result in a significant cure in those with relatively lower MIC of 1–4 µg/ml. Hence, exploring squalene gene mutations and *in vitro* susceptibility testing can direct the appropriate drug choice.[21, 22] Imran Majid et al. in their study observed that partial mycological clearance and relapse were high in cases treated with a standard dose of Terbinafine for 2 weeks.[23] Treatment failure with Terbinafine has led to the preference for Itraconazole over Terbinafine.

Several studies have shown low MICs to Itraconazole unlike Terbinafine, Griseofulvin, and Fluconazole; hence, resistance is unlikely.[24] Conventional Itraconazole 100 mg twice a day for 6–8 weeks, if used judiciously, can result in a complete cure. Super-bioavailable Itraconazole because of better bioavailability, predictable serum levels, and less inter-individual variability can be another option.[9] Griseofulvin and Fluconazole are used less often in the current scenario. Luliconazole, Sertaconazole, Eberconazole, Butenafine, Ciclopirox Olamine, and Whitefield's ointment can be used in addition, as per preference.[25] Both topical and systemic therapy needs to be continued for two weeks beyond clinical resolution. Frequent laboratory monitoring is required.[26]

CONCLUSION

Educating the patient at follow-up about hygiene, clothing and the importance of dusting and wet mopping the floor, will help reduce the spore load and infection. Finally, patients must be advised to report immediately if the lesions and symptoms recur. Strict adherence to general measures and avoidance of predisposing factors with judicious use of available treatment options can offer a complete cure.

Key Points

- Agent factors (emergence of *T. indotineae*), host factors (defective skin barrier), environmental factors (hot and humid climate, source of infection in soil, animals or humans) and drug related factors (defective absorption of itraconazole) may be responsible for relapse.
- General measures such as use of loose-fitting cotton clothes, restructuring kitchen environment, avoidance of sharing of fomites and clothes, washing linen in warm water and drying in sun is key to complete cure and prevention of relapse.
- Investigations such as KOH mount, fungal culture, *in vitro* susceptibility testing and detection of gene mutations must be done in cases of relapse.
- Updosing Terbinafine to 250 mg BID and use of Super Bioavailable Itraconazole may result in significant cure in resistant cases.

REFERENCES

1. Rajagopalan M, Inamadar A, Mittal A, Miskeen AK, Srinivas CR, Sardana K, et al. Expert consensus on the management of dermatophytosis in India (ECTODERM India). BMC Dermatology 2018;18(1):1–1.
2. Sharma R, Adhikari L, Sharma RL. Recurrent dermatophytosis: A rising problem in Sikkim, a Himalayan state of India. Indian J Pathol Microbiol 2017;60(4):541.

3. Bishnoi A, Vinay K, Dogra S. Emergence of recalcitrant dermatophytosis in India. The Lancet Infect Dis 2018;18(3):250–1.
4. Rengasamy M, Shenoy MM, Dogra S, Asokan N, Khurana A, Poojary S, et al. Indian Association of Dermatologists, Venereologists and Leprologists (IADVL) task force against recalcitrant tinea (ITART) consensus on the management of glabrous tinea (INTACT). Indian Dermatol Online J 2020;11(4):502.
5. Uhrlaß S, Verma SB, Gräser Y, Rezaei-Matehkolaei A, Hatami M, et al. *Trichophyton indotineae*—an emerging pathogen causing recalcitrant dermatophytoses in India and worldwide—a multidimensional perspective. J Fungi. 2022;8(7):757.
6. Verma S, Madhu R. The great Indian epidemic of superficial dermatophytosis: An appraisal. Indian J Dermatol. 2017;62(3):227.
7. Sardana K, Gupta A, Mathachan SR. Immunopathogenesis of dermatophytoses and factors leading to recalcitrant infections. Indian Dermatol Online J 2021;12(3):389.
8. Dogra S, Narang T. Emerging atypical and unusual presentations of dermatophytosis in India. Clinical Dermatol Rev. 2017;1(Suppl 1):S12–8.
9. Sardana K, Mathachan SR. Super bioavailable Itraconazole and its place and relevance in recalcitrant dermatophytosis: Revisiting skin levels of Itraconazole and minimum inhibitory concentration data. Indian Dermatol Online J 2021;12(1):1.
10. Lindsay J, Mudge S, Thompson III GR. Effects of food and omeprazole on a novel formulation of super bioavailability Itraconazole in healthy subjects. Antimicrob Agents Chemother 2018;62(12):e01723–18.
11. Wolverton SE, Wu JJ. Comprehensive dermatologic drug therapy. Elsevier Health Sciences; 2019.
12. Brüggemann RJ, Alffenaar JW, Blijlevens NM, Billaud EM, Kosterink JG, Verweij PE, et al. Clinical relevance of the pharmacokinetic interactions of azole antifungal drugs with other coadministered agents. Clin Infect Dis. 2009;48(10):1441–58.
13. Sardana K, Kaur R, Arora P, Goyal R, Ghunawat S. Is antifungal resistance a cause for treatment failure in dermatophytosis: A study focused on tinea corporis and cruris from a tertiary centre. Indian Dermatol Online J. 2018;9(2):90.
14. Ebert A, Monod M, Salamin K, Burmester A, Uhrlaß S, Wiegand C, et al. Alarming India-wide phenomenon of antifungal resistance in dermatophytes: a multicentre study. Mycoses 2020;63(7):717–28.
15. Rudramurthy SM, Shankarnarayan, Dogra S, Shaw D, Mushtaq K, Paul, et al. Mutation in the squalene epoxidase gene of *Trichophyton interdigitale* and *Trichophyton rubrum* associated with allylamine resistance. Antimicrob Agents Chemother. 2018;62(5):e02522–17.
16. Singh S, Verma P, Chandra U, Tiwary NK. Risk factors for chronic and chronic-relapsing tinea corporis, tinea cruris and tinea faciei: Results of a case–control study. Indian J Dermatol Venereol Leprol 2019;85:197.
17. Al-Khikani FH, Ayit AS. Major challenges in dermatophytosis treatment: Current options and future visions. Egyptian J Dermatol Venerol 2021;41(1):1.
18. Akhoundi M, Nasrallah J, Marteau A, Chebbah D, Izri A, Brun S. Effect of household laundering, heat drying, and freezing on the survival of dermatophyte conidia. J Fungi 2022;8(5):546.
19. Gautam M, Bhatia S. Mount the Menace!–Potassium hydroxide in superficial fungal infections. Indian J Paediatr Dermatol 2020;21(4):343–6.
20. Pihet M, Clément N, Kauffmann-Lacroix C, Nail-Billaud S, Marot A, Pilon F, et al. Diagnosis of dermatophytosis: An evaluation of direct examination using MycetColor® and MycetFluo®. Diagn Microbiol Infect Dis 2015;83(2):170–4.
21. Singh A, Masih A, Khurana A, Singh PK, Gupta M, Hagen F, et al. High terbinafine resistance in *Trichophyton interdigitale* isolates in Delhi, India harbouring mutations in the squalene epoxidase gene. Mycoses 2018;61(7):477–84.
22. Khurana A, Sardana K, Chowdhary A. Antifungal resistance in dermatophytes: Recent trends and therapeutic implications. Fungal Genet Biol 2019;132:103255.
23. Majid I, Sheikh G, Kanth F, Hakak R. Relapse after oral terbinafine therapy in dermatophytosis: A clinical and mycological study. Indian J Dermatol 2016;61(5):529.
24. Shaw D, Singh S, Dogra S, Jayaraman J, Bhat R, Panda S, et al. MIC and upper limit of wild-type distribution for 13 antifungal agents against a *Trichophyton mentagrophytes-Trichophyton interdigitale* complex of Indian origin. Antimicrob Agents Chemother2020;64(4):e01964–19.
25. Sahni K, Singh S, Dogra S. Newer topical treatments in skin and nail dermatophyte infections. Indian Dermatol Online J 2018;9(3):149.
26. Rengasamy M, Chellam J, Ganapati S. Systemic therapy of dermatophytosis: Practical and systematic approach. Clinical Dermatol Rev 2017;1(Suppl 1):S19–23.

CHAPTER **10**

Patient and Family Education for Dermatophytosis

• *Dattatray Gopal Saple* • *Sushrut N Save*

INTRODUCTION

Dermatophytosis presents to us a unique challenge in its management owing to its chronicity, relapsing and remitting course, psychosocial impact along with its ramifications on the quality of life as well as the family life of the individual.

According to the New Consensus Definition of Counseling 2020–21, *Counseling is defined as a professional relationship that empowers diverse individuals, families, and groups to accomplish mental health, wellness, education, and career goals"*.[1]

Therefore, according to this definition, we realize that counseling forms an integral part of the therapy of dermatophytosis, especially recalcitrant dermatophytosis, and the whole aim of counseling is to maximize the treatment response achieved using the available armamentarium of medications.

The current understanding of the tinea infection is slowly evolving and it is now being accepted as a chronic infection, which may be attributed to numerous factors including the concept of absent or defective cellular immunity in certain individuals which prevents them from mounting an effective response to dermatophytes.[2, 3] Hence as is the case with any chronic infection, an effective counseling therapy needs to be established to ensure proper compliance and adherence to the treatment regimen.[2, 3]

PATIENT COUNSELING (Our Perspective, A Proposed Working Indian Model)

Individual face-to-face counseling is required for every patient to emphasize the need to be compliant with the medications and complete the entire treatment course. Since the older treatment guidelines as per the western literature are no longer applicable, and often the medicines need to be taken for prolonged periods (up to 6 weeks) in order to ensure adequate cure, its essential to create a mindset for the patient wherein he remains adherent to the whole regimen.[4]

A minimum of 15–20 minutes should be allocated by a health care professional/trained staffer to every patient. It should be an educational-interactive session, wherein the patient should be explained about the gravity of the condition, skin-care methods, personal hygiene methods and regularity in intake of medicines. This counseling should be done mandatorily at every visit to ensure lesser patient dropout rates and adequate compliance.

It is also important to counsel the patients regarding the method of intake of administration including the dosing, e.g. the conventional Itraconazole preparations need to be taken on an empty stomach in order to maintain an acidic pH to enhance the bioavailability, however, this may not be applicable to the newer supra-bioavailable preparations. In contrast, the Fluconazole pharmacokinetics remain relatively insensitive to the intake of food and physiological changes in the gastrointestinal pH.[5]

As is the case with any medications, the side-effects of the prescribed medications should adequately be explained to the patient, and if the need be, relevant investigations should be advised periodically. For example, if any of the azoles or allylamines are being administered for a longer duration then the regular monitoring (every fortnightly for 6 weeks) of the liver function tests and serum creatinine should be performed.[4]

- It should be impressed upon the patient to avoid the use of any sort of over-the-counter creams, especially steroids, as the use of steroidal creams is considered as one of the root cause for fanning the wild-fire of recalcitrant dermatophytosis.
- Also, many geriatric patients are on polypharmacy owing to the underlying co-morbidities and hence in view of this, adequate drug history should be asked to avoid drug-drug interactions **(Table 10.1)** while prescribing the antifungals. In case of pediatric patients, adequate counseling should be imparted to the parents as well as the local guardian.

TABLE 10.1: Drug-drug interactions of Fluconazole, Itraconazole, and Terbinafine

Drugs	Fluconazole	Itraconazole	Terbinafine	Description
Statins	✓	✓	✓	Increases plasma levels and side effects of statins
Antacids	–	✓	–	Reduces Itraconazole absorption (administer 1h before or 2 h after)
H2-blockers/ Cimetidine	✓	✓	✓	• Reduces Fluconazole AUC and C_{max} • Reduces Itraconazole absorption • Reduces Terbinafine clearance by 33%
Proton-Pump Inhibitors (PPIs)	–	✓	–	Reduces Itraconazole absorption (administer 1 h before or 2 h after)
Warfarin	✓	✓	✓	• Increases anticoagulant effect, monitor prothrombin time (PT) INR values • Increase or decrease in PT
Rifampin/Isoniazid	✓	✓	✓	• Enhances metabolism of Fluconazole • Decreases Itraconazole levels and increases Isoniazid concentration • Terbinafine clearance increases by 100%
Hydrochlorothiazide	✓	–	–	Increases Fluconazole C_{max} and AUC
Benzodiazepines	✓	✓		Increases serum levels and thereby effects of Benzodiazepines
Tricyclic antidepressants (TCA)	✓	–	✓	Increases TCA concentration and its toxic effects
Zidovudine	✓	–	–	Increases Zidovudine AUC levels
Theophylline	✓	–	–	Increases C_{max}, half-life and AUC of theophylline
Sulfonylureas (SUs)	✓	–	–	Decreases metabolism and increases concentration of SUs

(Contd.)

TABLE 10.1: Drug-drug interactions of Fluconazole, Itraconazole, and Terbinafine *(Contd.)*

Drugs	Fluconazole	Itraconazole	Terbinafine	Description
Phenytoin	✓	✓	–	Increases phenytoin plasma concentration
Losartan	✓	–	–	Inhibits metabolism thus increases antihypertensive effect
Calcium Channel Blockers (CCBs)	–	✓	–	Inhibits metabolism of CCBs; increases edema and negative inotropic effects
Beta-blockers	–	–	✓	Decreases metabolism of beta-blockers, may require dose reduction
Cyclosporine	✓	✓	✓	• Increases C_{max}, half-life and AUC of Cyclosporine • Terbinafine increases Cyclosporine clearance by 15%
Corticosteroids	✓	✓	–	Decreases metabolism and increases toxicity of corticosteroids
Cisapride	✓	✓	–	Increases Cisapride concentration; cardiotoxicity may occur
Erythromycin/ Clarithromycin	–	✓	–	Increases Itraconazole concentration
Digoxin	–	✓	–	Increases Digoxin concentration and its effects/toxicity
Haloperidol	–	✓	–	Increases Haloperidol concentration and side effects
Oral hypoglycemic agents	–	✓	–	Increases hypoglycemia risk
Zolpidem	✓	✓	–	Increases plasma concentration and effects of Zolpidem, monitor plasma concentration, dose may need to be reduced
Dextromethorphan	–	–	✓	Increases Dextromethorphan concentration and its side effects
Monoamine oxidase inhibitors (MAOI) type B	–	–	✓	May require dose reduction of MAOIs

'✓': Significant drug interaction; '–': Drug interaction not reported commonly.
(INR: International normalized ratios; C_{max}: Maximum concentration of drug in plasma; AUC: Area under the curve–area under the plot of plasma concentration of a drug versus time).

- Personal hygiene measures are of utmost importance. Every patient should be advised to soak their clothes in hot boiling water before washing them, followed by proper ironing of the inner seams of the clothes. This practice should be followed at least for the initial couple of weeks. Apart from this, avoidance of tight/moist clothing and sharing of bed linen and towels/fomites are certain routine instructions which need to be given.
- Nails are a common reservoir for tinea and can result in recurrent tinea pedis and other tinea infections due to autoinoculation to other body parts, such as the hand, groin, and face. Special care of nail infections is important and should be looked for in every tinea patient and addressed accordingly. For patients having onychomycosis, appropriate

counseling should be done regarding the long duration of therapy (9–12 months for toenails and 4–6 months for finger nails) and consequently explained as to how the morphological appearance of the nails would take a similar timeline to show morphological improvement.
- All instructions for nail care written in table form should be handed over to the patient (**Appendix I**).

APPENDIX I

Instructions for patients with onychomycosis
- Trim the nails regularly
- Avoid walking barefoot in public places
- Avoid wearing wet socks
- Avoid using tight footwear
- Keep the foot dry

An assessment for overall obesity and excessive sweating should be also done to look for any trigger factors and associated lifestyle changes should be advised.

According to Saple et al., proper counseling and adherence to treatment regimen, ensured an 83% clinical and mycological cure rate.[6] Every patient is issued an educational pamphlet which allows them to go through all the points discussed in the counseling sessions once they go back home (**Appendix II**).

APPENDIX II

General instructions for patients with dermatophytoses
- Watch for decreased appetite, and report to us if there is any reduction in your appetite, nausea or vomiting.
- Treatment is for a long duration, so do not stop the treatment without asking the doctor.
- Do not apply harsh soaps to the affected area. Do not apply antiseptics such as dettol on the skin at all.
- Ask other members of the family if they have similar complaints. If at all they have similar complaints, then they need to get treated as well.
- Wash your daily clothes and undergarments separately with hot water and iron the seams of the clothes properly.
- Avoid use of topical steroid (cream) preparations.
- Oral anti-fungal agents to be avoided in pregnancy or planning pregnancy and lactation.
- Avoid close physical contact with family members and close contacts to avoid spread of infection.
- Avoid use of tight and synthetic clothes, prefer loose cotton garments.
- Change clothes including underclothes regularly.

FAMILY COUNSELING

Involvement of family members or even room-mates, in case of individuals staying away from their family, is extremely important. Close contacts of the patient should be counseled for the presence of tinea as well, which tends to be neglected at times and contributes to the recurrence of infection within the family/close-contacts. The family members should also be encouraged to keep a check on the drug-intake by the patient which ensures the patient compliance and adherence.

CONCLUSION

Although as busy clinicians, it is extremely difficult to find time for counseling, it is essential to implement this in our daily practice at it would complement our medical treatment. Although initially it may seem difficult to get things streamlined, but once initiated it would definitely work in the best interests of the tinea patients.

Key Points

- Dermatophytosis has now been accepted as a chronic infection
- Main stay of success is adequate adherence and compliance to therapy
- Counseling is the backbone of therapy to ensure adherence
- Counseling of family members is equally important to ensure complete clearance of infection
- A leaflet with instructions regarding cleanliness and other general measures should be handed over to the patient.

REFERENCES

1. Kaplan DM, Tarvydas VM, Gladding ST. 20/20: A vision for the future of counseling: The new consensus definition of counseling. J Couns Dev 2014;92:366–72.
2. Jones HE. Immune response and host resistance of humans to dermatophyte infection. J Am Acad Dermatol 1993;28(5 Pt 1):S12–S18.
3. Verma S, Vasani R, Reszke R, et al. Prevalence and clinical characteristics of itch in epidemic-like scenario of dermatophytoses in India: A cross-sectional study. J Eur Acad Dermatol Venereol 2020;34:180–3.
4. Rajagopalan M, Inamadar A, Mittal A, Miskeen AK, et al. Expert consensus on the management of dermatophytosis in India (ECTODERM India). BMC Dermatol 2018;18(1):6.
5. Zimmermann T, Yeates RA, Laufen H, Pfaff G, Wildfeuer A. Influence of concomitant food intake on the oral absorption of two triazole antifungal agents, itraconazole and fluconazole. Eur J Clin Pharmacol. 1994;46(2):147–50.
6. Saple DG, Save S, Tambe SA. Oral itraconazole and topical eberconazole therapy in the treatment of tinea cruris and corporis. Indian J Drugs Dermatol 2021;7:15–9.

CHAPTER 11

Therapeutic Ladder for Treatment for Dermatophytosis

• *Kabir Sardana*

INTRODUCTION

While it is evident that the main reason for lack of consistent response to terbinafine is mutation in the Erg1/SQLE, it is also evident that in some cases a higher dose might still be useful. Most clinicians are gravitating towards itraconazole and a myriad of irrational combinations.[1] The focus on research in the last 1 year is just on reporting "episodes of infection by *T. indotineae*" which does not add much to the solution nor does it give any answers, but does clog PubMed citations on the topic. The use of the term "indotinae" defies logic as there is no proof that the epidemic started in India and possibly if earlier isolates are collected and re-analysed using the latest molecular techniques this "new" species may have been in circulation in many parts of the world.

In India the issue is of relapse and also occasional failures to ITZ. Beyond quality and pellets and the role of SUBA ITZ, there is now a real issue of failure to our 2nd line drug and thus the need to understand the other mechanisms for resistance beyond SQLE.[2] We will examine this and suggest a treatment regimen based on the current scientific data.

THE FUNGAL SYNTHESIS PATHWAY

The focus of the major antifungal drugs is to target the ergosterol pathway as defects in ergosterol biosynthesis lead to impaired endocytosis, cell polarization, cell fusion and cell wall assembly. Thus a brief overview of the pathway and the varied steps is important to understand **(Fig. 11.1)**.

Firstly, two molecules of farnesyl-PP are used by the squalene synthase [ergosterol 9 (Erg9)] enzymes to form squalene, which is the precursor of all steroids. Secondly, the consecutive action of the squalene epoxidase **(Erg1)** and the lanosterol synthase enzymes results in conversion of squalene into lanosterol. In the further steps, lanosterol is transformed to zymosterol through a complex process involving various demethylation, reduction and desaturation reactions, which are catalyzed by lanosterol 14-α-demethylase **(Erg11)** (also known as Cyp51), C-14 reductase (Erg24) and C-4 demethylation complex (Erg25-Erg26-Erg27). Erg28 and Erg29 are likely to function in the C-4 demethylation complex reaction. Then, Erg6 converts zymosterol into fecosterol, followed by the formation of episterol by Erg2, which is finally desaturated and reduced by Erg3, Erg5 and Erg4 to ergosterol.

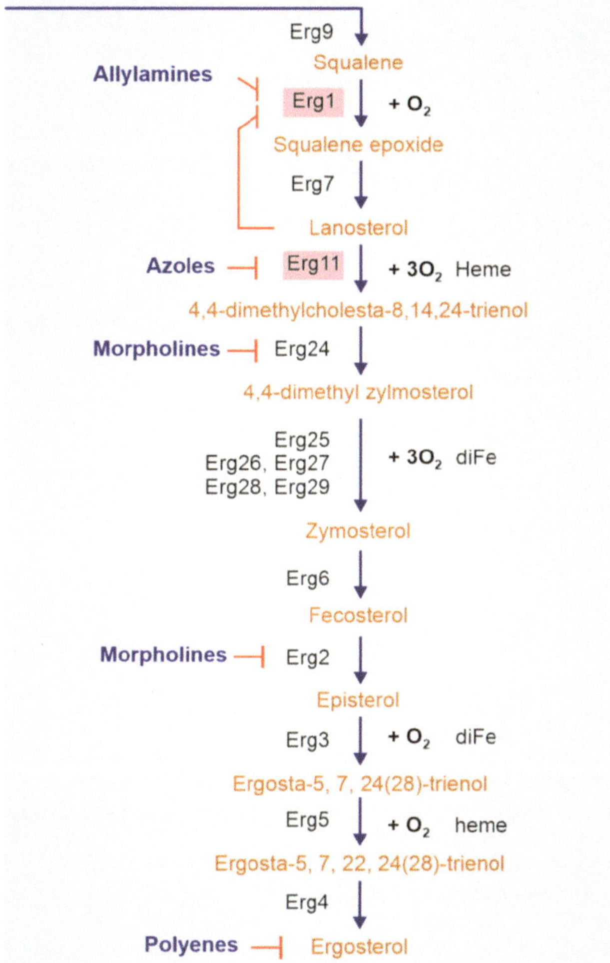

FIGURE 11.1: Ergosterol biosynthetic pathway in *S. cerevisiae* with gene loci that determine activity of enzymes and site of action of various drugs

Ergosterol is synthesized in the endoplasmic reticulum (ER), but is mostly transported to the plasma membrane (PM). **Erg1** and **Erg11** represent two ***rate-limiting steps*** in this part of the pathway (**Fig. 11.1**). This pathway is also dependent on oxygen and iron in multiple enzymatic steps.

A depiction of the site of action of the existent drugs is given in **Figure 11.2. Allylamines** are non-competitive inhibitors of squalene epoxidase (encoded by *Erg1* gene), while **azoles** target cytochrome P-450 enzyme–lanosterol 14-α-demethylase (encoded by *Erg11* gene)–by directly binding to the iron atom within the heme group of the enzyme. In case of dermatophytes, it was believed that fungal resistance to allylamines is not seen as these drugs target an early step in ergosterol biosynthesis, leading to compensatory mutations elsewhere in the pathway. Azole resistance amongst fungal pathogens is mediated by Erg11 mutations, but when this enzyme is inhibited, an alternate pathway catalyzed by Erg6, Erg25-Erg26-Erg27 and Erg3 is activated. Notably *T. indotineae* isolates also exhibit mutations in the sterol 14-α demethylase *Erg11B* gene apart from increase in *Erg11B* gene copies. This is a worrisome trend and if the drug is overused there is a high chance that there would be failure to Itraconazole.

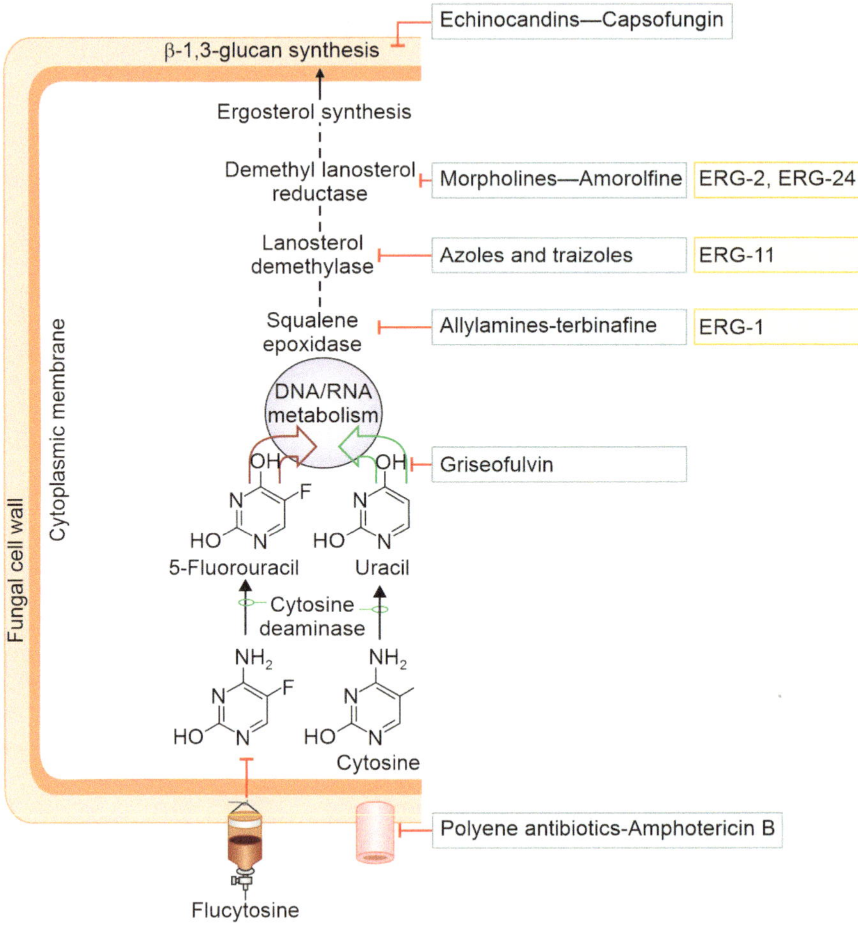

FIGURE 11.2: An overview of the site of action of varied antifungal drugs including drugs inhibiting cell wall, cell membrane and ergosterol synthesis. Most drugs approved for dermatophytes work on the ergosterol synthesis pathway

MECHANISMS FOR RESISTANCE

While there are varied resistance mechanisms **(Fig. 11.3)** we will focus on mutations and their implications and another dominant mechanism that has been missed by varied research groups that is Efflux pumps.

Efflux Pumps

Efflux pumps are an intrinsic defense mechanism that helps to extrude the antifungal drugs from the cell. This accounts for a gradual increase in MIC and is a possible cause of drug resistance and would effectively diminish the expected drug effect *in vivo*. This has been implicated in resistance toward azoles, and may be circumvented by certain efflux pump inhibitors. The major family that is instrumental in efflux is the ABC superfamily, which is evolutionarily conserved in both prokaryotes and eukaryotes **(Fig. 11.4)**.

There are three important members of the of ABC superfamily of transporters: Multidrug resistance (MDR), MDR-associated protein (MRP), and the pleiotropic drug resistance (PDR) families. Published data shows that some of these transporters including MDR 1/2,

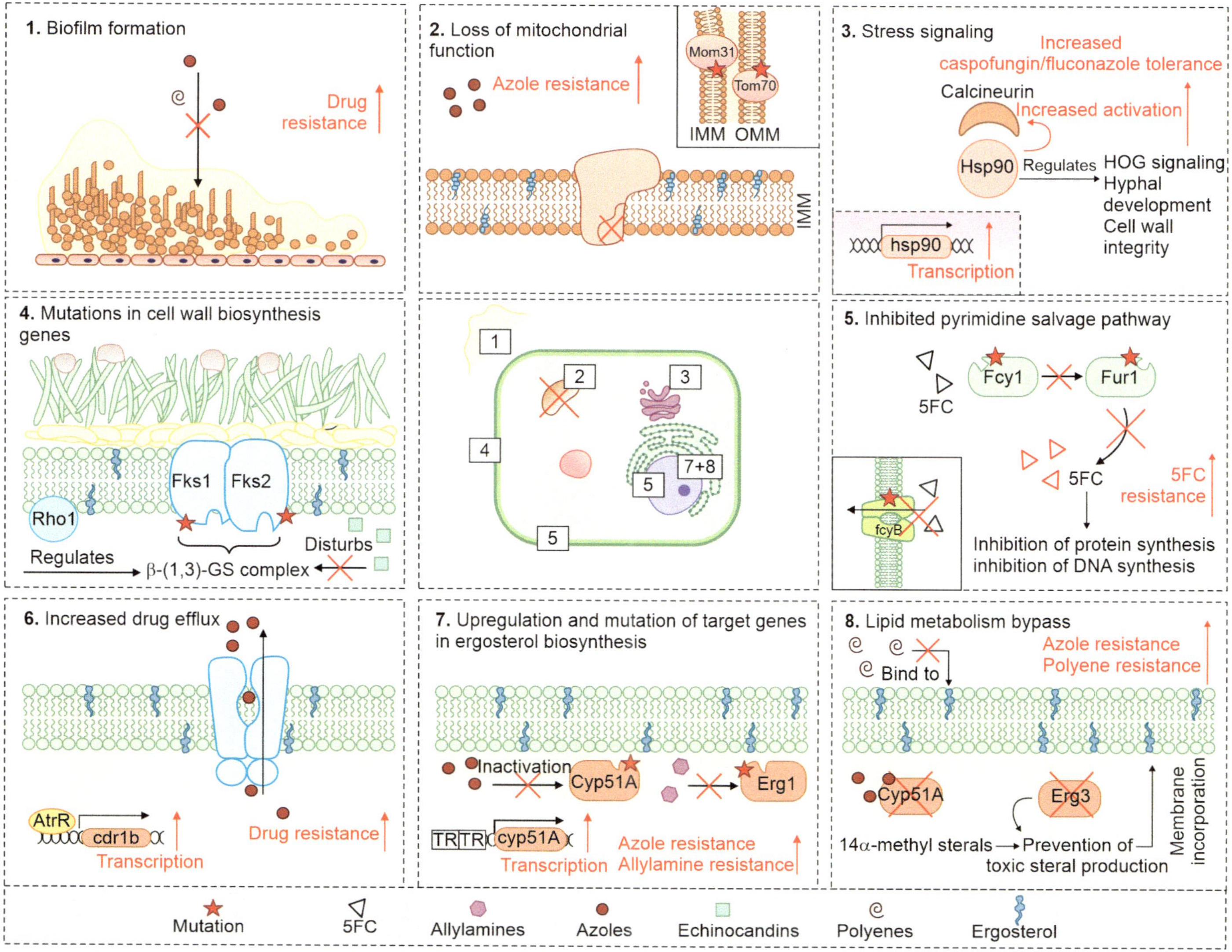

FIGURE 11.3: An overview of the varied known resistance mechanisms in fungi

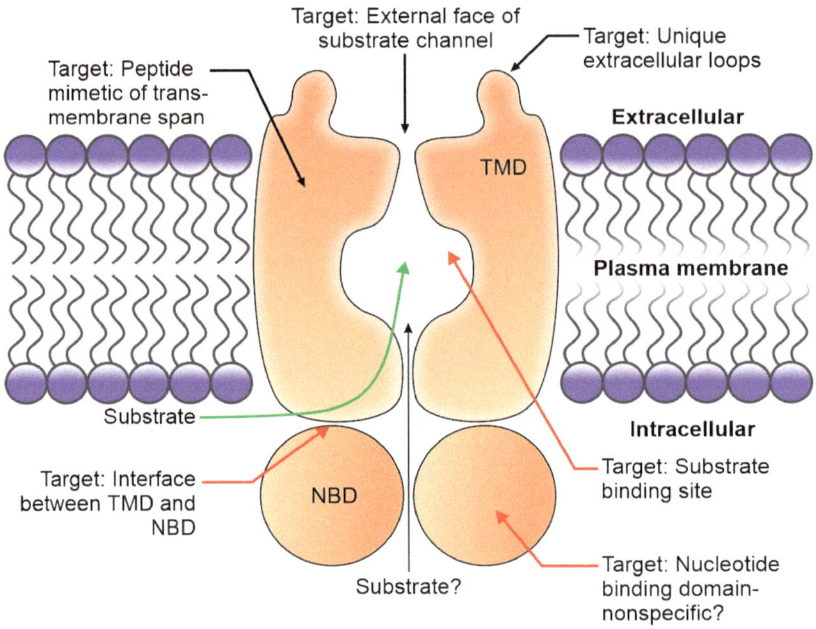

FIGURE 11.4: Possible drug targets of action on various parts of the fungal ABC efflux pumps (NBD: Nucleotide-binding domain; TBD: Transmembrane domain)

MFS, MDR4, and MDR5, and the pleiotropic drug resistance (PDR1) are overexpressed in dermatophytes under drug pressure.[3] TruMDR3 transports voriconazole and itraconazole, while TruMDR2 transports only itraconazole. Recently a second MFS transporter (TruMFS2) has also been implicated as an azole efflux pump in dermatophytes.[4]

Yamada et al.[5] reported TinMDR3 to be highly overexpressed in *T. indotineae* strains with low susceptibility to azole compounds (itraconazole MIC ≥0.5 mg/ml; voriconazole MIC ≥0.5 mg/ml). More recently, Bhattacharya et al. demonstrated mutations in *MDR1* and *MFS* genes of a *Trichophyton mentagrophyte interdigitale* complex strain, with high MICs to most antifungals, isolated from a patient who had failed both terbinafine and itraconazole.[6] This is the first study of efflux mechanisms in clinical failures as opposed to previous studies which were largely in laboratory strains. Thus the pressure of high dosage of ITZ, leads to activation of efflux pumps, which will negate the effect of the drug and hence, the dose of ITZ should be restricted to a maximum of 200 mg.[7]

Looking Beyond SQLE Mutations

The lack of response to terbinafine has been linked to mutations in the Erg1 gene. Amino acid substitutions at one of the four positions–L393, F397, F415, and H440–have been linked to terbinafine resistance in *Trichophyton* species.[8] The most common substitution in the emerging *T. indotineae* species reported worldwide is F397L (leading to MICs between 1 to >32 mg/L) followed by L393F (MIC range: 1 to 64 mg/L) and L393S (MIC range: 0.5 to 1 mg/L).[9]

With respect to itraconazole, in most of the strains of *T. indotineae* the MIC of ITZ was reported to be around 0.016 µg/ml (90%) while in 10% an increased MIC to ITZ (>0.05 µg/ml) was observed. Thus, it seems that the majority are still sensitive to ITZ. The strains with a high MIC also exhibited reduced susceptibility to VRC (>0.25 µg/ml), and it was presumed that an abnormal distribution of MICs was suggestive of resistance.[10] While resistance to azoles can be inferred from high MIC levels, but this is not the ideal method to define resistance to azoles, instead a proven Erg11 mutation with concomitant clinical failures is considered the preferred method to confirm azole resistance. A recent paper has described four different types of Erg11B mutants. All strains demonstrated different combinations of Erg1 and Erg11 genotypes. The authors concluded that resistance against terbinafine and azoles developed several times independently within the *T. indotineae* population.[11] The same group has shown that azoles upregulate varied defense mechanisms and exposure to itraconazole leads to overexpression of Erg11B which is more common than mutation and accounts for its possible failure.[12] A more recent paper also described Erg1, Erg3, Erg4, and Erg11 mutations in a multi-drug resistant isolate, identified as belonging to *Trichophyton mentagrophyte interdigitale* complex, from a patient who failed multiple oral antifungals.[6] Thus, clinical failures to azoles need to be corroborated with mutations or overexpression of *Erg 11* gene and efflux mechanisms.

A APPROACH TO TREATMENT

While basic measures include general measures and topical agents, such measures are at best adjuvant and do not always benefit as the new species necessitates administration of oral drugs. The bulwark of therapy is based on the use of oral itraconazole and terbinafine.

Overview of Individual Drugs in View of Prevalent Mutations

1. Terbinafine

While the increasing evidence of resistance has lead to a decrease in response to the drug, there are a substantial number of cases that do not have a mutation in SQLE. Also it has been shown that increasing dose/duration of TRB, even in the presence of *in vitro MICs* and *SQLE* gene mutations is a useful option. In about 70% patients, a prolonged course of TRB 250 mg QD (50% of cases, mean treatment duration–5.6 weeks) or shifting to 250 mg BID dose (a further 20% cases, mean total treatment duration–7.8 weeks) helped in cure and thus, higher TRB exposure could offset the effect of SQLE mutations in many patients.[13]

Terbinafine 250 mg/day would be useful in cases without mutations and that is a reason to preferentially use this drug due to safety across doses, low incidence of pharmacokinetic drug interactions and good patient tolerance.

2. Itraconazole

This drug is now the preferred oral drug but the dose and duration has varied across geographical areas and in many cases unnecessary high doses are prescribed.

A recent paper found that the duration needed for cure varies between 2 and 20 weeks with a mean treatment duration being 6.6 weeks. The treatment durations were 7.7 weeks with 100 mg/d, 7.2 weeks with 200 mg/d, and 5.2 weeks with 400 mg/d.[7] The week wise cure rates are depicted in the **Box 11.1**. The cost to achieve cure with 200 mg/d dose was 163%, and that with 400 mg/d was 220%, of the cost to achieve cure with a lower dose hence a lower dose would be a better option in a cost constrained environment. Weight based dose is not useful as this is primarily for pediatric age groups and extending it to adult case is pharmacologically incorrect. Notably the incorrect concept of weight based dosages have arisen out of the dose for onychomycosis, which is higher as the secretion of ITZ in the nail is not same as in the stratum corneum.

BOX 11.1: A summary of efficacy and the corresponding duration of Itraconazole monotherapy[7]

Time point	Doses-cure rate
2 weeks	100 mg–4.2% 200 mg–4.3% 400 mg–6.4%
4 weeks	100 mg–19.6% 200 mg–17.4% 400 mg–50%
8 weeks	100 mg–47.5% 200 mg–66.7% 400 mg–86%
12 weeks	100 mg–61.5% 200 mg–81.8% 400 mg–93%
16 weeks	100 mg–80% 200 mg–90.9% 400 mg–97.7%

Before switching or stopping ITZ, it must be borne in mind that cure with ITZ takes at least 6 to 8 weeks in most patients and shifting between drugs before this time may not be reasonable. We routinely use ITZ in a dose of 100 mg/d, and prescribe higher doses in patients with extensive disease, or in cases with inadequate response to this dose after at least 4 weeks of treatment.

A recent paper that has compared published data of ITZ *vs* TRB found that itraconazole 200 mg per day at fourth, eighth and the twelfth week achieved cure rates of 27.27%, 48.48% and 54.55%, respectively, which was significantly higher than terbinafine 250 mg per day (8.77%, 24.56% and 28.07%) and even 500 mg/d terbinafine.[14] Thus while ITZ is effective there seems to be a gap in cases that does not respond to the drug though our experience is much better than the review by Song G.

3. Other Drugs

Voriconazole: Voriconazole's use in dermatophytosis must be restricted in accordance with the principles of antifungal stewardship to minimize the risk for resistance amongst systemic fungal infections. Moreover existent data do not show that the MIC of the drug is lower than ITZ or it can circumvent Erg11 mutations. We have used the drug occasionally for recalcitrant limited *T. indotineae* infection and for extensive dermatophytoses in the setting of iatrogenic immunosuppression, but the efficacy and target site of action is identical to ITZ. Voriconazole has a narrow therapeutic window and a highly variable bioavailability, apart from being very expensive. Notably the latest study published from Bangladesh studied ITZ for 4 weeks, which is an inappropriate duration for ITZ, and concluded it as failure. Also a close reading of the paper showed that, complete cure was achieved in 47.4% of the patients being treated with voriconazole, which does not make the drug in any way superior to ITZ.[15] A recent study from Israel, used the drug in proven terbinafine-resistant cases and 3 responded to oral itraconazole 200 mg/day, with two responding only to oral voriconazole and one to oral itraconazole 400 mg/day. We probably need more real world data with concomitant mutational data to assess whether the lack of response is due to a curtailed duration of ITZ or actual resistance.[16]

Posaconazole: There are reports of successful treatment of tinea corporis with posaconazole but again we do not feel it is a viable or economical option. In fact in the case series on posaconazole, ITZ was given for 2 weeks before declaring it as a failure, which is an inappropriate duration to assess results.[17]

Fluconazole: There is sparse recent literature that show effectiveness of Fluconazole, but high *in vitro* MICs have been consistently observed with very low cure rates. Also a recent study (Berstecher N) showed that exposure to the drug leads to upregulation of Erg11b apart from activation of efflux pumps, which explains the consistent failure of the drug in dermatophytosis which was reported by the same author in 2020.[18] There is little utility of this drug in India and there is little real world efficacy.

Ketoconazole: The drug achieves cure-rates between 61% and 67% (doses between 200–400 mg/d) as per both past and recent literature, but the drug should be used as a reserve drug.[19] Notably ketoconazole could be used in case ITZ does not show a response after 4 weeks of therapy but is a 3rd line drug.

Griseofulvin: While early literature reported only modest efficacy with griseofulvin (cure rates 64.8%–69%), drug failures were increasingly reported in the 1980s. Recent literature on *T. indotineae* documents high MICs, and a very low cure rate of 14% was documented after 8 weeks of griseofulvin 10 mg/kg/d.[20] We do not recommend the use of griseofulvin for *T. indotineae* skin infections even though some note that in certain regions it seems to be effective. It does seem that wherever there is abundant hospital supply of the drug, clinicians administer the drug and the concomitant use of topical azoles may account for the response attributed to the drug.

What to do when the 1st and 2nd line drugs fail?

What happens when the first line drugs fail? This is all too a common issue and one should look at some simple measures like *compliance* and proper *duration* of the therapy before esoteric and expensive options like voriconazole and posaconazole.

Certain measures are listed in the **Table 11.1** below but any novel drug or regimen should be based on MIC data, minimum fungicidal concentration (MFC) assessment, checkerboard studies, serum and skin level of drugs and time kill studies, before attempting a clinical trial of monotherapy or combination therapy **(Fig. 11.5)**.

The use of two oral antifungals just on the "premise" of different modes of action is a irrational prescription with no mycological basis. Either a time kill assay or a checkerboard assay should be used to predict the ideal drug combinations **(Table 11.2)** and the existent combinations are listed below. The use of systemic combination therapies (different antifungals or retinoids) for *T. indotineae* is not backed by robust scientific evidence, highlighting the need for further research to validate synergistic combinations effective in real-life practice. Details of this concept are detailed in the Chapter 8 authored by Dr Adil, needless to say the incorrect "analogy" of combining drugs with different modes of action does not work unless tested in mycological models.

Closing Comments

The approach to treatment is depicted in **Figure 11.6** and notably topical agents by themselves do not help unless suitably combined with an oral drug based on synergy testing. Itraconazole, is now being increasingly preferred, but should be administered for

TABLE 11.1: Measures that can be adopted to treat dermatophyte infection[2]	
Using drugs with low MIC levels	• In case of terbinafine resistance (suggested by high *MIC* and *SQLE* gene mutations), itraconazole is an ideal oral drug though updosing terbinafine to 250 mg BD is option • MIC may be a good starting point and this is a singular reason why fluconazole and griseofulvin have fallen out of favor in India
Azoles with novel formulations	• SUBA itraconazole has a better pharmacokinetic profile than conventional pellet based itraconazole and may be prescribed (although it is approved only for deep fungal infections) • 50 and 65 mg formulations are approved globally and are equally effective • 100 mg and 130 mg are additionally available in India, though they are equally efficacious
Antifungal drug combinations	• Drug combinations based on *in vitro* synergy testing using checkerboard analysis is the basic minimum requirement before attempting combinations
Novel and experimental options	• Agents that target major antifungal drug resistance mechanisms • Efflux pump inhibitors, inhibitors of kinases, drugs that inhibit Hsp
Repurposed drugs	• Bisphosphonates • Statins • Calcineurin inhibitors • Calcium channel blockers • Natural plant products

TABLE 11.2: Data on varied combinations of antifungals based on published data and acceptable microbiological drug synergy models[2]

	Synergy	Model and Diagnosis
Sardana K, 2022	ITZ + LUZ, TER, KTZ	Clinical Failures *T. mentagrophytes/T. interdigitale*
Rocha et al., 2022	Sertraline (SRT) in combination with caspofungin (CASP)	*T. rubrum* biofilm and its biomass were studied
Sugiura et al., 2021	EFZ + TER 43.8%, EFZ + ITZ 12.5% LUZ + ITZ 31%	Onychomycosis *T. rubrum* and *T. interdigitale*
Laurent et al., 2017	AMF + ITZ/KTZ/MIZ/SER/SUL	*T. rubrum* was studied using sporulation
Tamura et al., 2014	AMF + ITZ	Study on 27 strains of dermatophytes
Santos et al., 2006	CCL + ITZ/KTZ	*T. rubrum, T. mentagrophytes* from Onychomycoses
Polak et al., 1993	AMF + ITZ/FLU/GRI/TER/KET	*T. mentagrophytes, T. rubrum* and *M. canis*

[AMF, amorolfine; BIZ, bifonazole; CCL, ciclopirox; CLO, chlorhexidine; EFZ, efinaconazole; FLU, fluconazole; GRI, griseofulvin; ITZ, itraconazole; LUZ, luliconazole; MIZ, miconazole; SER, sertaconazole; SUL, sulconazole; KTZ, ketoconazole; TER, terbinafine, PubMed search key words (antifungal, combinations, synergy, dermatophyte)].

6–8 weeks. Before declaring ITZ a "failure", clearance from all infected sites and (ideally) a negative potassium hydroxide smear examination (absence of hyphal fragment from all fields) should be ensured and this takes at least 6–8 weeks in most patients. Certain sites like buttocks should be examined as they prove to be the last to clear. The next line would still be Terbinafine, based on the fact that only 42–60% of patients harbor Terbinafine resistant species.[21, 22] Thus, in the rest, it would still be efficacious and this drug is a safer drug with less interactions as compared to ITZ.

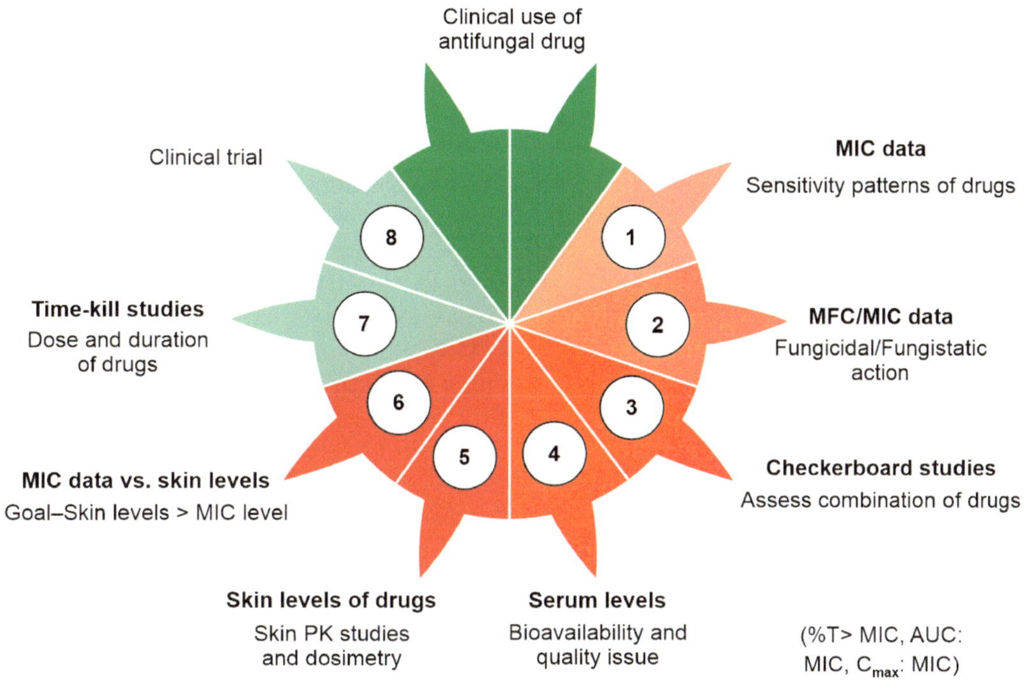

FIGURE 11.5: A diagram depicting the steps that determine the clinical use of antifungal drug(s) or combination, which should start clockwise from MIC data. [Sardana K, Mathachan SR. Br J Dermatol. 2021 Feb;184(2):376–377]

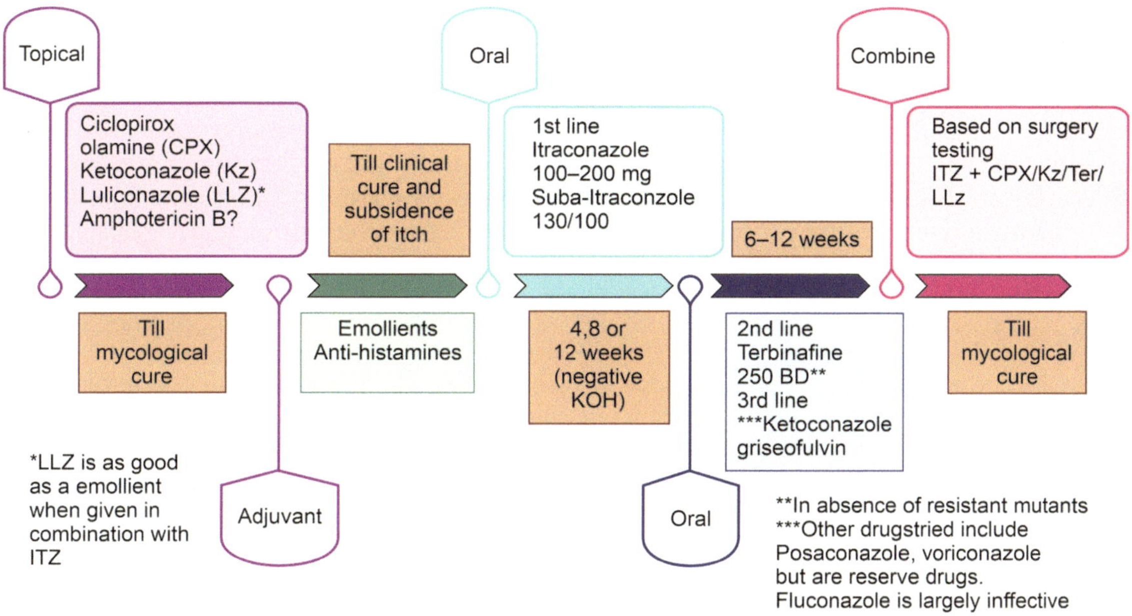

FIGURE 11.6: Step by step treatment of Tinea corporis

Remember that azole exposure can lead to resistance which may be specific to certain drugs in this class. Squalene epoxidase *erg1*^{Ala448Thr} mutants often show association with azole resistance. Several *T. indotineae* isolates demonstrate a heat-dependent increase of *Erg11B* transcripts combined with downregulation of *Erg1*, suggesting a protective role for *Erg11B* with persistent upregulation of *MFS1*. The addition of fluconazole or voriconazole has been shown to induce an enhanced expression of *Erg11A*, *MDR3* and, to a lesser extent, *Erg11B* and *Erg1* (Berstecher N). This explains the futility of giving these drugs in failure to ITZ. Here it is important to examine a study from Bangladesh, where resistance testing revealed terbinafine resistance in 49 and itraconazole "resistance" in 21 patients, even though the latter could not be explained by mutations in the *ERG11B* gene (Bhuiyan MSI). Notably resistance was defined by MIC cut off values (MIC > 0.5 µg/ml) and itraconazole (MIC > 0.25 µg/ml). While this study raises the spectre of ITZ failures, it also shows that using a MIC cut-off may not be a useful way of declaring resistance to ITZ. The presence of efflux pumps, that are overexpressed specially when azoles are administered explains the efficacy of a higher dose of ITZ (400 mg) in a certain subset of patients (Galili E). Also this shows that (Bhattacharyya A,) the fungi is able to surmount a "defense" to extrinsic oral "azole pressure" using multiple mechanisms and thus there is a need for efflux pump inhibitors. Notably in proven failures to ITZ with overexpression of Erg11, other azoles are unlikely to be useful as the site of action is similar to ITZ. Here lies the role of synergy testing that can lead to viable combinations evidenced by the fact that, even in clinical failures to terbinafine with SQLE mutations oral itraconazole and terbinafine (topical) were synergistic.[23]

A study (De Paepe R) that examined the geometric mean in TER resistant and susceptible strains found a clear increase in MIC-value for fluconazole, griseofulvin, naftifine and amorolfine, with the difference in GMs being significant for naftifine and amorolfine ($p = 0.05$). This aligns well with the prescription experience in India where these drugs have been found to be largely ineffective. Nevertheless presuming that efflux pumps are drug specific, in case of ITZ failures, oral KTZ, is a much cheaper option than voriconazole and can be used as last drug option in appropriate patient settings.

CONCLUSION

The approach given in the **Figure 11.6** is a real world regimen that can be followed, but there are certain cases that do fail to most measures and such cases, apart from relapses, will need investigations to assess mutations or upregulation of multiple gene pathways and possibly efflux pumps. Needless to say, the challenge of dermatophytosis will continue to be a issue in India unless we encourage more research into resistance mechanisms and drug trials based on established mycological testing.

Key Points

- In the current scenario of predominance of *T. indotineae* which frequently shows terbinafine resistance, Itraconazole is the preferred first line agent. A dose of 200 mg/day should be preferred over 400 mg/day keeping cost effectiveness and safety in mind.
- A prolonged treatment for 6 to 8 weeks with Itraconazole is needed before switching to another drug. Further, weight based dosages of itraconazole for adults is not scientific.
- A higher dose of terbinafine of 250 mg BD can be effective even for strains showing high MIC values for terbinafine or squalene epoxidase gene mutations.

(Contd.)

(*Contd.*)

- Griseofulvin and Fluconazole have shown high MIC values and have fallen out of favour as first line agents.
- Any novel drug or regimen should be based on MIC data, minimum fungicidal concentration, checkerboard studies, serum and skin levels of drug and time kill studies, before a clinical trial of the combination regimen or newer drug is attempted. The use of two systemic drugs in combination is not backed by any scientific rationale and should be avoided.

REFERENCES

1. Khurana A, Sharath S, Sardana K, Chowdhary A, Panesar S. Therapeutic Updates on the Management of Tinea Corporis or Cruris in the Era of *Trichophyton Indotineae*: Separating Evidence from Hype-A Narrative Review. Indian J Dermatol. 2023 Sep-Oct;68(5):525–540.
2. Sardana K, Sharath S, Khurana A, Ghosh S. An update on the myriad antifungal resistance mechanisms in dermatophytes and the place of experimental and existential therapeutic agents for *Trichophyton* complex implicated in tinea corporis and cruris. Expert Rev Anti Infect Ther. 2023;21(9):977–991.
3. Monod M, Feuermann M, Salamin K, et al. *Trichophyton rubrumazole* resistance mediated by a New ABC transporter, TruMDR3. Antimicrob Agents Chemother. 2019;63(11):e00863–19.
4. Yamada T, Yaguchi T, Maeda M, et al. Gene amplification of CYP51B: a New mechanism of resistance to azole compounds in *Trichophyton indotineae*. Antimicrob Agents Chemother. 2022;66(6):e0005922.
5. Yamada T, Yaguchi T, Maeda M, et al. Gene amplification of CYP51B: a New mechanism of resistance to azole compounds in *Trichophyton indotineae*. Antimicrob Agents Chemother. 2022;66(6):e0005922.
6. Bhattacharyya A, Sadhasivam S, Sinha M, et al. Treatment recalcitrant cases of tinea corporis/cruris caused by *T. mentagrophytes*–interdigitale complex with mutations in *ERG11 ERG 3, ERG4, MDR1MFS genes* & SQLE and their potential implications. Int J Dermatology. 2023;62(5):637–648.
7. Khurana A, Agarwal A, Agrawal D, et al. Effect of different itraconazole dosing regimens on cure rates, treatment duration, safety, and relapse rates in adult patients with tinea corporis/cruris: a randomized clinical trial. JAMA Dermatol. 2022;158(11):e223745.
8. Yamada T, Maeda M, Alshahni MM, et al. Terbinafine resistance of Trichophyton clinical isolates caused by specific point mutations inthe squalene epoxidase gene. Antimicrob Agents Chemother. 2017;61(7):e00115–17.
9. Chowdhary A, Singh A, Kaur A, et al. The emergence and world-wide spread of the species *Trichophyton indotineae* causing difficult-to-treat dermatophytosis: a new challenge in the management of dermatophytosis. PLOS Pathog. 2022;18(9):e1010795.
10. Khurana A, Sharath S, Sardana K, Chowdhary A. Clinico-mycological and therapeutic updates on cutaneous dermatophytic infections in the era of *Trichophyton indotineae*. J Am Acad Dermatol. 2024 Aug;91(2):315–323. doi: 10.1016/j.jaad.2024.03.024. Epub 2024 Apr 3. PMID: 38574764.
11. Burmester A, Hipler UC, Elsner P, et al. Point mutations in the squalene epoxidase erg1 and sterol 14-α demethylase erg11 gene of *T. indotineae* isolates indicate that the resistant mutant strains evolved independently. Mycoses. 2022;65(1):97–102.
12. Berstecher N, Burmester A, Gregersen DM, Tittelbach J, Wiegand C. *Trichophyton indotineae* $Erg1^{Ala448Thr}$ strain expressed constitutively high levels of sterol 14-α demethylase Erg11B mRNA, while transporter MDR3 and Erg11A mRNA expression was induced after addition of short chain azoles. J Fungi (Basel). 2024 Oct 22;10(11):731. doi: 10.3390/jof10110731. PMID: 39590650; PMCID: PMC11595479.
13. Khurana A, Masih A, Chowdhary A, et. al. Correlation of in vitro susceptibility based on MICs and squalene epoxidase mutations with clinical response to terbinafine in patients with tinea corporis/cruris. Antimicrob Agents Chemother 2018;62:e01038–18.
14. Song G, Kong X, Li X, Liu W, Liang G. Prior selection of itraconazole in the treatment of recalcitrant *Trichophyton indotineae* infection: Real-world results from retrospective analysis. Mycoses. 2024;67(1): e13663. doi: 10.1111/myc.13663. Epub 2023 Oct 26. PMID: 37882456.

15. Ali M, Ahmed N, Khan S, Kiran A. Efficacy of oral voriconazole versus oral itraconazole, in the treatment of dermatophyte infections. J Ayub Med Coll Abbottabad. 2024 Apr-Jun;36(2):294–298. doi: 10.55519/JAMC-02-12891. PMID: 39609968.
16. Galili E, Lubitz I, Shemer A, Astman N, Pevzner K, Gazit Z, Segal O, Lyakhovitsky A, Halevi S, Baum S, Barzilai A, Amit S. First reported cases of terbinafine-resistant *Trichophyton indotineae* isolates in Israel: Epidemiology, clinical characteristics and response to treatment. Mycoses. 2024 Nov;67(11):e13812. doi: 10.1111/myc.13812. PMID: 39547945.
17. Fernandez-Gonzalez P, García-Donoso C, Garcia-Mouronte E, Alejo Fernández-Baillo JL, De Nicolas-Ruanes B, Berna-Rico E, Perez-Ayala A, Gomez-Garcia de la Pedrosa E. *Trichophyton indotineae* extensive tinea: Successful posaconazole treatment in four cases from Spain. Clin Exp Dermatol. 2024 Oct 10:llae417. doi: 10.1093/ced/llae417. Epub ahead of print. PMID: 39387521.
18. Burmester A, Hipler UC, Uhrlaß S, Nenoff P, Singal A, Verma SB, Elsner P, Wiegand C. Indian *Trichophyton mentagrophytes* squalene epoxidase erg1 double mutants show high proportion of combined fluconazole and terbinafine resistance. Mycoses. 2020 Nov;63(11):1175–1180. doi: 10.1111/myc.13150. Epub 2020 Sep 23. PMID: 32725892.
19. Sharath S, Sardana K, Khurana A. Multi drug failure of tinea corporis to terbinafine, itraconazole and fluconazole; translating extensive Indian microbiological and resistance data to a trial of ketoconazole with remarkable efficacy. Indian J Dermatol Venereol Leprol. 2024 Jul 25:1-3. doi: 10.25259/IJDVL_497_2024. Epub ahead of print. PMID: 39152830.
20. Singh S, Chandra U, Anchan VN, et. al. Limited effectiveness of four oral antifungal drugs (fluconazole, griseofulvin, itraconazole and terbinafine) in the current epidemic of altered dermatophytosis in India: results of a randomized pragmatic trial. Br J Dermatol 2020; 183: pp. 840–6.
21. Bhuiyan MSI, Verma SB, Illigner GM, Uhrlaß S, Klonowski E, Burmester A, Noor T, Nenoff P. *Trichophyton mentagrophytes* ITS genotype VIII/*Trichophyton indotineae* infection and antifungal resistance in Bangladesh. J Fungi (Basel). 2024 Nov 5;10(11):768.
22. Bhuiyan MSI, Verma SB, Illigner GM, Uhrlaß S, Klonowski E, Burmester A, Noor T, Nenoff P. *Trichophyton mentagrophytes* ITS genotype VIII/*trichophyton indotineae* infection and antifungal resistance in Bangladesh. J Fungi (Basel). 2024 Nov 5;10(11):768.
23. Sardana K, Gupta A, Sadhasivam S, Gautam RK, Khurana A, Saini S, Gupta S, Ghosh S. Checkerboard analysis to evaluate synergistic combinations of existing antifungal drugs and propylene glycol monocaprylate in isolates from recalcitrant tinea corporis and cruris patients harboring squalene epoxidase gene mutation. Antimicrob Agents Chemother. 2021 Jul 16;65(8):e0032121. doi: 10.1128/AAC.00321-21. Epub 2021 Jul 16. PMID: 34097482; PMCID: PMC8284445.

CHAPTER 12

Treatment Protocol for Children

• Shashank Bhargava • Nidhi Gupta • Shaily Gupta

INTRODUCTION

Dermatophyte infection is one of the most common infections in children.[1] Tinea infections are transmitted through direct contact with infected humans or animals, as well as through contact with contaminated fomites or soil. In tropical countries, there has been a rise in tinea cases, accompanied by an increase in recurrent and recalcitrant infections.[2,3]

Tinea capitis is the most common dermatophyte infection in children with a prevalence of 26.9%.[4] It is caused commonly by *Trichophyton tonsurans* and *Microsporum canis*.[5] Tinea unguium, tinea corporis and tinea faciei are the other common types of fungal infection in children. The most common organisms isolated are *Microsporum audouinii* followed by *Trichophyton soudanense*.[4]

Children might get tinea infection through sharing of contaminated objects like towels or clothing from the infected individuals. Contact with pet animals further increases the risk of acquisition. With global warming, irrational use of over-the-counter creams containing potent steroids, resistance to terbinafine and increase in prevalence of *T. mentagrophytes* contrary to *T. rubrum* previously, there is increase in cases of failure to treatment. There is also shift from most common type of tinea from tinea capitis to tinea corporis. Situation is alarming as cases of extensive, chronic steroid modified tinea are now also seen in neonates and infants.[5]

Changes in trend of dermatophytosis makes it mandatory to give oral treatment in addition to topical therapies even in children in most cases.

GENERAL MEASURES

General measures are equally important for dermatophyte infections, as are medications **(Box 12.1)**.[6,7] Tinea pedis patients are advised to use open footwear instead of occlusive shoes as occlusion promotes sweating and fungal growth.

TREATMENT OF TINEA IN CHILDREN

The treatment of dermatophytosis in children largely depends on the type of fungal infection, age of the patient and symptoms; and consists of a combination of topical and oral medications.

BOX 12.1: General measures regarding tinea infection in children[7, 8]

- Tinea capitis is the most common type of dermatophyte infection in children. It can be transferred via contaminated combs also. Thus, sharing combs should be avoided or it should be disinfected with sodium hypochlorite 2%.[8]
- Pets, if any, should be examined and treated by veterinarians. *T. rubrum* has been reported to be present on carpets and public changing room floors, therefore protective footwear is advisable. Old footwear should be discarded. Parents should be counseled about keeping naphthalene balls in shoes of their children and enclosed in plastic bags for 3 days.[9]
- Nail trimming is advised and sharing nail cutters should be discouraged.[8, 10] Regular hair washing with gentle shampoo should be encouraged twice weekly. Any lesion over the scalp should not be scrapped off or shaved manually.

Treatment of Tinea Capitis

The treatment of tinea capitis depends on its subtype which can be:

a. *Inflammatory:* Kerion, favus
b. *Non-inflammatory:* Gray patch, black dot

It requires a combination of oral and topical as topical drugs cannot penetrate hair shafts.

Topical

Topical treatment with 1% selenium sulfide or 2% ketoconazole with or without zinc pyrithione is required to prevent spore transmission to other family members.[11, 12]

Topical treatment should be done twice or thrice weekly and should be kept for 5 mins.[13]

Oral

- Griseofulvin and Terbinafine are the first line of treatment in children greater than 2 years of age.[14] Griseofulvin has remained the preferred choice since many years and is more effective than Terbinafine in *Microsporum* species infection.[15] Micronized Griseofulvin in a dose of 20 mg/kg for at least 8 weeks is recommended.
- Terbinafine is better tolerated, safer, cost effective and equally efficacious as Griseofulvin in *Trichophyton* infection.[16, 17] However, Fleece et al. did not find any significant difference in adverse effects and tolerability of Griseofulvin and Terbinafine.[15] Recommended dose of Terbinafine is 62.5 mg/day for body weight <20 kg, 125 mg/day for 20–40 kg and 250 mg/day for >40 kg for 4 weeks. Shorter duration of therapy not only decreases cost of treatment but also improves patient's compliance and decreases chances of treatment resistance.
- Itraconazole remains the second line of treatment and can be given in doses of 50–100 mg/day for 2–4 weeks or 5 mg/kg/day for 4 weeks.
- Oral Ketoconazole is not recommended in children.[14]

Topical and oral antibiotics may be required in addition to antifungals in case of inflammatory favus or kerion.

Treatment of Cutaneous Tinea

Cutaneous tinea was considered less common in children in past years but recently there is changing trend towards this type of dermatophyte infection in children. Neonates, toddlers and children are these days presenting with extensive, steroid modified tinea.[6] Tinea corporis involving breasts and chest region in lactating mothers can be a source of infection in infants during breastfeeding. It is important to counsel the mothers about the safe breastfeeding practices. Adequate treatment should be undertaken in mothers as well. Cases of resistant and difficult to treat tinea is on rise due to multiple factors like shift in pathogen from *T. rubrum* to *T. mentagrophytes*, use of the counter creams containing steroid, increasing resistance to Terbinafine, prescription of antifungals in wrong dose and duration by quacks. In cases of tinea involving limited area (1–2 patches) topical therapy alone gave wonderful results in children as compared to adults, probably due to rapid turnover of skin in children. Topical medication used should be applied twice daily, 2 cm beyond margin and continued for 2 weeks after clinical clearance of lesion. This is known as rule of two.[6]

Terbinafine and butenafine are more effective then miconazole and clotrimazole due to fungicidal effect of these newer drugs.[18, 19] Children not responding to topical therapy or patients with extensive and steroid modified tinea require oral treatment along with topical medication.

Fluconazole is the preferred drug under two years of age. Above 2 years, Terbinafine, Itraconazole and Griseofulvin can be used.[20] Terbinafine is well tolerated and is the drug of choice for treatment in children above two years of age with no significant changes in liver function test.[21] Gupta et al. found Itraconazole to be safe in dose of 5 mg/kg/day with fewer serious side effects making it second line of treatment.[22, 23] Duration of treatment depends on site of involvement and clinical response. Longer duration of treatment than that is mentioned in the standard regimens, may be necessary in children with chronic/steroid modified/ recalcitrant dermatophytosis, based on the clinical response (**Table 12.1**). Antihistamines may be continued depending on the presence of itching.

Newer antifungals include drugs like Voriconazole, Posaconazole, Ravuconazole, Albaconazole, Isavuconazole. Their pediatric use is under study and requires large scale trials. They are largely limited to invasive fungal infections.

Treatment of Onychomycosis

Onychomycosis is not common in children with prevalence of <0.5% worldwide.[24] This is due to the fact that children have smaller surface area available for exposure to pathogens, lack of cumulative trauma, less exposure to pathogen and faster nail growth.[25] However, Sharma et el. reported tinea unguium as the most common fungal infection in girls aged 8–10 years as compared to tinea cruris in boys.[26] Distal and lateral subungual onychomycosis (DLSO) is the most common type of onychomycosis in children. It is commonly caused by *T. rubrum* and sometimes by *T. mentagrophytes*.[8] In onychomycosis various off label medications have been tried, although no medication is FDA approved.[27]

Topical therapy with ciclopirox olamine has shown to be effective, showing mycological cure in 70% patients and complete cure in 23% patients.[27] It is considered safe in children above 12 yrs of age. Topical therapies can be combined with systemic drugs resulting in 80% cure rate.[28] Treatment of onychomycosis with oral antifungals is considered safe.[29]

TABLE 12.1: Terminologies about cutaneous tinea

Type of tinea	Features
Chronic tinea	Persistent dermatophytosis which runs a prolonged course with periods of remissions and exacerbations. The period of chronicity in terms of duration and recurrences is, however, not well-defined
Tinea incognito	Steroid modified tinea
Recalcitrant tinea	Includes all cases of relapse, re-infection, recurrent and persistent cases

Terbinafine is the treatment of choice followed by Itraconazole and Fluconazole.[8] Terbinafine is administered as per the weight of the child:

- <20 kg: 62.5 mg/day
- 20–40 kg: 125 mg/day
- >40 kg: 250 mg/day

Treatment is given daily for 6 weeks in case of fingernail and for 12 weeks in case of toe nail infection. Itraconazole is the preferred second line drug, given as pulse therapy (5 mg/kg/day for one week every month), 2 pulses for fingernail and 3 pulses for toenail onychomycosis. Fluconazole is administered at a dose of 3–6 mg/kg once weekly for 12–16 weeks for finger nail infection and 18–26 weeks for toenail onychomycosis.

Griseofulvin is licensed for use in children but is not preferred due to lower efficacy and longer duration of treatment. Continuous therapy is more effective then pulsed therapy.[28] Oral therapy alone resulted in 80% cure rate in children.[28] Gupta et al. reported elevation in transaminase in one patient on Terbinafine, ataxia and fatigue in one patient each on Itraconazole and nail discoloration in one patient with ciclopirox olamine. Total percentage of adverse effect with medications was only 1.9% and most of the adverse effects were mild to moderate and transient.[27]

Newer Drugs

Topical agents namely, 5% tavaborole and 10% efinaconazole have received FDA approval for treatment of onychomycosis in elderly. In pediatric age group, once daily application for 48 weeks can prove beneficial because of the faster growth rate of nail in children.[9]

The various treatment modalities for different types of tinea in children have been summarized in **Table 12.2**.

LACUNAE IN KNOWLEDGE

The treatment of fungal infections has become increasingly challenging in the current era due to self-medication by patients, which has contributed to rising cases of resistance and treatment failure. Further studies and clinical trials are needed to evaluate the safety and efficacy of newer antifungal drugs in the pediatric population.

FUTURE DIRECTIONS

Current trends in fungal treatment are often associated with recurrence, reinfections, and prolonged treatment durations. The development of new formulations and drug delivery systems can improve antifungal penetration and enhance treatment outcomes. The pediatric population constitutes a significant group of susceptible individuals and, therefore, requires treatments that are effective, safe, have minimal side effects, are broad-spectrum, and are cost-effective.

CONCLUSION

Pediatric dermatophytosis is often seen as a worrisome condition by parents of the infected children. Aggressive use of over-the-counters medications should be strictly discouraged.

Localized lesions may be treated with topical antifungals alone. Oral medications like Griseofulvin provide good results in tinea capitis. Parents need to be counseled about the hygiene practices among their children. Adequate therapy based on age, site and type of infection is required. Treatment of affected family members should be advised to prevent recurrences.

TABLE 12.2: Summary of treatment for tinea capitis, onychomycosis and tinea infection of the skin

Therapy	T. capitis	Onychomycosis	Tinea (cutaneous)
Systemic therapy	**Griseofulvin:** Higher efficacy against *Microsporum* species *Dosage:* Weight <50 kg: 15–20 mg/kg/day for 6 to 8 weeks Weight >50 kg: 1 g/day for 6 to 8 weeks **Terbinafine:** Higher efficacy against *Trichophyton* species *Dosage:* Weight <20 kg: 62.5 mg/day for 2 to 4 weeks Weight 20–40 kg: 125 mg/day for 2 to 4 weeks Weight > 40 kg: 250 mg/day for 2 to 4 weeks **Itraconazole:** Effective against both *Trichophyton* and *Microsporum* species *Dose*: 50–100 mg/day for 4 weeks or 5 mg/kg/day for 2 to 4 weeks	**First choice:** *Terbinafine* (daily continuous): 62.5 mg/day for weight <20 kg 125 mg/day for weight 20 to 40 kg 250 mg/day for weight >40 kg, or 3–6 mg/kg/day, 6 weeks for fingernail and 12 weeks for toe nail onychomycosis **Second choice:** *Itraconazole:* Pulse therapy (5 mg/kg/day for one week every month), 2 pulses for fingernail and 3 pulses for toenail onychomycosis or 5 mg/kg/day for 2 to 3 months *Fluconazole:* 3–6 mg/kg once weekly for 12 to16 weeks for fingernail infection, and 18 to 26 weeks for toenail onychomycosis *Griseofulvin:* Above 1 month of age-10 mg/kg/day for 6 to 9 months in fingernail and 12 to 18 months in toenail onychomycosis	**First choice:** *Terbinafine*: For 2 to 4 weeks 62.5 mg/day for weight <20 kg, 125 mg/day for weight 20 to 40 kg, 250 mg/day for weight >40 kg), or 3–6 mg/kg/day *Itraconazole:* 5 mg/kg/day for 1to 2 weeks *Griseofulvin:* >1 month of age 10–20 mg/kg/day for 2 to 4 weeks
Topical therapy	2% ketoconazole or 1–2.5% selenium sulfide or 1–2% zinc pyrithione or 2.5% povidone iodine shampoos	Ciclopirox 8% OD, Amorolfine 5% once/week, Efinaconazole 10% OD, Tavaborole 5% OD for 48 weeks	Azoles once or twice daily for 2 to 4 weeks Terbinafine 1% twice daily for 2 weeks

Key Points

- Tinea infection in children can be more contagious through sharing of contaminated objects.
- Treatment depends on site and type of fungal infection.
- A combination of topical as well as oral medications may be required.
- Proper counselling with age appropriate therapy can prove beneficial.

REFERENCES

1. Smith SD, Relman DA. Dermatophytes. In: Wilson WR, Sande MA, (eds). Current diagnosis and treatment in infectious diseases. New York, NY: McGraw-Hill Professional; 2001:777–8.
2. Havlickova B, Czaika VA, Friedrich M. Epidemiological trends in skin mycoses worldwide. Mycoses 2008;51:2–15.
3. Sahoo AK, Mahajan R. Management of tinea corporis, tinea cruris, and tinea pedis: A comprehensive review. Indian Dermatol Online J 2016;7:77–86.

4. Andrews D, Burns M. Common tinea infections in children mark.*Wake* Forest University School of Medicine, Winston-Salem, North Carolina, 2008;77:10.
5. VermaS, Madhu R. The great Indian epidemic of superficial dermatophytosis: An appraisal. Indian J Dermatol 2017;62:227–36.
6. Hay RL, Ashbee RH. Fungal infections. In: Griffiths CEM (ed). Rook's Textbook of Dermatology, 9th ed. New Delhi: Wiley-Blackwell; 2016;32:1–55.
7. Ameen M, Lear JT, Madan V, Mohd Mustapa MF,Richardson M. British Association of Dermatologists' guidelines for the management of onychomycosis 2014. Br J Dermatol 2014;17:937–58.
8. Kaul S, Yadav S, Dogra S. Treatment of dermatophytosis in elderly, children, and pregnant women. Indian Dermatol Online J 2017;8:310–8.
9. Maulingkar SV, Pinto MJ, Rodrigues S. A clinico-mycological study of dermatophytoses in Goa, India. Mycopathologia 2014;178:297–301.
10. Schieke SM, Garg A. Superficial fungal infection. In: Goldsmith LA(ed). Fitzpatrick's Dermatology in General Medicine, 8th edn. Palantino: McGraw-Hill; 2012.pp.2277–96.
11. Fuller LC, Barton RC, MohdMustapa MF, Proudfoot LE, Punjabi SP, Higgins EM. British Association of Dermatologists' guidelines for the management of tineacapitis 2014. Br JDermatol 2014;171:454–63.
12. Givens TG, Murray MM, Baker RC. Comparison of 1% and 2.5% selenium sulfide in the treatment of tinea capitis. Arch Pediatr Adolesc Med 1995;149(7):808–11.
13. Pickering LK. Tinea capitis. In: Pickering LK (ed). Red Book: 2006 Report of the Committee on Infectious Diseases. Elk Grove Village, Ill: American Academy of Pediatrics; 2006:654–6.
14. Fleece D, Gaughan JP, Aronoff SC. Griseofulvin versus terbinafine in the treatment of tinea capitis: Ameta-analysis of randomized, clinical trials. Pediatrics. 2004;114(5):1312–5.
15. Friedlander SF, Aly R, Krafchik B, et al. Terbinafine in the treatment of *Trichophyton* tinea capitis: Arandomized, double-blind, parallel-group, duration-finding study. Pediatrics. 2002;109(4):602–7.
16. Ergin S, Ergin C, Erdogan BS, Kaleli I, Evliyaoglu D. An experience from an outbreak of tinea capitis gladiatorum due to *Trichophyton tonsurans.*Clin Exp Dermatol. 2006;31(2):212–214.
17. Piraccini BM, Starace M, Bruni F. Onychomycosis in children. Expert Rev Dermatol 2012;7:569–78.
18. Feldstein S, Totri C, Friedlander SF. Antifungal therapy for onychomycosis in children. Clin Dermatol 2015;33:333–9.
19. Sharma H, Chawla RK. Clinico-epidemiological profile of dermatophyte infections in children at a tertiary care hospital in Mathura. Asian J Med Res 2019;8(2):DT08-DT10.
20. Gupta AK, Mays RR, Versteeg SG, Shear NH, Friedlander SF. Onychomycosis in children: Safety and efficacy of antifungal agents. Pediatr Dermatol 2018;00:1–8.
21. Gupta AK, Paquet M. Systemic antifungals to treat onychomycosis in children: A systematic review. Pediatr Dermatol 2013;30:294–302.
22. Huang PH, Paller AS. Itraconazole pulse therapy for dermatophyte onychomycosis in children. Arch Pediatr Adolesc Med 2000;154:614–8.
23. Jones TC. Overview of the use of terbinafine (Lamisil) in children. Br J Dermatol 1995;132:683–9.
24. Warshaw EM, Fett DD, Bloomfield HE, et al. Pulse versus continuous terbinafine for onychomycosis: A randomized, double-blind, controlled trial. J Am Acad Dermatol. 2005;53(4):578–4.
25. Hart R, Bell-Syer SE, Crawford F, Torgerson DJ, Young P, Russell I. Systematic review of topical treatments for fungal infections of the skin and nails of the feet. BMJ1999;319(7202):79–82.
26. Davis R, Balfour JA. Terbinafine. A pharmacoeconomic evaluation of its use in superficial fungal infections. Pharmacoeconomics. 1995; 8(3):253–69.
27. Rengasamy M, Shenoy MM, Dogra S, Asokan N, Khurana A, Poojary S, et al. Indian Association of Dermatologists Venereologists and Leprologists (IADVL) task force against recalcitrant tinea (ITART) consensus on the management of glabrous tinea (INTACT). Indian Dermatol Online J 2020;4:502–19.
28. Filho ST, Cucé LC, Foss NT, Marques SA, Santamaria JR. Efficacy, safety and tolerability of terbinafine for tineacapitis in children: Brazilian multicentric study with daily oral tablets for 1, 2 and 4 weeks. J Eur Acad Dermatol Venereol 1998;11:141–6.
29. Chen S, Sun KY, Feng XW, Ran X Lama J, Ran YP. Efficacy and safety of itraconazole use in infants. World J Pediatr 2016;12:399–407.

CHAPTER 13

Treatment of Dermatophytic Infections in Special Conditions

• *Ananta Khurana* • *Sinu Rose Mathachan*

INTRODUCTION

Dermatophytoses being a very common cutaneous infection, often poses challenges in management when presenting in special population groups such as pregnancy, pediatric age, etc. While details of the various topical and systemic modalities of treatment of dermatophytoses have been covered in the respective chapters, this chapter highlights the management considerations in certain special patient groups/conditions like pregnancy, lactation, pediatric and elderly patients, renal dysfunction and liver diseases. A summary for pregnancy, hepatic and renal dysfunction is provided in **Table 13.1**. Further details are given in individual sections.

PREGNANCY

Prescribing any drug during pregnancy requires careful assessment of maternal benefit and fetal risks, including fetal loss, congenital malformations, organ toxicity, and prematurity. In addition to the pharmacodynamics, pharmacokinetics and intrinsic antifungal activity of a given drug, specific parameters to be considered are the period of gestation, level of fetal drug

TABLE 13.1: Summary of preferred treatment for certain special patient groups

Condition	Preferred drug
Pregnancy	Topicals preferred; First line: Clotrimazole, miconazole Second line: Terbinafine Systemic: Terbinafine–safety of standard dosing regimens recently established
Lactation	Topicals preferred; First line: Clotrimazole Second line: Miconazole Systemic: Ketoconazole
Pediatric	Same drugs as adults; with weight based dosing
Hepatic dysfunction	Cautious use of fluconazole (safer than others)
Renal dysfunction	Itraconazole: Dose adjustment with GFR <10 ml/min Fluconazole with dose adjustments with GFR <50 ml/min Terbinafine with dose adjustments with GFR <50 ml/min

exposure and maternal physiological pharmacokinetic changes.[1] The drug pharmacokinetics may be altered by many factors like vomiting, increased gastric pH, increased cardiac output and increased intestinal blood flow. Increased intra- and extravascular blood flow and reduced serum albumin concentration enhance the distribution of unbound drugs. Finally, increased renal filtration/elimination and increased (3A4, 2D6, 2C9, 2A6) or decreased (1A2, 2C19) cytochrome activities can modify drug clearance. Fetal exposure relies on the drug's ability to cross the placenta, depending on the stage of pregnancy (placental maturation with enhanced fetal exposure in later term) and on intrinsic drug parameters (liposolubility, molecular weight, protein binding).[2–4]

Information on drug safety during pregnancy can be accessed from certain online resources such as Teratogen Information System (TERIS); the European Network of Teratology Information Services (ENTIS); an American equivalent of ENTIS, known as the Organization of Teratology Information Specialists (OTIS); the International Centre for Birth Defects Surveillance and Research (ICBDSR) and REPROTOX.

The widely used drug pregnancy classification systems include the United States Food and Drug Administration (US FDA), European *Farmaceutiska Specialiteter i Sverige* (FASS or Swedish Catalogue of Approved Drugs) and the Australian Drug Evaluation Committee (ADEC) systems (**Table 13.2**). However, following much criticism, the US FDA system was abolished in 2014 and is to be replaced gradually by a new system called pregnancy and lactation labelling rule (PLLR) with narrative-based labelling requirements.[5]

We wish to highlight a few points which the reader must keep in mind while interpreting the following tables regarding pregnancy categorizations of US FDA (and other systems). According to the US FDA system, new drugs are readily classified as category B based on negative animal studies and lack of human data. Following an "innocent until proven guilty" policy, drugs remain in category B unless future data indicates risk in animal or human fetuses.[6] If, however, there are animal studies showing fetal risk, but no human studies to refute this conclusion, or if there is a paucity of both human and animal data, drugs are assigned to category C. When controlled studies are lacking, established medications may be labeled category C, despite decades of use in pregnant women with few or no reports of adverse effects. Therefore, rating under pregnancy category B or C can be inaccurate and misleading. It is recommended to exercise caution when considering therapy for a pregnant patient with a newer medication labeled as category B, and alternatively, one may consider established category C medications with little or no evidence of adverse effects as a therapeutic option.[7]

Topical Antifungals (Table 13.3)

The pregnancy safety evidence regarding the various topical antifungals is presented below:

Miconazole

Miconazole cream was evaluated in two studies from the Hungarian case–control surveillance of congenital abnormalities, which compiled 22843 newborns/fetuses with congenital abnormalities and 38151 control newborns, from 1980 to 1996. Treatment during the first trimester did not increase the risk of congenital abnormalities (OR 0.9, range 0.6–1.6).[8] Further, data of 2236 women exposed in first trimester did not have an increased association with cardiovascular defects, oral clefts, and spina bifida.[9] Additional data obtained from the same program (1985–1990) found no linkage with congenital defects among 7266 newborns exposed during the first trimester. Thus, miconazole is safe in pregnancy and may be used as first line agent.

TABLE 13.2: Comparison of pregnancy labelling by US FDA, FASS, ADEC		
US FDA	**FASS**	**ADEC**
A—Clinical data show no evidence of risk to the fetus	A—Reliable clinical data indicate no evidence of disturbance of the reproductive process	A—Extensive clinical experience in pregnant women and women of child-bearing age has shown no increase in the frequency of malformations or other harmful effects on the fetus
B—Clinical data are limited or not available, but animal studies show no evidence of risk to the fetus, or clinical data show no evidence of risk to the fetus, but animal studies show adverse effects to the fetus	B—Clinical experience of use in pregnant women is limited or insufficient. Classification is based on animal data, by allocation to 3 subgroups (B:1, B:2, and B:3) B:1—Animal experiments have not given evidence of an increased incidence of fetal damage; similar to FDA category B B:2—Animal experiments are inadequate; similar to FDA category C B:3—Reproduction toxicity studies in animals have revealed an increased incidence of fetal damage, the significance of which is considered uncertain in humans; similar to FDA category C	B—Human data are lacking or inadequate. Limited use in pregnant women and women of child-bearing age has shown no increase in the frequency of malformation or other harmful effects on the human fetus Classification is based on available animal data into 3 subcategories (B:1, B:2, and B:3). *Note:* Allocation to category B does not imply greater safety than category C B:1—Studies in animals have not shown evidence of an increased occurrence of fetal damage; similar to FDA category B B:2—Studies in animals are inadequate or lacking, but available data show no evidence of an increased occurrence of fetal damage; similar to FDA category C B:3—Studies in animals have shown evidence of an increased occurrence of fetal damage, the significance of which is considered uncertain in humans; similar to FDA category C
C—Clinical data are not available and animal studies are not available, or clinical data are not available, but animal studies show adverse effects to the fetus	C—Data suggest pharmacologic effects may have adverse effects on the reproductive process	C—Drugs which, owing to their pharmacologic effects, have caused or may be suspected of causing, harmful effects on the human fetus or neonate without causing malformations. These effects may be reversible
D—Positive evidence of risk to the fetus from clinical data	D—Data indicate an increased incidence of malformations in humans	D—Drugs which have caused, are suspected to have caused, or may be expected to cause, an increased incidence of human fetal malformations or irreversible damage. These drugs may also have adverse pharmacologic effects. *Note:* Drugs in category D are not absolutely contraindicated in pregnancy. In some cases, the D category has been assigned on the basis of suspicion
X—Contraindicated based on animal studies or clinical data		X—Contraindicated in pregnancy

(US FDA: The United States Food and Drug Administration; FASS: Swedish Catalogue of Approved Drugs; ADEC: Australian Drug Evaluation Committee)

TABLE 13.3: Pregnancy categorization of topical antifungals

Topical drug	US FDA	FASS	ADEC	PLLR rating
Clotrimazole	B	A	A	Compatible
Miconazole	C			Compatible
Nystatin	C – topical A – vaginal	A	A	–
Terbinafine	B	B:1	B1	–
Ciclopirox	B	A	–	Probably compatible
Selenium sulfide	C	A, B:3	–	–
Luliconazole	C	–	–	Probably compatible
Amphotericin B	B	–	–	–
Ketoconazole	C	–	–	–
Oxiconazole	B	–	–	Probably compatible
Naftifine	B	–	–	Low-risk

(US FDA: The United States Food and Drug Administration; FASS: Swedish Catalogue of Approved Drugs; ADEC: Australian Drug Evaluation Committee; PLLR: Pregnancy and lactation labelling rule)

Clotrimazole

0.5% of topically applied clotrimazole is absorbed systemically.[10] Animal studies with high doses did not cause teratogenicity.[10] Hungarian case-control surveillance of congenital abnormalities (1980–1992) dataset did not find any association between vaginal or topical clotrimazole use and congenital anomalies. A large surveillance study of 2624 exposed newborns and other smaller studies also reported no adverse fetal outcomes from clotrimazole use.[11–13] Thus, topical clotrimazole is safe in pregnancy, and some authors consider it a first-line topical medication for cutaneous mycoses in pregnancy.[14, 15]

Oxiconazole

Animal studies using doses up to 57 times the typical human doses based on mg/m^2 did not report fetal harm.[16] No studies or reports of oxiconazole in human pregnancies have been published. The use of topical oxiconazole is permitted after other safer alternatives, such as clotrimazole and miconazole.

Luliconazole

Pregnancy safety data in humans is lacking. No embryofetal toxicity or malformations were noted in animal studies except increased incidence of skeletal variation in rats at 3 times the maximum recommended human dose (MRHD).[17, 18]

Ketoconazole

Animal studies using doses 10 times the oral MRHD reported fetal syndactylia and oligodactyly.[18] Studies or reports of topical ketoconazole use in human pregnancies are lacking. Oral ketoconazole use has however been associated with decreased androgen production and reports of limb malformation and hydrops fetalis.[19] Thus, in presence of safer alternatives, topical ketoconazole should not be used in pregnancy.

Terbinafine

Topical terbinafine demonstrates minimal absorption after topical use. Data on human exposures is still sparse. A prospective follow-up study of 23 pregnant women exposed to topical terbinafine did not report teratogenic potential above the baseline risk of 1–3%.[20] In a recent real-world, routine clinical practice study on a cohort of 1,650,649 pregnancies[21] no increased risk of major malformation and spontaneous abortion was observed with topical terbinafine use in pregnancy compared with unexposed pregnancies.

Naftifine

6% of the topical 1% cream is absorbed systemically. Animal studies using 12–150 times the recommended topical dose demonstrated no fetal harm.[22] Although human studies are lacking, no problems have been reported from topical use.[23] Limited application is likely safe.

Ciclopirox

Animal studies have not demonstrated any fetotoxicity or teratogenicity. Human studies are lacking but the drug is likely safe for topical use during pregnancy.[23]

Amorolfine

The drug has poor systemic absorption and has not shown deleterious effects in animals. It may be, hence, used during pregnancy.[24]

Nystatin

Nystatin is poorly absorbed orally, if at all, and has long been categorized as category A by US FDA. A surveillance study reported 489 newborns exposed to nystatin during the 1st trimester and 1881 newborns at any time in pregnancy, and found no association with congenital malformations such as oral clefts, cardiovascular defects, spina bifida, polydactyly, limb reduction defects, and hypospadias.[25] Four other studies also concluded that topical nystatin is safe in pregnancy.[26–28] However, a possible association between hypospadias and nystatin was reported in another case-control study. Recent Hungarian data also raises the possibility of a slightly increased risk of hypospadias in exposed fetuses, although otherwise safe. Accordingly, it may be prudent to avoid its use during the critical period for this malformation (8–14 weeks of gestation).[24]

Selenium Sulphide

No animal or human studies are available. However, short-term use over limited areas may be considered safe.[29]

Salicylic Acid

Although not an antifungal, the drug is used to enhance fungal clearance along with the conventional anti-fungals and is hence mentioned here. Following topical application, about 9–25% of the dose is systemically absorbed.[30,31] A large prospective study of 50,282 pregnant women did not report any adverse events.[32] But, when used in the 3rd trimester, salicylic acid can cause premature closure of ductus arteriosus and oligohydramnios.[33] Therefore, avoid widespread use in the 3rd trimester, application over large surface areas for prolonged time periods, or application under occlusive dressings at any time during pregnancy, as this may enhance systemic absorption.[34]

Systemic Antifungals (Table 13.4)

Terbinafine

Oral reproduction studies did not find any evidence of embryo-fetotoxicity in rabbits and rats administered up to 23 times the maximum recommended human dose.[35] It is not known whether terbinafine crosses the human placenta. There is limited data on human exposure. A follow-up on 54 women gestationally exposed to terbinafine (26 oral and 23 topical), with 24 exposures occurring during the first trimester and with a mean duration of exposure being 32±9 days, reported no increased risk for major malformations above the baseline risk.[19] More recently, in a large study published in 2020 on a cohort of oral and topical terbinafine-exposed pregnancies (n = 891 and 3174 respectively), no significant differences in the risk of major malformations or spontaneous abortion between oral terbinafine-exposed, topical terbinafine-exposed, and unexposed pregnancies (n = 40650) were identified.[21] Although the duration of use is not mentioned, since terbinafine's use is largely restricted to dermatophytic infections, it may be presumed that the exposures defined entailed standard dosage regimens recommended for cutaneous and nail infections. The authors concluded that terbinafine can be used relatively safely in both oral and topical formulations during pregnancy.

Itraconazole

Itraconazole has been shown to be embryotoxic and teratogenic in rodents, inducing craniofacial and rib abnormalities.[35] However, a prospective study involving 229 women exposed to itraconazole, including 198 during the first trimester [daily doses ranged from 50 to 800 mg (median of 200 mg) for a median of 3 days (range 1–90)], failed to identify any increased risk of fetal malformations.[36] Another study on 206 women exposed during the first trimester also did not find an increased risk of malformations (mean daily dose of 182+63 mg for a mean of 6.9+6.4 days). An increase in early fetal loss was however reported.[37] A recent meta-analysis with pooled data from various previous reports, including 1311 pregnant women who used itraconazole during pregnancy, found no significant association of itraconazole exposure with birth defects, but concluded that the small risk of eye defects in the itraconazole-exposed population should be investigated cautiously.[38] No increase in rates of spontaneous abortion, or stillbirth were observed with itraconazole exposure. The PLLR system classifies itraconazole as low-risk during pregnancy. Importantly, the available data is largely on short-term exposure during pregnancy and the risks may not be similar for longer use.

TABLE 13.4: Pregnancy categorization of systemic antifungals

Systemic drug	US FDA	FASS	ADEC	PLLR Rating
Griseofulvin	C	–	B3	Moderate–high risk
Fluconazole	C/D	B:3	D	Moderate–high risk
Ketoconazole	C	B:3	B3	Probably compatible
Itraconazole	C	B:3	B3	Low-risk
Terbinafine	B	B:1	B1	Low-risk

(USFDA: The United States Food and Drug Administration; FASS: Swedish Catalogue of Approved Drugs; ADEC: Australian Drug Evaluation Committee)

Fluconazole

Fluconazole readily crosses the placenta and has shown teratogenic and embryotoxic effects at high doses in animals.[39] Oral fluconazole treatment has been linked to a distinct pattern of birth defects in five infants of mothers who were treated for severe fungal infections with 400–800 mg daily during most or all of the first trimester of pregnancy.[40–43] Similar defects have been observed in animals exposed to systemic azole antifungal agents.[44–46] In 2011, the US FDA issued a drug-safety announcement concerning the possible teratogenic risks conferred by long-term, high-dose fluconazole treatment. The FDA pregnancy category for fluconazole was consequently changed from C (adverse fetal effects in animals and no adequate human data) to D (evidence of human fetal risk, but benefits may warrant use), with the exception of the use of fluconazole at a single dose of 150 mg, for the treatment of vaginal candidiasis.[47] A recent meta-analysis including 14,534 pregnant women who used fluconazole also indicated that oral fluconazole exposure during pregnancy might slightly increase the risk of congenital heart defects and limb defects relative to the general population.[38]

Griseofulvin

Griseofulvin is carcinogenic, embryotoxic, and teratogenic in rodents at 3–45 times the human dose.[35] A retrospective study compared 38,151 normal pregnancies and 22,843 pregnancies with birth defects in relation to their exposure to griseofulvin (reported in 7 and 21 cases, respectively) and did not find any association with any birth defect or with any excess of conjoined twins, as reported previously.[48, 49] There is limited human data to support its use in pregnancy, especially in the first trimester.

Ketoconazole

It is unclear to what extent ketoconazole crosses the placenta; however, ketoconazole has been shown to be embryotoxic and teratogenic at high doses (80 mg/kg/day) in animals (2 times the human recommended dose).[50] In addition, doses one fourth that of normal human doses have caused prolonged labor in rats.[50] Finally, ketoconazole inhibits gonadal and adrenal steroid synthesis in humans. This inhibition could potentially alter sex organ differentiation in the human fetus.[50] Thus in view of the theoretical risk, it is not recommended to be used during pregnancy.

To summarize, it is advisable to treat localized dermatophytoses with only topicals throughout pregnancy (**Table 13.5**). Amongst these, clotrimazole and miconazole have most well established safety profiles and should be preferred. Dermatophytic nail infections can be treated with topical ciclopirox or amorolfine as these have favorable safety profiles during pregnancy. Among oral anti-fungals, terbinafine now has large dataset which supports a safe use in pregnancy including first trimester use. However, the higher doses as used in current context may not be similarly safe. Itraconazole is also labelled low-risk as per the new PLLR rating.

TABLE 13.5: Treatment of dermatophytoses in pregnancy

Topicals	**First line:** Clotrimazole, miconazole **Second line:** Terbinafine **For onychomycosis:** Ciclopirox, amorolfine
Systemic	Terbinafine now has adequate safety data for use in early pregnancy (Concern: Effect of higher doses and longer durations as used in current context not clear)

LACTATION

Topical Antifungals (Table 13.6)[51]

Clotrimazole

The amount of clotrimazole absorbed systemically from the skin and vagina is negligible and thus the drug is safe during lactation.[52]

Ciclopirox

Although there are no reported cases of ciclopirox use during lactation, the systemic absorption is extremely low, at only 1.3%, even when applied under occlusion, indicating minimal exposure to infants via breast milk.

Terbinafine

Less than 5% of topical terbinafine is absorbed systemically, and thus it is likely safe in lactation. Application around nipple area should be avoided.

Selenium Sulfide

Selenium is a vital element that is typically excreted in breast milk. Although, there is concern that excessive exposure may inhibit milk production, animal studies examining toxic-level exposures have not shown significant changes. Additionally, there have been no reported cases of adverse effects when used during lactation.[53]

Systemic Antifungals (Table 13.7)

Fluconazole

In a study of 96 breastfeeding mothers, fluconazole intake was associated with adverse events in 7 infants, including flushed cheeks, abdominal pain, possible diarrhea, mucous feces, tiredness, and eczema.[54a, 54b] However, other studies have not found any significant adverse effects.[55, 56] The relative infant dose (RID), which is an important parameter for predicting medication safety during breastfeeding, is generally considered safe, if it is less than 10%. In a report, breast milk concentrations of fluconazole after oral administration of 150 mg were measured as 2.93 μg/ml, 2.66 μg/ml, 1.76 μg/ml, and 0.98 μg/ml at 2 hours, 5 hours, 24 hours, and 48 hours, respectively. The estimated RID in this case was 17%.[57] However, it should be noted that RIDs calculated in this study used the highest level of fluconazole in breast milk, which is an overestimate as infants would not be exposed to this amount with each feeding.

TABLE 13.6: Lactation categorization of topical antifungals

Topical drug	Newer rating (PLLR)
Clotrimazole	Compatible
Miconazole	Probably compatible
Oxiconazole	Probably compatible
Efinaconazole	Probably compatible
Ciclopirox	Probably compatible
Tavaborole	Probably compatible
Luliconazole	Probably compatible
Oxiconazole	Probably compatible
Naftifine	Probably compatible

TABLE 13.7: Lactation categorization of systemic antifungals

Topical drug	Newer rating (PLLR)
Fluconazole	Probably compatible
Griseofulvin	Moderate high-risk
Itraconazole	Moderate high-risk
Ketoconazole	Probably compatible
Terbinafine	Probably compatible
Voriconazole	Moderate high-risk
Amphotericin	Probably compatible

In reality, the amounts excreted into breast milk are less than the neonatal fluconazole dosage. Therefore, fluconazole is generally considered compatible with breastfeeding. However, if the mother is receiving a high dose or prolonged treatment (weeks to months), monitoring the infant's liver function should be considered.

Itraconazole

Limited data suggests that maternal itraconazole levels in breast milk is lower than the recommended 5 mg/kg daily dose for treating infants. Based on available data, it is estimated that fully breastfed infants between 3 and 12 months of age would receive only 1.48% of the mother's weight-adjusted dosage of itraconazole, resulting in a plasma concentration of 0.77% of the mother's plasma concentration.[58] However, it should be noted that itraconazole may concentrate within nursing infants, and therefore alternative imidazole derivatives are preferred,[52] despite no reported adverse effects from exposure through breast milk. The PLLR has classified itraconazole under the moderate high-risk group.

Terbinafine

Terbinafine is transferred to breast milk, with the child receiving approximately 4% of the maternal dose. Considering that terbinafine is prescribed for long periods of time, and there are no available human data on infantile toxicities, the risk may be significant enough to recommend avoiding its use during lactation.[51] Limited information however indicates that oral maternal doses of 500 mg daily produce low levels in milk and would not be expected to cause any adverse effects in breastfed infants, especially, if the infant is older than 2 months.[59] The PLLR has also given a rating of probably compatible with breastfeeding.

Griseofulvin

Griseofulvin has tumorigenic potential and could hamper neonatal development. Griseofulvin should be avoided while breastfeeding.[51]

Ketoconazole

Limited data exists on ketoconazole excretion in human milk. In a study by Moretti et al., it was found that even when the infant was breastfed constantly during the time when the drug concentration in milk was highest, the maximum exposure was estimated to be only 1.4% of the mother's dose per body weight, which is considered minimal. Therefore, maternal monotherapy with ketoconazole is suggested to be compatible with breastfeeding.[60] Taking the dose just before the infant's longest sleep period or avoiding breastfeeding from 2 to 5 hours after the dose can further minimize the infant's exposure to ketoconazole.[61] The American Academy of Pediatrics (AAP) classifies ketoconazole as safe to use during lactating.[62]

TABLE 13.8: Treatment of dermatophytoses in lactation	
Topicals	**First line:** Clotrimazole **Second line:** Miconazole Ketoconazole shampoo or topical use (except on breast or nipples)[61]
Systemic	Ketoconazole is found to be safe during lactation Avoid other systemic antifungals

To summarize, it is advisable to treat dermatophytoses with only topicals during lactation (**Table 13.8**). Amongst these, clotrimazole and miconazole have most well established safety profiles and should be preferred. All oral anti-fungals should ideally be avoided throughout lactation. However, if needed, ketoconazole is considered safer to use while lactating.[62]

PEDIATRIC AGE GROUP

Pediatric antifungal use has been most widely described with respect to tinea capitis, and has been covered in the respective section in this manual. There are reports and a few good reviews[63–65] available on pediatric onychomycosis (OM), while dermatophytoses of the glabrous skin in children is scantly covered in literature.

Pediatric OM is being increasingly recognized and several studies from around the world have estimated a prevalence ranging from 0.2% to 2.6% (significantly less than adults).[66–68] Children are less likely to develop onychomycosis than adults due to their faster nail growth, smaller nail surface area, reduced time spent in environments containing pathogens, reduced likelihood of trauma and subsequent colonization, reduced prevalence of tinea pedis, and rarity of co-morbid predisposing conditions, like pre-existing nail disorders and impaired circulation.[66] It is more common in children with Down syndrome and HIV-AIDS or other immune deficiencies. Similar to adults, the most common presentation in children is distal subungual onychomycosis, and toenails are affected more commonly than fingernails. The most likely causative organism is the dermatophyte *Trichophyton rubrum*, followed by other dermatophytes including: *Trichophyton mentagrophytes*, *Microsporum canis*, *Trichophyton tonsurans*, and rarer dermatophytes such as *Trichophyton equinum*.[69–71] *Candida* is a less common cause and generally associated with perionyxis.[63] It is important to perform laboratory confirmation of OM in children, and to examine affected children for concomitant tinea pedis. As familial disease often occurs, it is important to check parents and siblings as well for onychomycosis and tinea pedis. Treatment options are the same as adults with topical (ciclopirox and amorolfine) and systemic (terbinafine, itraconazole and fluconazole) drugs. There is no data on the use of newer topical drugs tavaborole and efinaconazole in children. Children are more likely to respond to topicals as their nails are thin and grow faster than adults.[72] Oral therapy is often required when multiple nails are involved, more than 50% of the distal nail plate is affected, or when topical penetration may be suboptimal. Complete cure rates obtained for the systemic antifungals (Terbinafine/Itraconazole) in children are largely similar or slightly higher than rates observed in the adult population.[65] Addition of topical treatment to systemic drugs, increases the cure rate of pediatric OM from 70.8 to 80%, according to a recent meta-analysis, and may be added in older children who are more likely to adhere to this.[65] However, OM in children recurs more often than in adults.[72] None of the treatments is currently US FDA-approved for onychomycosis in children. Terbinafine is FDA-approved for the treatment of pediatric tinea capitis. Fluconazole is used off-label to treat onychomycosis in adults and children, but is FDA-approved for candidiasis in children, and considered very safe to use. Although rarely significant, some experts recommend a complete blood count and liver function tests prior to starting systemic antifungals in children. Surgical modalities in terms of debridement and avulsion can be used in combination.[63] There is no data on the use of laser and other devices in pediatric OM.

Terbinafine

Dosing is weight-based with a dose of 62.5 mg for children weighing less than 20 kg, 125 mg for children between 20 and 40 kg, and 250 mg for children weighing more than 40 kg.[73] The clearance of terbinafine is about 40% higher in children compared to adults.[74] It has been used for the same durations as in adults, in continuous dosing for 6 weeks for fingernails and 12 weeks for toenails. A systematic review of pediatric OM reported a pooled complete clearance rate of 78.8% with oral terbinafine, higher than that reported in adults.[65] The pooled efficacy of terbinafine combined with a topical antifungal (ciclopirox or amorolfine) was 90%.[65] The drug has a good safety profile in children with only occasional adverse events like acute urticaria, anorexia, epigastric pain, tiredness, vesiculopustular eruption, and agranulocytosis.[65] In adults, there have been rare reports of serious hepatic toxicity, which usually occurred in patients with pre-existing liver disease. Therefore, by extension systemic terbinafine is not recommended in a child with underlying liver disease.

Itraconazole

This has been used in the doses of 3–5 mg/kg/day, as a continuous therapy for 2–4 months, or in a pulsed regimen (in doses ranging from 3–7 mg/kg/day) similar to adults (1 week/month, 2–3 pulses),[65] if weighing more than 50 kg, an adult dose of 200 mg/day is given.[75] It has a broader spectrum of activity than terbinafine and is useful in candidal and non-dermatophytic mould infections as well. A systematic review of pediatric studies on OM found the complete cure rate for itraconazole to be 68.4% in the pulsed regimen and 85.7% for the continuous regimen.[65] Itraconazole is well tolerated in the pediatric patients, with most reported adverse effects being transient and mild. The reported adverse effects include fatigue, gastritis, headache, dizziness, sleepiness and liver function test abnormalities. Itraconazole's potential for drug interactions, though less significant in children, must be kept in mind. It is advisable to order a liver function test in case of continuous dosage for more than one month, with concomitant use of other hepatotoxic drugs. Finally, by extrapolation from the adult literature, its use in the setting of congestive cardiac failure is to be avoided.

Other systemic drugs used less often are **griseofulvin** (daily dosing) and **fluconazole** (daily/weekly/alternate day). Griseofulvin has been used in doses of 10 mg/kg/day or conventional dosing of 250 mg/day, for 2–12 months, with pooled efficacy of 6.3%.[65] Fluconazole has been used in very few reports, in doses of 50–100 mg/day or 300 mg once weekly or 100 mg on alternate days, and durations ranging from 40 days (with continuous dosing) to 4 months (with weekly dosing) with a pooled complete clearance rate of 66.7%. Fluconazole is relatively safe in pediatric patients, gastrointestinal toxicity being the most common adverse event. Hepatotoxicity, renal dysfunction, and rash have been reported rarely. It is important to be aware of drug interactions with fluconazole in pediatric patients being co-prescribed other systemic drugs.[63]

Tinea of the glabrous skin, hitherto considered uncommon is being increasingly seen over the past few years (**Fig. 13.1**). We have been seeing tinea corporis/cruris in children as young as 6 months. Affected children mostly have affected parents, and hence family history should be asked for specifically. Although the presentation is generally classical, difficulties may arise in the setting of atopic eczema. Further, tinea corporis in atopics may have staphylococcal superinfection.[76]

Tinea cruris can occur in both sexes but is more frequent in teenage boys.[77] It often occurs in conjunction with tinea pedis, because the fungus is autologously spread upwards while

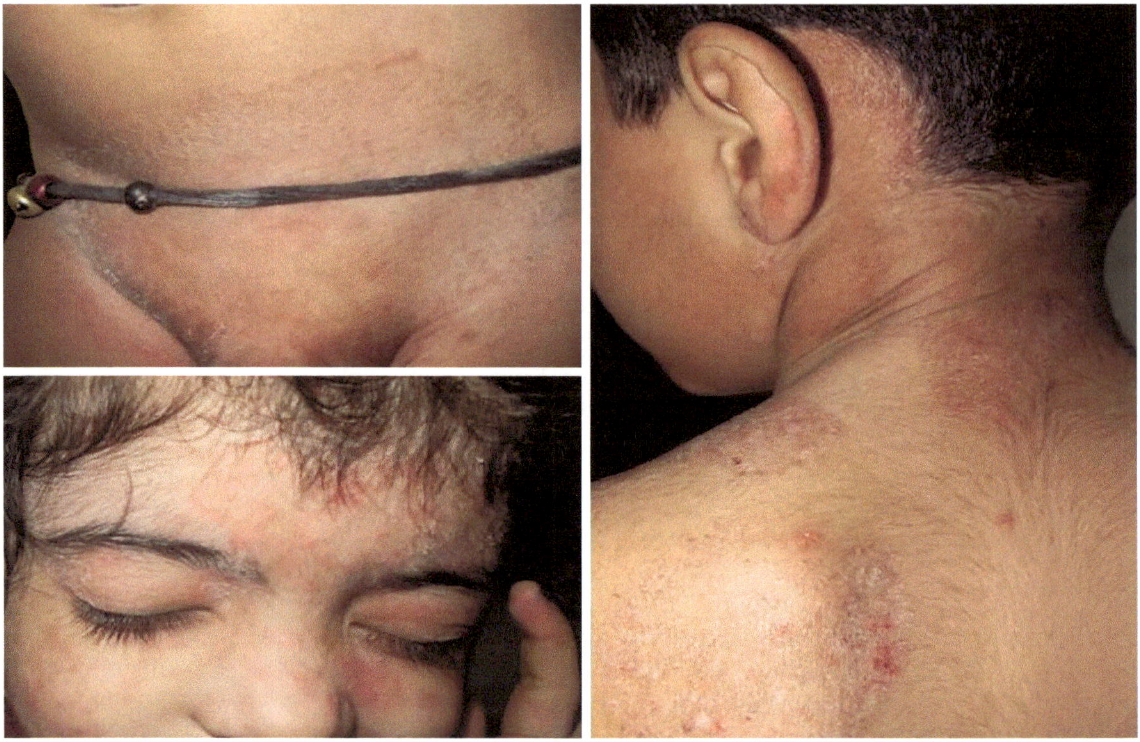

FIGURE 13.1: The spectrum of dermatophytoses being commonly seen in the pediatric age group in the recent times

putting on pants and undergarments. Other risk factors include obesity, excessive sweating or participation in athletics. Tinea pedis, or athlete's foot, commonly presents in adolescents, but is rare in prepubertal children. Occlusive footwear may be a predisposing factor.

There are not many reports dealing with tinea corporis/cruris/pedis in the pediatric age group, but the treatment remains essentially the same. There is often a history of self-medication using the topicals prescribed to adults in the household. In general, children are likely to respond better with topical alone due to their rapid skin turnover. Azoles and terbinafine may be used in the same way as adults.[77] Systemic antifungals may be added if there is extensive involvement **(Table 13.9)**. Related safety concerns have been previously addressed in OM section. The drugs need to be continued for as long as it takes for clearance to be achieved.

TABLE 13.9: Use of antifungal drugs in children (for onychomycosis and tinea corporis/cruris/pedis)

Drug	Dosage
Terbinafine	<20 kg: 62.5 mg 20–40 kg: 125 mg >40 kg: 250 mg *OR* 3–6 mg/kg/day
Itraconazole	3–5 mg/kg/day
Fluconazole	6 mg/kg/day
Griseofulvin	10–20 mg/kg/day

LIVER DISEASE (Table 13.10)

Hepatic dysfunction alters the metabolism of certain drugs and drugs with propensity to cause of hepatic damage should be avoided/used with caution in this setting. Hepatotoxicity has been consistently reported for all dermatologically important antifungal agents, and may range from mild abnormalities in liver function tests to fatal fulminant hepatic failure. But, the risk of liver injury requiring or not requiring treatment discontinuation is generally low (<2%) for all treatment regimens.[79]

Terbinafine

The clearance of terbinafine is decreased by approximately 50% in cirrhotic, compared to normal volunteers. However, the C_{max}, T_{max} and absorption half-life of terbinafine in patients with liver dysfunction were identical to healthy volunteers. For dermatologic view point, terbinafine use should be avoided in the setting of a pre-existing liver disease due to its potential to cause a severe drug-induced liver injury (DILI). Minor elevations in serum transaminases may develop in <1% of patients, which may be asymptomatic and can resolve without stopping the drug.[80] DILI due to terbinafine is a rare and idiosyncratic reaction which usually occurs within the first 6 weeks of therapy. It has an incidence of 1 in 50,000 to 120,000 prescriptions.[81] The reaction can be hepatocellular or cholestatic. But, it typically evolves into a usually prolonged cholestatic pattern and may progress to the vanishing bile duct syndrome.[82] The reaction is potentially organ- and life-threatening and hence it is a good practice to inform the patients about it at the time of starting treatment.[83] The US FDA and the British National Formulary (BNF) both recommend a baseline LFT prior to starting treatment with terbinafine and the BNF further recommends repeat measurements every 4–6 weeks of treatment. However, a recent critical appraisal of existing literature reported that DILI due to terbinafine is generally symptomatic, with presenting complaints of jaundice/icterus, flu-like symptoms or pruritus, and hence recommended a change in the BNF guidelines of performing repeat LFTs at 4–6 weeks.[81] We would like to mention here that we have observed marked elevations of liver enzymes without any clinical symptoms and hence routinely perform LFTs when the use of drug exceeds 4 weeks.[83,84]

Itraconazole

Liver dysfunction has rarely been reported with dermatologic use in otherwise healthy people. Tucker et al. administered itraconazole in doses up to 400 mg/day for durations up to 1 year, for deep and superficial mycoses and reported mild (<2 fold) transient increase in liver enzymes in 4 patients, but the treatment was not discontinued in any.[85] In patients receiving pulsed itraconazole, an asymptomatic increase in liver enzymes has been reported in 1.7–2% of patients.[86] The elevated enzymes usually return to normal either spontaneously or following discontinuation of treatment. There are rare isolated reports of symptomatic hepatotoxicity

TABLE 13.10: Antifungal drug use with hepatic dysfunction

Drug	Remark
Terbinafine	Avoid in acute or chronic liver disease (safer than azoles and griseofulvin)
Ketoconazole	Avoid in acute or chronic liver disease
Griseofulvin	Avoid in acute or chronic liver disease
Itraconazole	Avoid; use with serum drug level monitoring
Fluconazole	Safer than others; BUT cautious use; dose adjustments not advised

with continuous dosing for dermatological indications and in most of these symptoms resolved within several weeks to months after discontinuation.[87] Fatal hepatitis is also rarely reported with pulsed regimen.[88, 89] As itraconazole is predominantly metabolized in the liver, it is recommended that liver function monitoring be done in patients with pre-existing hepatic function abnormalities or those who have experienced liver toxicity with other medications.[90] A pharmacokinetic study conducted in 6 healthy and 12 cirrhotic subjects who were administered a single 100 mg dose of itraconazole as capsule showed a statistically significant reduction in mean C_{max} (47%) and a two-fold increase in the elimination half-life (37±17 hours vs. 16±5 hours) of itraconazole in cirrhotic subjects compared with healthy subjects. However, overall exposure to itraconazole, based on AUC, was similar in cirrhotic patients and in healthy subjects. Data are not available in cirrhotic patients during long-term use of itraconazole. Further in such cases, treatment with itraconazole is discouraged unless there is a serious or life-threatening situation where the expected benefit exceeds the risk of exacerbating hepatic dysfunction and if used, monitoring drug concentrations in serum are recommended.

Fluconazole

A cautious use is advised in patients with liver dysfunction.[91] But, fluconazole has an overall low incidence of hepatotoxicity and a better hepatic safety profile, compared to other anti-fungals. Dose adjustments are not routinely recommended with use in liver dysfunction. Instances of fatal hepatic reactions occur primarily in patients with serious underlying medical conditions (predominantly AIDS or malignancy) and often while taking multiple concomitant medications. Its hepatotoxicity has usually, but not always, been reversible on discontinuation of therapy.

Ketoconazole

Use of ketoconazole is contraindicated in a patient with acute or chronic liver disease. Liver toxicity of this antifungal azole is well documented with an overall rate of 3.6–4.3%, but there is no clear correlation with dosing, and lower rates (1.4%) are reported in children.[92] Due to its hepatotoxic side effects (along with endocrine dysregulation, and drug interactions), oral ketoconazole was withdrawn from the European and Australian markets in 2013. Similarly, strict restrictions and cautionary advisements for hepatic function monitoring, have been added to oral ketoconazole labelling in the US and Canada.

Comparison of hepatotoxicity of the various antifungals: There have been few comparative analyses on relative hepatotoxicity of antifungals.[93] A meta-analysis of the safety of oral antifungals in the treatment of superficial dermatophytosis and onychomycosis estimated the pooled probability of discontinuing terbinafine (250 mg per day) because of DILI at 0.34% (95% CI: 0.09–0.6); the corresponding rates were 0.70 (95% CI: 0.33–1.06) for continuous itraconazole (200 mg/day) and 1.22 (95% CI: 0.00–5.30) for continuous fluconazole at 50 mg/day.[93]

In another meta-analysis, among dermatologically important antifungals, most cases of DILI were attributed to terbinafine (n = 422; 27 with LF), followed by fluconazole (n = 412; 31 with LF), itraconazole (n = 182; 4 with LF) and ketoconazole (n = 94; 6 with LF).[80] The corresponding reporting odds ratios for liver failure were highest among ketoconazole users (4.22; 95% CI: 1.88–9.45), followed by fluconazole (3.46; 2.42–4.93), and terbinafine users (3.39; 2.32–4.96).[94]

Thus, it is not advisable to use a systemic antifungal for treatment of dermatophytoses in patients with pre-existing liver disease.[95] The risk for drug-induced hepatotoxicity increases with concomitant alcohol intake, old age, drugs with significant hepatic metabolism and a daily dosage of antifungal drug exceeding 50 mg. Further, dermatologist must keep the inherent hepatotoxicity of antifungals in mind, especially during prolonged use, and liver function test monitoring is recommended for patients who receive multiple medications, who are elderly, who are on long-term treatment, or who have a previous history of liver cell damage.[96]

KIDNEY DISEASE (Table 13.11)

Terbinafine

In patients with renal impairment (creatinine clearance <50 ml/min), the clearance of terbinafine is decreased by approximately 50% compared to normal volunteers. Appropriate dose adjustments are advised.[95]

Itraconazole

It is primarily metabolized in the liver. Not much data is available on long-term use in renal insufficiency. Itraconazole needs dose adjustment only in the case of glomerular filtration rate (GFR) <10 ml/min. Drug exposure is unaffected in those on dialysis.[98]

Fluconazole

The pharmacokinetics of fluconazole are markedly affected by reduction in renal function. There is an inverse relationship between the elimination half-life and creatinine clearance.[91] However, there is no need to adjust single-dose therapy for vaginal candidiasis because of impaired renal function. In patients with impaired renal function who will receive multiple doses, an initial loading dose of 50–400 mg should be given. After the loading dose, the daily dose (according to indication) should be based on the creatinine clearance (ml/min); with normal regular dosing with clearance of >50 ml/min and in patients on dialysis; and 50% of the dose if clearance <50 ml/min and patient is not on dialysis.[90]

CARDIAC DISEASES

There are cardiac concerns with the use of the following anti-fungals:

Itraconazole

It should not be administered in patients with evidence of ventricular dysfunction, such as congestive heart failure (CHF) or a history of CHF.[89] Reversible edema of the extremities is reported in 0.4–3.5% of patients, and mild hypertension has been reported with high doses (60 mg/day) in several patients.[97, 98] There are isolated reports of Conn's syndrome (hypokalemia, edema and hypertension) and ventricular fibrillations due to hypokalemia.[99]

TABLE 13.11: Antifungal drug use with renal dysfunction

Drug	Remark
Terbinafine	Clearance reduced; dose adjustment advised
Itraconazole	Not much data; drug levels may be reduced (but not with dialysis) Dose adjustment with GFR<10 ml/min
Ketoconazole and voriconazole	Do not require dose adjustment
Fluconazole	PK markedly affected Single dose: No change If multiple doses: Loading with 50–400 mg; further doses depending on creatinine clearance (see text)

Ketoconazole

It can prolong the QT interval, leading to dysrhythmias. Co-administration of the following drugs with ketoconazole is contraindicated: Dofetilide, quinidine, pimozide, cisapride, methadone, disopyramide, dronedarone, ranolazine. Ketoconazole can cause elevated plasma concentrations of these drugs, which may prolong the QT interval, sometimes resulting in life-threatening ventricular dysrhythmias, such as torsades de pointes.[100]

Fluconazole

It can increase the plasma levels of terfenadine, astemizole, quinidine, pimozide and cisapride, leading to QT interval prolongation; hence, co-administration is to be avoided.[91]

GERIATRIC AGE GROUP (Table 13.12)

Use of antifungals in the elderly must take into account their co-morbidities and other drugs the patient is on. Pharmacokinetics of fluconazole has been shown to be altered in the elderly with higher values of C_{max}, AUC and mean terminal half-life compared with normal young male volunteers, possibly due to the decreased kidney function expected in the elderly.[91] Azoles have prominent drug interactions due to inhibition of CYP3A4 enzymes and hence, terbinafine may be a better drug to use. Pulsed regimens should be preferred over continuous regimens wherever appropriate. And needless to say topicals must be preferred wherever possible.

Prominent and clinically significant drug interactions with the three most commonly used antifungals are as follows:

Fluconazole

It has been shown to increase the levels of the following drugs which geriatric patients may commonly be on: oral hypoglycemic tolbutamide, glipizide and glyburide; rifabutin; tacrolimus; cisapride; terfenadine (at ≥400 mg); voriconazole; midazolam; zidovudine; cyclosporine and warfarin. Interestingly, fluconazole co-administration can increase the C_{max} of terbinafine by 52% and its AUC levels by 69%.[91] The diuretic hydrochlorothiazide drugs can increase fluconazole's serum levels.[91]

Itraconazole

Concomitant administration of itraconazole with with cisapride, oral midazolam, nisoldipine, pimozide, quinidine, dofetilide, triazolam and levacetylmethadol (levomethadyl) is contraindicated.[88] HMG-CoA-reductase inhibitors metabolized by CYP3A4, such as lovastatin and simvastatin as well as ergot alkaloids metabolized by CYP3A4 such as dihydroergotamine, ergometrine (ergonovine), ergotamine and methylergometrine are also contraindicated with itraconazole.[89]

TABLE 13.12: Treatment of dermatophytoses in the elderly

Prefer: • Topicals over systemic • Terbinafine over azoles • Pulsed regimens over continuous	**Consider:** • Reduced renal function (altered fluconazole PK) • Peripheral vascular compromise (may complicate treatment for OM) • Co-morbidities
Watch out for: • Drug interactions • Toxicities	

Terbinafine

Drug interactions are much less with terbinafine. However, terbinafine is an inhibitor of the CYP450 2D6 isozyme and drugs predominantly metabolized by the CYP450 2D6 isozyme should not be used. These drugs include: Tricyclic antidepressants, selective serotonin reuptake inhibitors, beta-blockers, antiarrhythmics class 1C (e.g. flecainide and propafenone) and monoamine oxidase inhibitors Type B.[96]

Griseofulvin

Evidence suggests low potential use of griseofulvin in the elderly patient due to its low cure rates and high relapse rates. It is also associated with prolonged duration of treatment, especially in onychomycosis, since, it persists for only a short duration (~2 weeks) after the treatment is discontinued. Griseofulvin should be administered with caution with warfarin type anticoagulant and barbiturates as it enhances their metabolism and decreases their therapeutic activity.[97]

CONCLUSION

This chapter highlights the management of dermatophytic infections in special populations, including pregnant women, lactating mothers, children, elderly patients, and those with cardiac, hepatic, or renal conditions. Topical antifungals are preferred for their minimal systemic absorption, especially in pregnancy, lactation and elderly patients. Systemic antifungals require careful use with regular monitoring and dose adjustments, particularly in patients with hepatic, cardiac or renal impairments.

Key Points

1. **Pregnancy:**
   - Topical antifungals like clotrimazole and miconazole are preferred.
   - Terbinafine has sufficient safety data for early pregnancy but should be used cautiously at higher doses.
   - Systemic antifungals are generally avoided unless absolutely necessary.
2. **Lactation:**
   - Clotrimazole and miconazole are safe topical options.
   - Systemic antifungals like ketoconazole may be considered, but others are avoided.
3. **Pediatric patients:**
   - Children respond well to topical antifungals due to faster skin and nail growth.
   - Terbinafine, itraconazole, and fluconazole are effective but require weight-based dosing.
4. **Hepatic dysfunction:**
   - Fluconazole is safer compared to other systemic antifungals.
   - Monitoring liver function tests is essential due to the hepatotoxic potential of antifungals.
5. **Renal dysfunction:** Dose adjustments are required for drugs like itraconazole, terbinafine, and fluconazole based on glomerular filtration rate.
6. **Cardiac conditions:**
   - Itraconazole is contraindicated in patients with ventricular dysfunction, such as congestive heart failure, due to the risk of worsening symptoms.
   - Ketoconazole and fluconazole can prolong the QT interval, increasing the risk of dysrhythmias, particularly when combined with other QT-prolonging medications.
7. **Elderly patients:**
   - Prefer topical treatments over systemic options.
   - Terbinafine is favored due to fewer drug interactions.

REFERENCES

1. Chow AW, Jewesson PJ. Pharmacokinetics and safety of antimicrobial agents during pregnancy. Rev Infect Dis 1985;7:287–313.
2. Forfar JO, Nelson MM. Epidemiology of drugs taken by pregnant women: Drugs that may affect the fetus adversely. Clin Pharmacol Ther 1973;14:632–42.
3. Hebert MF, Ma X, Naraharisetti SB, et al. Are we optimizing gestational diabetes treatment with glyburide? The pharmacologic basis for better clinical practice. Clin Pharmacol Ther 2009;85:607–14.
4. Tracy TS, Venkataramanan R, Glover DD, et al. Temporal changes in drug metabolism (CYP1A2, CYP2D6 and CYP3A activity) during pregnancy. Am J Obstet Gynecol 2005;192:633–9.
5. Gupta AK. Systemic antifungal agents. Wolverton Comprehensive Dermatologic drug therapy. 3rd edition USA, Elsevier's, 2013. p98–120
6. Millsop JW, Heller MM, Murase JE. Safety classification systems used in dermatological medication risk counseling of pregnant and lactating patients: A case for an evidence-based approach. Dermatol Ther 2013;26:347–53.
7. Wilmer E, Chai S, Kroumpouzos G. Drug safety: Pregnancy rating classifications and controversies. Clin Dermatol. 2016;34:401–9.
8. Czeizel AE, Kazy Z, Puho E. Population-based case-control teratologic study of topical miconazole. Congenit Anom (Kyoto) 2004;44:41–5.
9. Rosa F, Baum C, Shaw M. Pregnancy outcomes after first-trimester vaginitis drug therapy. Obstet Gynecol 1987;69:751–5.
10. Schering Corporation. Lotrisone cream package insert. 2009. Available at:http://www.accessdata.fda.gov/drugsatfda_docs/label/2009/020010s021lbl.pdf. (last accessed 2016 October 25)
11. Tan C, Good C, Milne L, Loudon J. A comparative trial of six days therapy with clotrimazole and nystatin in pregnant patients with vaginal candidiasis. Postgrad Med J 1974;50:102–5.
12. Haram K, Digranes A. Vulvovaginal candidiasis in pregnancy treated with clotrimazole. Acta obstetricia et gynecologica Scandinavica 1978;57:453–5.
13. Frerich W, Gad A. The frequency of Candida infections in pregnancy and their treatment with clotrimazole. Curr Med Res Opin 1977;4:640–4.
14. Hale EK, Pomeranz MK. Dermatologic agents during pregnancy and lactation: an update and clinical review. Int J Dermatol 2002;41:197-203.
15. King CT, Rogers PD, Cleary JD, Chapman SW. Antifungal therapy during pregnancy. Clin Infect Dis 1998;27:1151–60.
16. Pharma Derm. Oxistat package insert. 2014. Available at: https://dailymed.nlm.nih.gov/dailymed/drugInfo.cfm?setid=b87a89d2-6e45-4eb8-be2c-7f55f34d61e5.
17. https://www.accessdata.fda.gov/drugsatfda_docs/label/2013/204153s000lbl.pdf, (accessed on 24/12/2024
18. https://www.accessdata.fda.gov/drugsatfda_docs/label/2013/018533s040lbl.pdf. (accessed 2017 October 5)
19. Lind J. Limb malformations in a case of hydrops fetalis with ketoconazole use during pregnancy. Arch Gynecol 1985;237:398.
20. Sarkar M, Rowland K, Koren G. Pregnancy outcome following gestational exposure to terbinafine: A prospective comparative study. Clin Mol Teratol 2003;67:390.
21. Andersson NW, Thomsen SF, Andersen JT. Evaluation of association between oral and topical terbinafine use in pregnancy and risk of major malformations and spontaneous abortion. JAMA dermatology. 2020;156(4):375–83.
22. Merz Pharmaceuticals. Naftin package insert. 2013. Available at: http://www.naftin.com/wpcontent/uploads/NAFTIN-Cream-2-PI.pdf.
23. Leachman SA, Reed BR. The use of dermatologic drugs in pregnancy and lactation. Dermatol Clin 2006;24:167–97.
24. Pilmis B, Jullien V, Sobel J, Lecuit M, Lortholary O, Charlier C. Antifungal drugs during pregnancy: an updated review. J Antimicrob Chemother 2015;70:14–22.

25. Briggs G. Drugs in pregnancy and lactation: A reference guide to fetal and neonatal risk. 10th ed. Philadelphia, PA: Lippincott Williams & Wilkins, 2014.
26. Culbertson C. Monistat: A new fungicide for treatment of vulvovaginal candidiasis. Am J Obstet Gynecol 1974;120:973–6.
27. Davis J, Frudenfeld J, Goddard J. Comparative evaluation of Monistat and Mycostatin in the treatment of vulvovaginal candidiasis. Obstet Gynecol 1974;44:403–6.
28. Wallenburg HC, Wladimiroff JW. Recurrence of vulvovaginal candidiasis during pregnancy: Comparison of miconazole vs nystatin treatment. Obstet Gynecol 1976;48:491–4.
29. Patel VM, Schwartz RA, Lambert WC. Topical antiviral and antifungal medications in pregnancy: A review of safety profiles. J Eur Acad Dermatol Venereol. 2017;31:1440–6.
30. Morra P, Bartle WR, Walker SE, Lee SN, Bowles SK, Reeves RA. Serum concentrations of salicylic acid following topically applied salicylate derivatives. Ann Pharmacother 1996;30:935–40.
31. Schwarb F, Gabard B, Rufli T, Surber C. Percutaneous absorption of salicylic acid in man after topical administration of three different formulations. Dermatology 1999;198:44–51.
32. Slone D, Siskind V, Heinonen OP, Monson RR, Kaufman DW, Shapiro S. Aspirin and congenital malformations. Lancet 1976;1:1373–5.
33. Klebanoff MA, Berendes HW. Aspirin exposure during the first 20 weeks of gestation and IQ at four years of age. Teratology 1988;37:249–55.
34. Lam J, Polifka JE, Dohil MA. Safety of dermatologic drugs used in pregnant patients with psoriasis and other inflammatory skin diseases. J Am Acad Dermatol 2008;59:295–315.
35. Briggs GG, Freeman RK, Yaffe SJ. Drugs in pregnancy and lactation: A Reference guide to fetal and neonatal risk. Philadelphia: Lippincott Williams & Wilkins, 2011.
36. Bar-Oz B, Moretti ME, Bishai R, et al. Pregnancy outcome after in utero exposure to itraconazole: A prospective Cohort study. Am J Obstet Gynecol 2000;183:617–20.
37. De Santis M, Di Gianantonio E, Cesari E, et al. First-trimester itraconazole exposure and pregnancy outcome: A prospective cohort study of women contacting teratology information services in Italy. Drug Saf Int J Med Toxicol Drug Exp 2009;32:239–44.
38. Liu D, Zhang C, Wu L, Zhang L, Zhang L. Fetal outcomes after maternal exposure to oral antifungal agents during pregnancy: A systematic review and meta-analysis. Int J Gynaecol Obstet. 2020;148(1):6–13.
39. Vlachadis N, Iliodromiti Z, Vrachnis N. Oral fluconazole during pregnancy and risk of birth defects. N Engl J Med 2013;369:2061.
40. Aleck KA, Bartley DL. Multiple malformation syndrome following fluconazole use in pregnancy: Report of an additional patient. Am J Med Genet 1997;72:253–6.
41. Lee BE, Feinberg M, Abraham JJ, Murthy AR. Congenital malformations in an infant born to a woman treated with fluconazole. Pediatr Infect Dis J 1992;11:1062–4.
42. Lopez-Rangel E, Van Allen MI. Prenatal exposure to fluconazole: An identifiable dysmorphic phenotype. Birth Defects Res a Clin Mol Teratol 2005;73:919–23.
43. Pursley TJ, Blomquist IK, Abraham J, Andersen HF, Bartley JA. Fluconazole-induced congenital anomalies in three infants. Clin Infect Dis 1996;22:336–40.
44. Tiboni GM, Marotta F, Del Corso A, Giampietro F. Defining critical periods for itraconazole-induced cleft palate, limb defects and axial skeletal malformations in the mouse. Toxicol Lett 2006;167:8–18.
45. Mineshima H, Fukuta T, Kato E, et al. Malformation spectrum induced by ketoconazole after single administration to pregnant rats during the critical period—comparison with vitamin A-induced malformation spectrum. J Appl Toxicol 2012;32:98–107.
46. Tiboni GM, Giampietro F. Murine teratology of fluconazole: evaluation of developmental phase specificity and dose dependence. Pediatr Res 2005;58:94–9.
47. Food and Drug Administration. Use of long-term, high-dose diflucan (fluconazole) during pregnancy may be associated with birth defects in infants. 2011 (http://www.fda.gov/Drugs/DrugSafety/ ucm266030.htm)
48. Rosa FW, Hernandez C, Carlo WA. Griseofulvin teratology, including two thoracopagus conjoined twins. Lancet 1987;1:171.
49. Czeizel AE, Me´tneki J, Kazy Z, et al. A population-based case—control study of oral griseofulvin treatment during pregnancy. Acta Obstet Gynecol Scand 2004; 83: 827–31.

50. Cottreau JM, Barr VO. A review of antiviral and antifungal use and safety during pregnancy. Pharmacotherapy. 2016;36:668–78.
51. Butler DC, Heller MM, Murase JE. Safety of dermatologic medications in pregnancy and lactation: Part II. Lactation. Journal of the American Academy of Dermatology. 2014;70(3):417–e1.
52. Briggs GG, Freeman RK, Yaffe SJ. Drugs in pregnancy and lactation, 8th ed. Philadelphia (PA): Lippincott Williams & Wilkins; 2008.
53. Willhite CC. Selenium teratogenesis. Species-dependent response and influence on reproduction. Ann N Y Acad Sci 1993;678:169–77.
54. Moorhead AM, Amir LH, O'Brien PW, Wong S. A prospective study of fluconazole treatment for breast and nipple thrush. Breastfeed Rev 2011;19(3):25–9.
54b. Solís-Arias MP García-Romero MT. Onychomycosis in children. A review. Int J Dermatol. 2017;56:123–130.
55. Chetwynd EM, Ives TJ, Payne PM, Edens-Bartholomew N. Fluconazole for postpartum candidal mastitis and infant thrush. J Hum Lact 2002;18(2):168–71.
56. Bodley V, Powers D. Long-term treatment of a breastfeeding mother with fluconazole-resolved nipple pain caused by yeast: a case study. J Hum Lact 1997;13(4):307–11.
57. Force RW. Fluconazole concentrations in breast milk. Pediatr Infect Dis J 1995;14(3):235–6.
58. Drugs and lactation database (LactMed®) [Internet]. Bethesda (MD): National Institute of Child Health and Human Development; 2006-. Itraconazole. [Updated 2022 Sep 19]. Available from: https://www.ncbi.nlm.nih.gov/books/NBK500573/
59. Drugs and Lactation Database (LactMed®) [Internet]. Bethesda (MD): National Institute of Child Health and Human Development; 2006–. Terbinafine. 2018 Oct 31.
60. Moretti ME, Ito S, Koren G. Disposition of maternal ketoconazole in breast milk. American Journal of Obstetrics and Gynecology. 1995;173(5):1625–6.
61. Drugs and Lactation Database (LactMed®) [Internet]. Bethesda (MD): National Institute of Child Health and Human Development; 2006-. Ketoconazole. [Updated 2021 Nov 15]. Available from: https://www.ncbi.nlm.nih.gov/books/NBK501228/
62. American Academy of Pediatrics Committee on Drugs. Transfer of drugs and other chemicals into human milk. Pediatrics 2001;108:776–89.
63. Friedlander SF, Totri C. Antifungal therapy for onychomycosis in children. Clin Dermatol. 2015;33:333–9.
64. Totri CR, Feldstein S, Admani S, Friedlander SF, Eichenfield LF. Epidemiologic analysis of onychomycosis in the San Diego pediatric population. Pediatr Dermatol. 2017;34:46–49.
65. Gupta AK, Paquet M. Systemic antifungals to treat onychomycosis in children: A systematic review. Pediatr Dermatol. 2013;30:294–302.
66. Gupta AK, Sibbald RG, Lynde CW, et al. Onychomycosis in children: Prevalence and treatment strategies. J Am Acad Dermatol 1997;36:395–402.
67. Kim DM, Suh MK, Ha GY. Onychomycosis in children: An experience of 59 cases. Ann Dermatol 2013;25:327–334.
68. Gunduz T, Metin DY, Sacar T, et al. Onychomycosis in primary school children: Association with socioeconomic conditions. Mycoses 2006;49:431–3.
69. Aly R, Hafeez ZH, Rodwell C, et al. Rapid response to *Trichophyton tonsurans* induced onychomycosis after treatment with terbinafine. Int J Dermatol 2002;41: 357–9.
70. Ploysangam T, Lucky AW. Childhood white superficial onychomycosis caused by *Trichophyton rubrum*: Report of seven cases and review of the literature. J Am Acad Dermatol 1997;36:29–32.
71. Nicholls DS, Midgley G. Onychomycosis caused by *Trichophyton equinum*. Clin Exp Dermatol 1989;14:464–5.
72. Eichenfield LF, Friedlander SF. Pediatric onychomycosis: The emerging role of topical therapy. J Drugs Dermatol. 2016;16:105–9.
73. Gupta AK, Skinner AR. Onychomycosis in children: A brief overview with treatment strategies. Pediatr Dermatol. 2004;21:74–9.
74. Nejjam F, Zagula M, Cabiac MD, Guessous N, Humbert H, Lakhdar H. Pilot study of terbinafine in children suffering from tinea capitis: Evaluation of efficacy, safety and pharmacokinetics. Br J Dermatol 1995;132:98–105.

75. Gupta AK, Cooper EA, Ginter G. Efficacy and safety of itraconazole use in children. Dermatol Clin. 2003;21:521–35.
76. Veraldi S, Schianchi R, Pontini P, Gorani A. The association of isoconazole-diflucortolone in the treatment of pediatric tinea corporis. J Dermatolog Treat. 2017;19:1–2.
77. Hawkins DM, Smidt AC. Superficial fungal infections in children. Pediatr Clin North Am. 2014;61:443-55.
78. Paloni G, Valerio E, Berti I, Cutrone M. Incognito. J Pediatr 2015;167:1450–e2.
79. Chang CH, Young-Xu Y, Kurth T, Orav JE, Chan AK. The safety of oral antifungal treatments for superficial dermatophytosis and onychomycosis: A meta-analysis. Am J Med. 2007;120:791–8.
80. Liver Tox: Clinical and research information on drug-induced liver injury: drug record: terbinafine. http://livertox.nlm.nih.gov/Terbinafine. httm accessed on 2/11/2017
81. Kramer ON, Albrecht J. Clinical presentation of terbinafine-induced severe liver injury and the value of laboratory monitoring: A critically appraised topic. br j dermatol. 2017. doi: 10.1111/bjd.15854. [Epub ahead of print]
82. Ajit C, Suvannasankha A, Zaeri N, Munoz SJ. Terbinafine-associated hepatotoxicity. Am J Med Sci 2003;325:292–5.
83. Khurana A, Sardana K, Bhardwaj V. Response to 'clinical presentation of terbinafine-induced severe liver injury and the value of laboratory monitoring: A critically appraised topic'. Br J Dermatol. 2017. doi: 10.1111/bjd.16134.
84. Guidance for industry, drug-induced liver injury: Premarketing Clinical Evaluation (2009).
85. Tucker RM, Williams PL, Arathoon EG, Stevens DA. Treatment of mycoses with itraconazole. Ann N Y Acad Sci. 1988;544:451–70.
86. De Doncker P. Itraconazole and terbinafine in perspective: from petri dish to patient. J Eur Acad Dermatol Venereol. 1999;12 (Suppl 1):S10-6; discussion S17.
87. Pettit NN, Pisano J, Weber S, Ridgway J. Hepatic failure in a patient receiving itraconazole for pulmonary histoplasmosis-case report and literature review. Am J Ther. 2016;23:e1215–21.
88. Srebrnik A, Levtov S, Ben-Ami R, Brenner S. Liver failure and transplantation after itraconazole treatment for toenail onychomycosis. J Eur Acad Dermatol Venereol. 2005;19:205–7.
89. https://www.accessdata.fda.gov/drugsatfda_docs/label/2009/020083s040s041s044lbl.pdf (accessed 3/11/2017).
90. Tuccori M, Bresci F, Guidi B, Blandizzi C, Del Tacca M, Di Paolo M. Fatal hepatitis after long-term pulse itraconazole treatment for onychomycosis. Ann Pharmacother. 2008;42(7):1112–7.
91. https://www.accessdata.fda.gov/drugsatfda_docs/label/2011/019949s051lbl.pdf (accessed 4/11/2017)
92. Yan JY, Nie XL, Tao QM, Zhan SY, Zhang YD. Ketoconazole associated hepatotoxicity: A systematic review and meta-analysis. Biomed Environ Sci 2013;26:605–10.
93. Phillips P, Shafran S, Garber G, et al. Multicenter randomized trial of fluconazole versus amphotericin B for treatment of candidemia in non-neutropenic patients. Canadian Candidemia Study Group. Eur J Clin Microbiol. Infect Dis 1997;16:337–45.
94. Raschi E, Poluzzi E, Koci A, Caraceni P, Ponti FD. Assessing liver injury associated with antimycotics: Concise literature review and clues from data mining of the FAERS database. World J Hepatol 2014;6:601–12.
95. https://www.accessdata.fda.gov/drugsatfda_docs/label/2012/020539s021lbl.pdf (accessed 5/11/2017)
96. Thomas J, Parthasaradhi A, Bajaj AK, Girdhar M, Ghoshal A, Haq R, et al. Expert consensus on management of dermatophytosis in elderly patients, patients with comorbidities, and immunocompromised status: an Indian perspective. International Journal of Research. 2021;7(1):141.
97. Grant SM, Clissold SP. Itraconazole. A review of its pharmacodynamic and pharmacokinetic properties and therapeutic potential in superficial and systemic mycoses. Drugs 1989;37:310–344.
98. Rosen T. Debilitating edema associated with itraconazole therapy. Arch Dermatol 1994;130:260–271.
99. Nelson MR, Smith D, Erskine D et al. Ventricular fibrillation secondary to itraconazole induced hypokalemia. J Infect 1993;26:348.
100. https://www.accessdata.fda.gov/drugsatfda_docs/label/2014/018533s041lbl.pdf (accessed on 5/11/2017)

CHAPTER 14

What We Still Need to know about the New Species—*Trichophyton Indotineae*

• Shukla Das • Richa Anjleen Tigga

INTRODUCTION

An age-old nemesis of morbidity of skin and its appendages is the entity of "Dermatophytosis". This superficial infection is caused by the fungal agents–dermatophytes which show affinity towards the keratin layer of skin and its appendages. The three Genera of dermatophytes—*Trichophyton, Epidermophyton* and *Microsporum* adhere to the skin surface and invade this first line of defense with the help of enzymes and metabolic products, causing eruption of circular, erythematous and pruritic skin lesions termed "tinea".

Since 2015, many articles have brought to light the change in epidemiological pattern of the causative pathogens of tinea of the glabrous skin (tinea corporis/cruris/faciei). The predominant species causing this infection in India has shifted from *Trichophyton rubrum* to *Trichophyton indotineae*.[1] Influence of external factors like suboptimal drug dosing and steroid misuse have been claimed as possible contributors to this shift, although the views are speculative at best.

Dermatologists face new hurdles in the treatment of dermatophytosis with the infections now being chronic, recalcitrant and resistant to standard antifungal treatment.[2–4] There have also been increasing reports on drug resistance especially to terbinafine over the past few years.[5–7] While a lot of literature now exists on resistance to terbinafine mediated by mutations in the gene of the target enzyme squalene epoxidase (SQLE), prevalence of resistance across azole family of drugs has also been reported.[7] In the current times with advent of new techniques, the causative agent has also undergone nomenclature changes.

TAXONOMY

Since 1841, when the studies of Robert Remak and David Gruby laid ground for the dermatophyte taxonomy, the use of conventional approach and molecular techniques to examine the relatedness of species has changed the taxonomy of dermatophytes **(Fig. 14.1)**.[8] The conventional approach is based on clinical appearance, cultural characteristics, microscopy and physiology. The molecular techniques vary from use of the ribosomal small and large subunits as markers to use of variable rDNA ITS region.

In 2016, new terminologies based on the internal transcribed spacer (ITS) regions 1 and 2 of ribosomal DNA (rDNA) and partial large subunit (LSU), the ribosomal 60S protein, and fragments of b-tubulin and translation elongation factor 3 were suggested by de Hoog et al.[8]

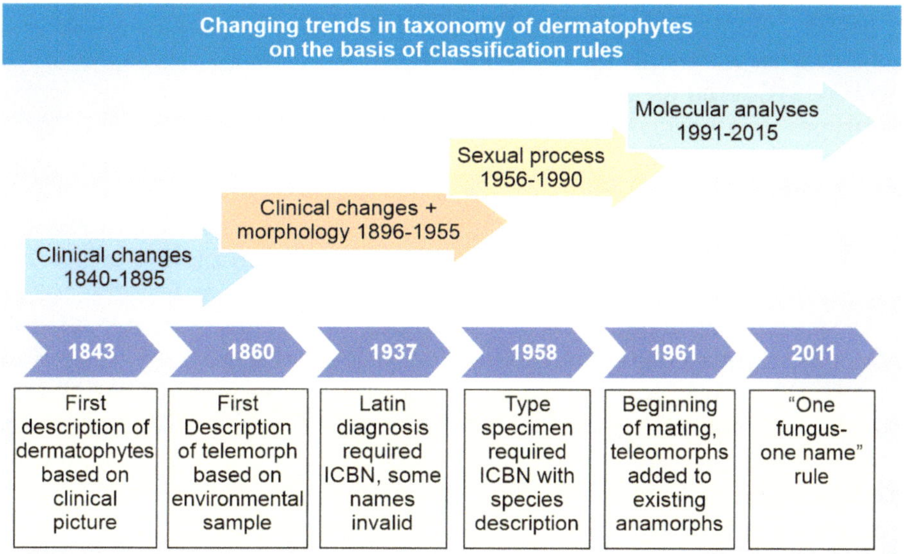

FIGURE 14.1: Changing trends in taxonomy of dermatophytes on the basis of classification rules

Time	Nomenclature	Taxonomy on basis of classification rules
Before 2016	*"Trichophyton mentagropytes/Trichophyton interdigitale* complex" = *"Trichophyton interdigitale"*	Previously based on Morphological characteristics, followed by genetic differentiation on sequencing for rDNA ITS
2016	Zoophilic *Trichophyton mentagrophytes* Anthropophilic *Trichophyton interdigitale*	Sequencing for rDNA ITS and partial LSU, the ribosomal 60s protein, and fragments of b-tubulin and translation elongation factor 3
2017	*Trichophyton mentagrophytes* ITS genotype VIII	Sequencing the Internal Transcribed Spacer (ITS) region of the rDNA
2020	*Trichophyton mentagrophytes* ITS genotype VIII= *Trichophyton indotineae*	• Multigene phylogeny • Using high mobility group (HMG) • A box genes in addition to the Internal Transcribed Spacer genes used by Nenoff

FIGURE 14.2: Timeline of change in nomenclature to the current "*Trichophyton indotineae*"

The term "*T. mentagrophytes/T. interdigitale* complex" was introduced which led to an update of the dermatophyte taxonomy.[9] Later, in 2020, Kano et al. identified the highly terbinafine-resistant *T. interdigitale* like strains from a Nepali patient and an Indian patient with tinea corporis and suggested that it be considered a new species—*T. indotineae*.[10] *Trichophyton indotineae* is considered an anthropophilic clonal offshoot of *Trichophyton mentagrophytes* genotype VIII.[10, 11] **Figure 14.2** shows the timeline of the change in nomenclature of the new *T. indotineae* species.

THE NEW SPECIES: *TRICHOPHYTON INDOTINEAE*

Trichophyton indotineae is the only genotype amongst the clades of *Trichophyton mentagrophytes* genotype to be considered as a new species.[1, 10, 11] 'Cryptic species' or 'molecular siblings' classify genotypes in a species.[12] *Trichophyton indotineae/Trichophyton mentagrophytes* ITS genotype VIII is a "clonal offshoot" of the *T. mentagrophytes/T. interdigitale* complex, with molecular and phenotypic differences seen in patients presenting with chronic virulent dermatophytosis. This classification as a new species has significance in recognizing this troubling entity as a "difficult-to-treat" pathogen. The clinical picture of the *Trichophyton indotineae* infection is that of chronic recalcitrant relapsing tinea lesions, not adequately responding to standard dose regimens of terbinafine, as used in the past.[13] A significant rise in the number of such cases has been reported in the country since 2014.[14] Infection with this species has spread beyond India and cases have also been detected in various countries of Asia and Europe with isolated reports also from Australia, South and North America.[15–17] This epidemiological spread has become a matter of concern for dermatologists and mycologists everywhere.

Microbiological analysis is difficult due to similarities between *Trichophyton indotineae* and *T. mentagrophytes/T. interdigitale* complex in morphology.[18] On growth in culture media, colonies of *Trichophyton indotineae* are similar to that of *Trichophyton mentagrophytes/ Trichophyton interdigitale* as both are fast-growing with central beige-stained, flat colonies with white periphery on the obverse side **(Fig. 14.3)**. Under microscope, both species demonstrate round microconidia, cigar-shaped macroconidia, chlamydospores and spiral hyphae in microscopy **(Fig. 14.4)**.

Molecular analysis, however, enables us to differentiate between the two species. Tang et al. observed that based on molecular characteristics, *T. mentagrophytes s. str.* and *T. interdigitale s. str.* can be distinguished (with difficulty) from each other, but that these are unambiguously different from *T. indotineae* by sequences of the *HMG* gene, while ITS sequencing cannot reliably differentiate the two.[11] This suspicion is supported by the antifungal susceptibility

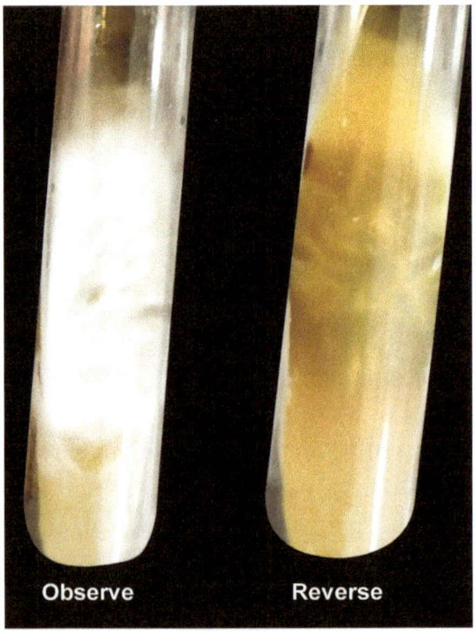

FIGURE 14.3: Growth of *Trichophyton indotineae* on culture media

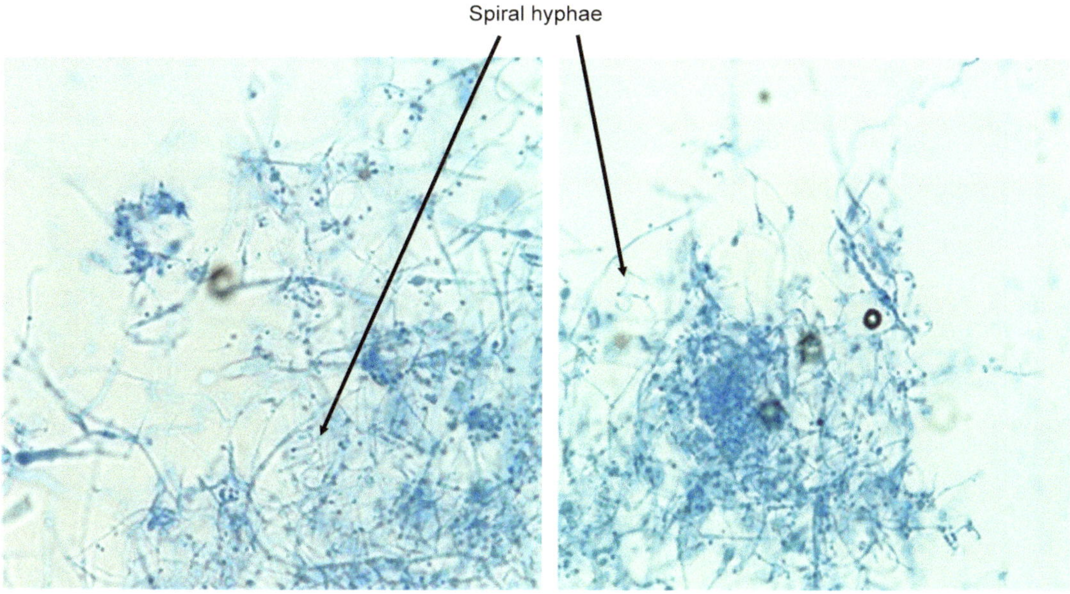

FIGURE 14.4: Lactophenol cotton blue (LPCB) mount showing clavate to spherical microconidia, macroconidia and spiral hyphae

testing showing high minimum inhibitory concentration (MIC) value (4–32 mg/L) for terbinafine **(Fig. 14.5)**.[19] High level of terbinafine resistance associated with mutations in its molecular target, squalene epoxidase (SQLE/Erg1) has been observed, along with high MIC values for terbinafine in *T. indotineae*.[20] Single point mutations *Leu393Phe* or *Phe397Leu* in the SQLE gene have been observed in the isolates with high terbinafine MIC.[5, 21]

Ebert et al. in their study on *T. mentagrophytes* ITS Type VIII (*T. indotineae*) observed reduced susceptibility to triazoles in the isolates was associated with the amino acid substitution *Ala448Thr* at the C-terminus of the squalene epoxidase.[7]

Three single nucleotide polymorphisms (SNPs) at position 94 (C), 125 (T) and 462 (T) in the ITS region help in differentiating and identifying *Trichophyton indotineae*.[10, 21]

WHAT DOES THE NEW SPECIES MEAN FOR DERMATOLOGISTS?

1. Dermatologists in their day-to-day practice would benefit by knowing that with the ever-changing taxonomical nomenclature of dermatophytes, *Trichophyton mentagrophytes* genotype VIII and the species *Trichophyton indotineae* are the same.
2. When the practicing dermatologist encounters a patient with chronic recalcitrant dermatophytosis, difficult to treat with terbinafine as well as azoles, it should be a hint to both the dermatologist and microbiologist to go for antibiotic susceptibility testing and molecular confirmation of *Trichophyton indotineae*. This dermatophyte should also prompt the dermatologist to enquire about past drug history of sub-optimal non-compliant antifungal therapy and overuse and abuse of over-the counter fixed dose combination creams containing steroids (clobetasol, beclomethasone).[22]

Systemic and local antifungals should be used in a judicious and rational manner in cases of multidrug resistant *Trichophyton indotineae* infections. It may benefit to use systemic and topical antifungals together, based on demonstration of *in vitro* synergism on checkerboard

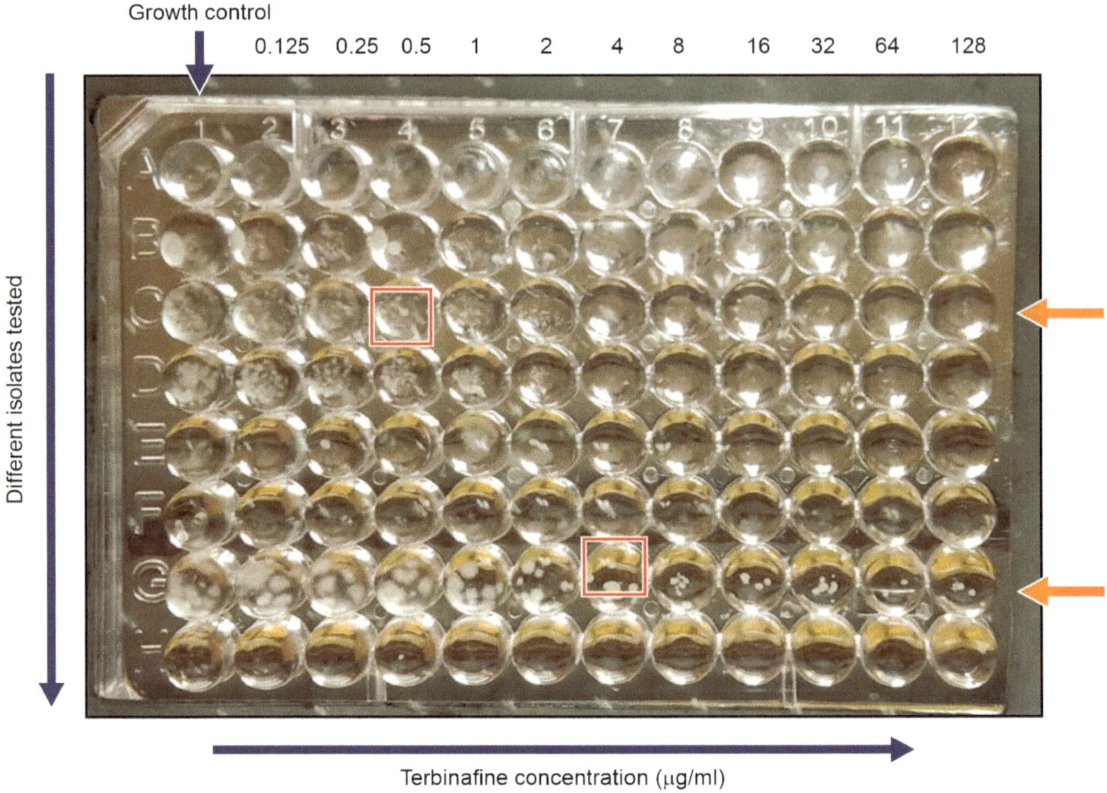

FIGURE 14.5: Antifungal sensitivity testing of the isolates against terbinafine showing high MICs

studies, although the same has not been proven in trials to be of any benefit[23] and a recent study failed to show supremacy of topical luliconazole-oral itraconazole combination treatment over itraconazole given alone.[24] Also, systemic combinations of itraconazole and terbinafine have not shown a superior efficacy as compared to itraconazole alone.[25]

LACUNAE IN KNOWLEDGE

- There is a need for detailed analysis of genomic features likely to be associated with virulence, pathogenicity and treatment response variability of *T. indotineae*.
- We have only a few antifungals in our armamentarium to fight the infection and these need to be used judiciously so as to derive maximum benefit out of them for longer times. The situation also demands increase in research efforts for newer drugs which could counter the infection.

FUTURE DIRECTIONS

We need to strengthen rapid molecular diagnostics for detecting *Trichophyton indotineae* so as to facilitate appropriate treatment and to slow down the situation from taking epidemic proportion. We need to study the virulence factors of *T. indotineae* which make the disease caused by it to assume chronic nature and leads to frequent relapses.[23] We also need to undertake research to understand the slow clinical responses to itraconazole, a drug to which the species is largely susceptible.[26]

CONCLUSION

Chronic recalcitrant relapsing dermatophytosis due to *Trichophyton indotineae* has become a public health nuisance due to its multidrug resistant nature.[27] Conscious efforts from different stakeholders (Practicing dermatologists/clinicians, microbiologists/mycologists, policy holders) to facilitate early detection and treatment of infection and to assist further research to aid in development of new treatment and diagnostic modalities is the need of the hour.

Key Points

- Be vigilant of tinea lesion non-responsive to antifungal therapy.
- Ensure proper judicial antifungal dosing with compliance to complete therapy.
- Stay updated with changing mycological terminology.
- Take support of mycologist to detect early and treat the disease rationally.
- Refer to centers with availability of advance research modalities for troubleshooting in such recalcitrant cases.

REFERENCES

1. Verma SB, Panda S, Nenoff P, Singal A, Rudramurthy SM, Uhrlass S, et al. The unprecedented epidemic-like scenario of dermatophytosis in India: II. Diagnostic methods and taxonomical aspects. Indian J Dermatol Venereol Leprol 2021;87(3):326–32.
2. Rengasamy M, Shenoy MM, Dogra S, Asokan N, Khurana A, Poojary S, et al. Indian association of dermatologists, venereologists and leprologists (IADVL) task force against recalcitrant tinea (ITART) consensus on the management of glabrous tinea (INTACT). Indian Dermatol Online J 2020;11(4):502.
3. Dogra S, Uprety S. The menace of chronic and recurrent dermatophytosis in India: Is the problem deeper than we perceive? Indian Dermatol Online J 2016;7(2):73.
4. Sardana K, Kaur R, Arora P, Goyal R, Ghunawat S. Is antifungal resistance a cause for treatment failure in dermatophytosis: A study focused on tinea corporis and cruris from a tertiary centre? Indian Dermatol Online J 2018;9(2):90.
5. Singh A, Masih A, Khurana A, Singh PK, Gupta M, Hagen F, et al. High terbinafine resistance in *Trichophyton interdigitale* isolates in Delhi, India harbouring mutations in the squalene epoxidase gene. Mycoses 2018;61(7):477–84.
6. Uhrlaß S, Verma SB, Gräser Y, Rezaei-Matehkolaei A, Hatami M, Schaller M, et al. *Trichophyton indotineae*—An emerging pathogen causing recalcitrant dermatophytoses in India and worldwide—A multidimensional perspective. J Fungi 2022;8(7):757.
7. Ebert A, Monod M, Salamin K, Burmester A, Uhrlaß S, Wiegand C, et al. Alarming India-wide phenomenon of antifungal resistance in dermatophytes: A multicentre study. Mycoses 2020;63(7):717–28.
8. de Hoog GS, Dukik K, Monod M, Packeu A, Stubbe D, Hendrickx M, et al. Toward a novel multilocus phylogenetic taxonomy for the dermatophytes. Mycopathologia. 2017;182:5–31
9. Nenoff P, Verma SB, Uhrlaß S, Burmester A, Gräser Y. A clarion call for preventing taxonomical errors of dermatophytes using the example of the novel *Trichophyton mentagrophytes* genotype VIII uniformly isolated in the Indian epidemic of superficial dermatophytosis. Mycoses 2019;62(1):6–10.
10. Kano R, Kimura U, Kakurai M, Hiruma J, Kamata H, Suga Y, et al. *Trichophyton indotineae* sp. nov.: A new highly terbinafine-resistant anthropophilic dermatophyte species. Mycopathologia 2020;185:947–58.
11. Tang C, Kong X, Ahmed SA, Thakur R, Chowdhary A, Nenoff P, et al. Taxonomy of the *Trichophyton mentagrophytes/T. interdigitale* species complex harboring the highly virulent, multiresistant genotype *T. indotineae*. Mycopathologia 2021;186:315–26.
12. de Hoog GS, Chaturvedi V, Denning DW, Dyer PS, Frisvad JC, Geiser D, et al. Name changes in medically important fungi and their implications for clinical practice. J Clin Microbiol. 2015;53(4):1056–62.

13. Khurana A, Masih A, Chowdhary A, Sardana K, Borker S, Gupta A, et al. correlation of *in vitro* susceptibility based on mics and squalene epoxidase mutations with clinical response to terbinafine in patients with tinea corporis/cruris. Antimicrob Agents Chemother 2018;62(12):e01038–18.
14. Kumar P, Ramachandran S, Das S, Bhattacharya SN, Taneja B. Insights into changing dermatophyte spectrum in India through analysis of cumulative 161,245 cases between 1939 and 2021. Mycopathologia 2023;188:183–202.
15. Ngo TMC, Ton Nu PA, Le CC, Ha TNT, Do TBT, Tran TG. First detection of *Trichophyton indotineae* causing tinea corporis in central Vietnam. Med Mycol Case Rep 2022;36:37–41.
16. Nenoff P, Verma SB, Ebert A, Süß A, Fischer E, Auerswald E, et al. Spread of terbinafine-resistant *Trichophyton mentagrophytes* type VIII (India) in Germany—"the tip of the iceberg? J Fungi (Basel) 2020;6:207.
17. Posso-De Los Rios CJ, Tadros E, Summerbell RC, Scott JA. Terbinafine resistant *Trichophyton indotineae* isolated in patients with superficial dermatophyte infection in Canadian patients. J Cut Med Surg 2022;26:371–6.
18. Nenoff P, Uhrlaß S, Verma SB, Panda S. *Trichophyton mentagrophytes* ITS genotype VIII and *Trichophyton indotineae*: A terminological maze, or is it? Indian J Dermatol Venereol Leprol 2022;88(5):586–9.
19. Singh A, Singh P, Meis JF, Chowdhary A. *In vitro* activity of the novel antifungal olorofim against dermatophytes and opportunistic moulds including *Penicillium* and *Talaromyces* species. J Antimicrob Chemother 2021;76(5):1229–33.
20. Kumar P, Das S, Tigga R, Pandey R, Bhattacharya SN, Taneja B. Whole genome sequences of two *Trichophyton indotineae* clinical isolates from India emerging as threats during therapeutic treatment of dermatophytosis. 3 Biotech 2021;11(9):402.
21. Yamada T, Maeda M, Alshahni MM, Tanaka R, Yaguchi T, Bontems O, et al. Terbinafine resistance of *Trichophyton* clinical isolates caused by specific point mutations in the squalene epoxidase gene. Antimicrob Agents Chemother 2017;61: e00115–17.
22. Sardana K, Gupta A, Sadhasivam S, Gautam RK, Khurana A, Saini S, et al. Checkerboard analysis to evaluate synergistic combinations of existing antifungal drugs and propylene glycol monocaprylate in isolates from recalcitrant tinea corporis and cruris patients harboring squalene epoxidase gene mutation. Antimicrob Agents Chemother 2021;65:e00321–21.
23. Khurana A, Sharath S, Sardana K, et al. Therapeutic updates on the management of tinea corporis or cruris in the era of *Trichophyton indotineae*: Separating evidence from hype—A narrative review. Ind J Dermatol 2023;68:525–40.
24. Rana DK, Shah TS, Rohit MH, Patel NH, Khadela AD, Oza YP, Padhiyar JK. Evaluation of the benefit of the addition of 1% topical luliconazole versus topical bland emollient to the systemic itraconazole therapy for the management of disseminated dermatophytosis: A randomised control trial. Mycoses 2024;67:e13681. https://doi.org/10.1111/myc.13681
25. Singh SK, Subba N, Tilak R. Efficacy of terbinafine and itraconazole in different doses and in combination in the treatment of tinea infection: A randomized controlled parallel group open labeled trial with clinico-mycological correlation. Indian J Dermatol 2020;65:284–89.
26. Khurana A, Agarwal A, Agrawal D, Panesar S, Ghadlinge M, Sardana K, et al. Effect of different itraconazole dosing regimens on cure rates, treatment duration, safety, and relapse rates in adult patients with tinea corporis/cruris: A randomized clinical trial. JAMA Dermatol 2022;158(11):1269–78.
27. Chowdhary A, Singh A, Kaur A, Khurana A. The emergence and worldwide spread of the species *Trichophyton indotineae* causing difficult-to-treat dermatophytosis: A new challenge in the management of dermatophytosis. PLoS Pathog 2022;18:e1010795.

CHAPTER 15

Prospects for New Drug Development Against Dermatophytes

• *Rashmi Jindal*

INTRODUCTION

Dermatophytoses of skin, hair, and nails are one of the most common fungal infections world-wide affecting all ages, races, genders, and socio-economic status.[1] Despite being ubiquitous, the search for an ideal antifungal that is broad-spectrum, fungicidal and has minimal toxicity continues. At present, five main classes of antifungals are available having different modes of action. But each has its own limitations necessitating the need for better alternatives (**Table 15.1**).[2–4] Most useful antifungal agents against dermatophytes are azoles. Benzimidazole was the first azole identified in 1944 to have antifungal activity. Now, there are about 23 antifungal azoles available in the market most widely used being clotrimazole, fluconazole, itraconazole, miconazole and luliconazole.[5,6]

The relentlessly increasing antifungal resistance and emergence of new fungal strains has established an unmet therapeutic need for new agents. Understanding the mechanisms of drug resistance can pave the way to find suitable alternatives. Drug resistance can develop because of the following mechanisms: (also *see* Chapter 2)

- Change in drug targeting molecules: Modification in drug targets or their overexpression renders the drug ineffective.

TABLE 15.1: Five main classes of antifungals currently available

S. No.	Class	Mechanism of action	Limitations
1.	Echinocandins	Inhibits synthesis of 1,3-β-D glucan resulting in cell lysis	• No oral formulation • Active only against yeast and moulds
2.	Allylamines	Inhibits squalene epoxidase	• Emerging drug resistance
3.	Polyenes	Increase cell membrane permeability by binding to ergosterol	• No oral formulation • Dose related nephrotoxicity • Infusion reactions
4.	Azoles	Inhibits ergosterol synthesis by inhibiting lanosterol 14-α-demethylase	• Emerging drug resistance • Hepatotoxicity • Drug interactions • Erratic oral absorption
5.	Flucytosine	Selectively interferes with fungal nucleic acid synthesis	• Rapid development of resistance • Bone marrow suppression

- Reduction in drug concentration: Due to increase efflux (membrane efflux pumps) or decreased cell permeability.
- Alterations in metabolic pathways.
- Adaptations in cell wall.
- Biofilm formation.

SLOW PROGRESS IN DRUG DEVELOPMENT

In contrast to development of new antimicrobials, development of new antifungals has been slow and restricted primarily because of the similar eukaryotic mechanism used by fungal pathogens and humans, limiting availability of pathogen specific targets. Since the beginning of 21st century, only few new antifungal agents have been approved by FDA **(Table 15.2)**.[7] Dermatophytoses though more prevalent, receive less attention in terms of focus on new drug development, mainly because of less mortality. However, the associated morbidity is significant.

APPROACH TO NEW DRUG DEVELOPMENT

Approaches for development of new antifungals can focus on improving efficacy of old targets, developing new targets or developing better formulations with increased bioavailability and stability **(Table 15.3)**.[8] Certain drugs used in diverse indications have also been repurposed because of their anti-fungal properties.

TABLE 15.2: Recently FDA approved antifungals

S. No.	Drug	Class	Route of administration	Approved on	Approved for
1.	Luliconazole (1%)	Azole	Topical	November 2013	Tinea cruris, tinea corporis, tinea pedis
2.	Efinaconazole (10%)	Azole	Topical	June 2014	Toenail onychomycosis
3.	Tavaborole (5%)	Oxaborole	Topical	July 2014	Toenail onychomycosis
4.	Isavuconazole	Triazole	Oral/intra-venous	March 2015	Invasive fungal infection (Aspergillosis, mucormycosis)
5.	Ibrexafungerp	Triterpenoid	Oral/intra-venous	June 2021	Vulvo-vaginal candidiasis
6.	Oteseconazole (VT-1161)	Tetrazole	Oral	2022	Vulvo-vaginal candidiasis, onychomycosis, tinea pedis

TABLE 15.3: Approaches for development of new anti-fungal agents

Old targets with improved efficacy	Novel targets	Repurposing of drugs	Better formulations	Natural products
• Rezafungin • Tolsura • VT-1161 (Oteseconazole) • MAT 2203	• Ibrexafungerp • Fosmanogepix • Olorofim • Nikkomycin • T-2307 • VL-2397 • Aureobasidin • Turbinmicin	• Sertraline • Tamoxifen • AR-12	• Amphotericin B cochleate • Super-bioavailability itraconazole • Novel topical drug delivery systems	• *Kalopanax pictum* • Clove oil • M14 acridone • Chitosan • *Nephthea* sp.

Improving Efficacy of Old Targets

Drugs including rezafungin, oteseconazole, VT-1129 and VT-1598 act on similar fungal biosynthesis pathways as the existing classes, but with additional advantages **(Fig. 15.1)**. ***Rezafungin*** is an echinocandin with increased stability, solubility and half-life allowing once a week dosing.[13] VT-1161 (***Oteseconazole***), VT-1129 and VT-1598 are novel azole-like compounds with better affinity for fungal CYP51, improving their side effect profile.[7, 12] Oteseconazole has been found effective against *Trichophyton* species and are used for treatment of onychomycosis and tinea pedis.[7] Monoclonal antibodies have also been investigated as potential antifungals. H5K1 is a humanised monoclonal antibody specific for 1,3-β-D glucan and is found effective against *C. auris in vitro*.[14]

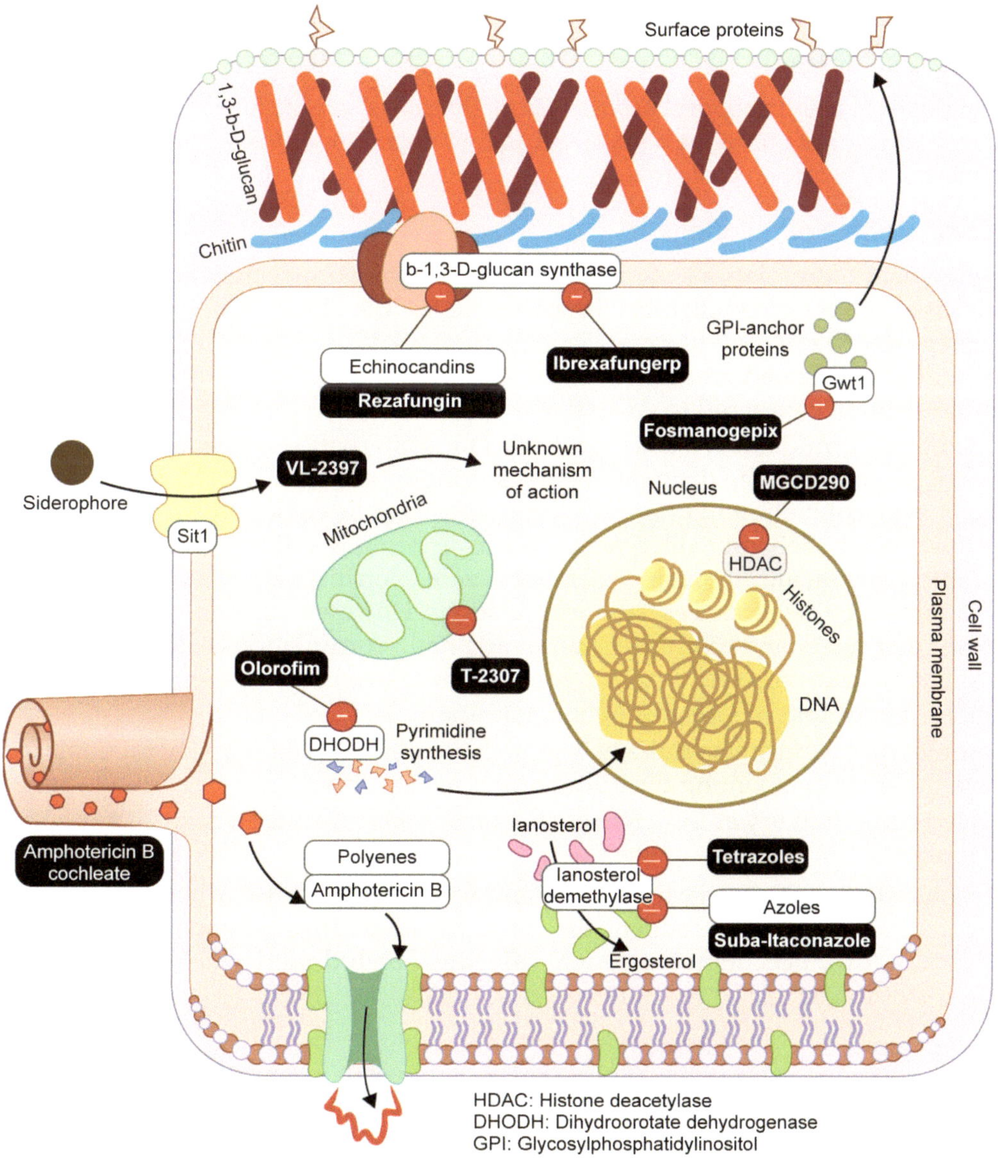

FIGURE 15.1: Molecular targets of the antifungal drugs

Identifying Novel Drug Targets

Antifungal agents having novel drug targets are also under development **(Fig. 15.1)**.[7–12] ***Fosmanogepix*** inhibits fungal glycosylphosphatidylinositol-1 production that is important for the integrity of cell wall mannoproteins.[15, 16] It has a broad spectrum of activity and is effective against yeast and mould, with over 90% bioavailability. ***Nikkomycin-Z*** is a chitin synthase inhibitor.[17] ***Ibrexafungerp*** is a triterpenoid that inhibits 1,3-β-D glucan synthase similar to echinocandins.[18] T-2307 is arylamidine that inhibits fungal mitochondria synthesis.[19] ***Olorofim*** is an orotomide acting by inhibiting dihydro-orotate dehydrogenase required for pyrimidine biosynthesis.[20] However, most of these drugs are being evaluated for invasive fungal infections. Riparin III an alkaloid containing an amide group has been found to be fungicidal against dermatophytes with additional inhibitory action on dermatophyte biofilms. Acridone M14 is another experimental drug found effective against dermatophytes.[21]

Repurposing of Drugs

The advantages of using a repurposed drug is likely lack of safety issues.[7] Isolated experiments have shown efficacy of quinoline derivatives against dermatophytosis, however future studies are warranted to establish their role.[22]

Developing Better Formulations

Developing better formulations of existing drugs aim to optimize their benefits and alleviate their toxicities. Super-bioavailability itraconazole (SUBA-ITRA) is being used widely and scores over itraconazole by having a better bioavailability (173%) and less interpatient variability.[23] Encochleated amphotericin B (AMB) is a nanocrystal AMB being studied for oral administration compared to AMB that needs to be given intravenously.[24]

Novel topical formulations that are liposome, niosome, nano-emulsion or solid lipid nano-particle based, improve the drug delivery resulting in better efficacy. These nanoparticles alter the pharmacokinetic and pharmacodynamic properties of the drug making them more stable allowing for their controlled release, thus improving efficacy and reducing toxicity. Many antifungals including miconazole, econazole, clotrimazole, itraconazole, terbinafine and AMB have been developed as nano-formulations. However, further studies are warranted to confirm their safety and efficacy. Additionally nano-formulations can help overcome the development of antifungal resistance.[25] Some of these mechanisms are:

- Combining multiple antifungals in one nano-particle.
- Liposomes and dendrimers quickly fuse with the plasma membrane of microbial cell and release the drug overcoming the efflux pump mechanism.
- Targeted drug delivery at local site ensures faster killing of the fungus before resistance development.

The major challenges in marketing of nano-formulations is their high production cost, physical instability and immunogenicity. Lipid based gel formulations of AMB have been used topically for mucocutaneous fungal infections including dermatophytosis and have shown good efficacy.[26]

Natural Products

Use of medicinal plants is well-established in ancient medicine. A number of antifungal drugs including polyenes and griseofulvin have connection with natural products. Plants and their derivatives have been used for development of new antifungal agents. *Fructus Psoraleae, Folium Eucalypti Globuli, Citrus bergamia* and *Brazilian Copaiba oil* are some of the plant products found useful in treating diverse species causing dermatophytosis.[27] The Red sea coral *Nephthea* sp. potentially inhibits the CYP51 enzyme in dermatophytes and has shown anti-dermatophyte activity in laboratory studies.[28] Clove oil was also shown to have strong antifungal effect against dermatophytes in *in vitro* studies and in cows when applied topically.[29] Chitosan, a non-toxic, biodegradable polymer found in *Mucoracea* fungi, demonstrates protective activity against dermatophytes by inhibiting their proteases and can be a potential alternate to conventional antifungal agents.[30] Acridones are alkaloids found in *Rutaceae* plants and a novel acridone M14 was found to have antidermatophytic activity in clinical isolates.[31]

CONCLUSION

The evidence of patient need in terms of increasing incidence of fungal diseases reinforces new antifungal drug development, but this has to be supported by adequate innovation and funding. Further the innovation gaps because of discovery-approval delay needs to be minimized. With better focus on quality research, we hope to have promising antifungals available for commercial use soon.

Key Points

- Dermatophytoses of skin, hair and nail are one of the most common fungal infections worldwide affecting all ages, races, genders and socioeconomic status.
- Development of resistance to available antifungals is on the rise necessitating need for innovation of better alternatives.
- Approaches for development of new antifungals can focus on improving efficacy of old targets, developing new targets or developing better formulations with increased bioavailability and stability.
- Focussed research supported by adequate funding is the need of the hour.

REFERENCES

1. Gnat S, Nowakiewicz A, Zięba P. Taxonomy of dermatophytes–The classification systems may change but the identification problems remain the same. Postępy Mikrobiologii—Advancements of Microbiology 2019;58:49–58.
2. Rauseo AM, Coler-Reilly A, Larson L, Spec A. Hope on the Horizon: Novel fungal treatments in development. Open Forum Infect Dis 2020;7(2):ofaa016
3. Fernandez de Ullivarri M, Arbulu S, Garcia-Gutierrez E, Cotter PD. Antifungal peptides as therapeutic agents. Front Cell Infect Microbiol 2020;10:105.
4. Hasim S, Coleman JJ. Targeting the fungal cell wall: Current therapies and implications for development of alternative antifungal agents. Future Med Chem 2019;11:869–83.
5. Teixeira MM, Carvalho DT, Sousa E, Pinto E. New antifungal agents with azole moieties. Pharmaceuticals (Basel) 2022;15:1427.
6. Kane A, Carter DA. Augmenting azoles with drug synergy to expand the antifungal toolbox. Pharmaceuticals 2022;15:482.
7. Cui X, Wang L, Lü Y, Yue C. Development and research progress of anti-drug resistant fungal drugs. J Infect Public Health 2022;15:986–1000.
8. Pianalto KM, Alspaugh JA. New horizons in antifungal therapy. J Fungi (Basel) 2016;2:26.
9. McCarty TP, Pappas PG. Antifungal Pipeline. Front Cell Infect Microbiol 2021;11:732223.
10. Li D, She X, Calderone R. The antifungal pipeline: The need is established. Are there new compounds? FEMS Yeast Res 2020;20:foaa023

11. Hoenigl M, Sprute R, Egger M, Arastehfar A, Cornely OA, Krause R, et al. The antifungal pipeline: Fosmanogepix, Ibrexafungerp, Olorofim, Opelconazole, and Rezafungin. Drugs 2021;81:1703–29.
12. Gintjee TJ, Donnelley MA, Thompson GR 3rd. Aspiring antifungals: Review of current antifungal pipeline developments. J Fungi (Basel) 2020;6:28.
13. Sandison T, Ong V, Lee J, Thye D. Safety and pharmacokinetics of CD101 IV, a novel echinocandin, in healthy adults. Antimicrob Agents Chemother 2017;61:e01627–16.
14. Di Mambro T, Vanzolini T, Bruscolini P, Perez-Gaviro S, Marra E, Roscilli G, et al. A new humanized antibody is effective against pathogenic fungi *in vitro*. Sci Rep 2021;11:19500.
15. Miyazaki M, Horii T, Hata K, Watanabe NA, Nakamoto K, Tanaka K, et al. In vitro activity of E1210, a novel antifungal, against clinically important yeasts and molds. Antimicrob Agents Chemother 2011;55:4652–8.
16. Tsukahara K, Hata K, Nakamoto K, Sagane K, Watanabe NA, Kuromitsu J, et al. Medicinal genetics approach towards identifying the molecular target of a novel inhibitor of fungal cell wall assembly. Mol Microbiol 2003;48:1029–42.
17. Larwood DJ. Nikkomycin Z-Ready to Meet the Promise? J Fungi (Basel) 2020 30;6(4):261.
18. Ghannoum M, Long L, Larkin EL, Isham N, Sherif R, Borroto-Esoda K, et al. Evaluation of the antifungal activity of the novel oral glucan synthase inhibitor SCY-078, singly and in combination, for the treatment of invasive aspergillosis. Antimicrob Agents Chemother 2018;62:e00244–18.
19. Abe M, Nakamura S, Kinjo Y. Efficacy of T-2307, a novel arylamidine, against ocular complications of disseminated candidiasis in mice. J Antimicrob Chemother 2019;74:1327–32.
20. Negri CE, Johnson A, McEntee L, Box H, Whalley S, Schwartz JA, et al. Pharmacodynamics of the novel antifungal agent F901318 for acute sinopulmonary aspergillosis caused by *Aspergillus flavus*. J Infect Dis 2018;217:1118–27.
21. Silva EP, Rocha MAND, Silva RNM, Moura-Mendes J, Sousa GR, de Souza-Ferrari J, et al. Antifungal and antibiofilm activity of Riparin III against dermatophytes. J Fungi (Basel) 2023;9:231.
22. da Rosa Monte Machado G, Diedrich D, Ruaro TC, Zimmer AR, Lettieri Teixeira M, de Oliveira LF, et al. Quinolines derivatives as promising new antifungal candidates for the treatment of candidiasis and dermatophytosis. Braz J Microbiol. 2020;51:1691–1701.
23. Sardana K, Mathachan SR. Super bioavailable itraconazole and its place and relevance in recalcitrant dermatophytosis: Revisiting skin levels of itraconazole and minimum inhibitory concentration data. Indian Dermatol Online J 2021;12:1–5.
24. Santangelo R, Paderu P, Delmas G, Chen Z-W, Mannino R, Zarif L, et al. Efficacy of oral cochleate-amphotericin B in a mouse model of systemic candidiasis. Antimicrob Agents Chemother 2000;44:2356–60.
25. Sousa F, Ferreira D, Reis S, Costa P. Current insights on antifungal therapy: Novel nanotechnology approaches for drug delivery systems and new drugs from natural sources. Pharmaceuticals (Basel) 2020;13(9):248.
26. Sahni K, Singh S, Dogra S. Newer topical treatments in skin and nail dermatophyte infections. Indian Dermatol Online J 2018;9:149–58.
27. Soares LA, de Cássia Orlandi Sardi J, Gullo FP, de Souza Pitangui N, Scorzoni L, Leite FS, et al. Anti dermatophytic therapy–prospects for the discovery of new drugs from natural products. Braz J Microbiol 2014;44:1035–41.
28. Hassan NH, El-Hawary SS, Emam M, Rabeh MA, Abdelmohsin UR, Selim NM. Potential inhibitors of CYP51 enzyme in dermatophytes by red sea soft coral *Nephthea* sp.: In silico and molecular networking studies. ACS Omega 2022;7:13808–17.
29. Eman-Abdeen E, El-Diasty EM. Antifungal activity of clove oil on dermatophytes and other fungi. Int J Advanced Res 2015;3:1299–305.
30. Lopes AI, Tavaria FK, Pintado ME. Application of Chitosan in the control of fungal infections by dermatophytes. Ann Appl Microbiol Biotechnol J 2017;1:1006.
31. de Oliveira DBC, Silva LB, da Silva BV, Borges TC, Marques BC, dos Santos MB, et al. A novel acridine with anti-fungal properties against *Candida* spp. and dermatophytes, and antibiofilm activity against *C. albicans*. J Appl Microbiol 2019;127:1362–72.

CHAPTER 16

Vaccines for Dermatophyte Infections

• Dipali Rathod • Ruchi Hemdani

INTRODUCTION

Menace of dermatophytosis continues to grow with higher incidence of recalcitrant, drug resistant cases being reported frequently. Treating these infections is a challenge with the limited therapeutic options available to us. In the current scenario, control of dermatophyte infections in the form of a vaccine would be an effective therapeutic strategy to prevent the disease burden altogether both in humans and animals. An efficient vaccine against dermatophyte must prevent the clinical disease, its transmission to other subjects and environment. There have been attempts in the past to develop such a vaccine against dermatophyte infection and non-approved commercial vaccines only for animals[1,2] exist due to differences in their dermatophyte infection from humans (**Table 16.1**). However, there is no vaccine for preventing or treating dermatophytosis in humans. Animal vaccination campaigns have been held in Western countries with both favorable and contradictory responses.[1] There is limited available data on vaccines in dermatophyte infection as the basic immunopathogenesis of dermatophytes is yet to be clearly elucidated. These knowledge gaps are being bridged gradually with ongoing studies and we have tried to briefly explain current status on immunology of dermatophyte infection in this chapter with its extrapolation to vaccines in dermatophytosis.

PREMISE FOR A VACCINE IN DERMATOPHYTES

Dermatophytes are obligatory parasites (except geophilic species). They do not reproduce, do not produce conidia in environment, and are not a part of the normal cutaneous flora. Dermatophyte infections are not life threatening and occur in immunocompetent individuals as well.[1] These characteristics favor the development of a useful vaccine against

TABLE 16.1: Differences between animal and human dermatophyte infection

Characteristic	Animal dermatophyte infection	Human dermatophyte infection
Age group	Clinical infection often seen in young	At all ages
Reinfection following recovery/ clearance	Rare, both from original species or another one	Frequent, both by original species
Existing and upcoming vaccines	Present	None
Types of vaccines available	Killed, live, recombinant	None

dermatophyte infections, but not much work has been done by researchers in this subject in past. With the recent ongoing molecular characterization of antigenic determinants in different dermatophyte species, it is expected that an efficient vaccine will be developed to tackle human dermatophytosis in addition to the new ones being tried for animal infections.

Immune Response Against Dermatophytes[1, 3] (Fig. 16.1)

In order to develop a vaccine against dermatophytes, it is essential to understand the immune response in natural dermatophyte infection. In a nutshell, dermatophyte antigens are recognized, processed, and presented in conjunction with major histocompatibility complex (MHC) molecules on the surface of antigen presenting cells (APCs), which set the immune cascade into action with the help of cytokines which may amplify the presentation of antigens or cause the proliferation of various subsets of lymphocytes (Th1/Th2).[4, 5] Past studies have shown that a specific immune response is induced with dermatophyte infection.

Cell Mediated Response

This is the prime immune response mediated by key cytokines IL-12 and IFN-gamma from the Th1 lymphocytes axis and effector cells (macrophages and neutrophils), thereby clearing infection and offering efficient protection against dermatophyte infection. Findings supporting protective role are: the association of delayed type hypersensitivity (DTH) skin tests to *Trichophyton* with highly inflamed lesions and resistance to reinfection.[6] The intensity of immune response varies according to the dermatophyte species, the host species, and the physiopathological status of the host.

Innate Immune Response

The role of humoral immune response is proposed to be negligible with specific antibodies against dermatophytes conferring little protection as demonstrated by immediate hypersensitivity (IH) skin tests being associated with chronic infection. The interaction of various components (cellular and enzymatic) of innate immunity like keratinocytes, Langerhans cells, neutrophils, macrophages, proteases, LL32 cathelicidin, defensins, and antibodies produced upon dermatophyte exposure, is still an enigma which needs further research. The antigens/proteins and receptors involved in this interaction may serve as potential targets and aid vaccine development.

Induction of T helper type-2 (Th2) cells after dermatophyte exposure causes IL-4 production which acts on B cells and leads to antibody formation (IgE, IgG) and establishes chronic

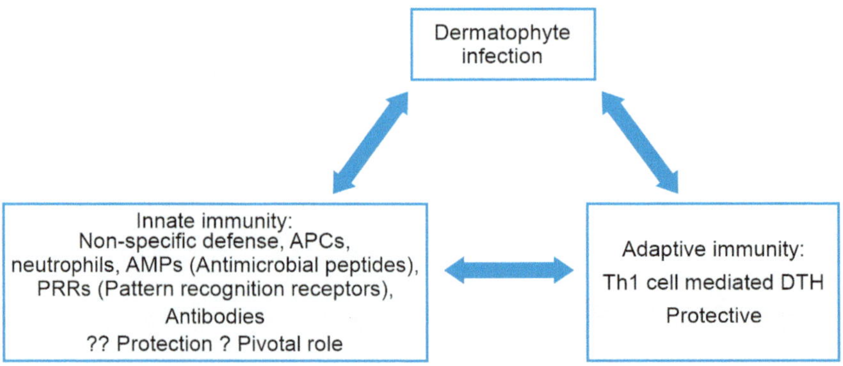

FIGURE 16.1: Immune interactions in dermatophyte infection

lesions. Chronic and recurrent infections are commonly seen with *T. rubrum* infection in immunocompetent host. These are correlated with deficient DTH only to *T. rubrum* (selective immune defect: Cell-mediated responses to other antigens being normal), elevated specific IgE and IgG4, and IgE mediated immediate hypersensitivity. It has been proposed that active suppression of cell-mediated immunity to *Trichophyton* antigens is mediated by suppressor T lymphocytes and inhibitory serum factors via modulation of cell-mediated responses.

Duality of the Immune Response to Dermatophytes (Table 16.2)[3]

Type-1 cells and Type-2 cells antagonize each other and a mutual exclusion phenomenon is said to exist. However, *Trichophyton* species, have the ability to elicit diverse immune responses. This unusual dichotomy between Th1 and Th2 subsets exists with a single Trichophyton protein, as established by eliciting both immediate and delayed hypersensitivity upon intradermal test in different individuals with Trichophyton antigens with differing clinical response. Clinical application of this will help in development of antidermatophyte vaccine.

TABLE 16.2: Skin test results with Trichophyton

Features	Immediate hypersensitivity	Delayed type hypersensitivity
Clinically	Chronic lesion	Acute, highly inflamed lesions
Resolution	Not seen	Spontaneous
Re-infection	Can occur	Resistance to re-infection
Antibody titres	High	Low
Immune response	Humoral	Cell mediated
Subset of T lymphocyte	Th2	Th1

Virulence Factors of Dermatophytes

Identification of the fungal virulence factors and their role in infection, adhesion and invasion of epidermis is the key to understanding the immunopathogenesis in dermatophytes. These are important antigenic determinants modulating the host immune response[7] and their molecular characterization is thus important for vaccine development. Few virulence factors that have been fully characterized are shown in **Box 16.1** while structural antigens like cell wall glycoproteins are yet poorly characterized.

BOX 16.1: Virulence factors that have been fully characterized

- Endoproteases (Sub3 and Mep3 of *M. canis*)
- *Trichophyton* antigens: Protein IV (cultures of both *T. rubrum* and *T. tonsurans*) and *T. rubrum* serine proteinase belonging to the class D sub-family of sub-tilases
- Regulatory genes like DNR1 of *M. canis* and *PACC* of *T. rubrum*
- Exo-keratinases (*T. verrucosum, T. mentagrophytes,* and *M. canis*)

BASIC PRINCIPLES OF A VACCINE AGAINST DERMATOPHYTE

A vaccine is a form of augmented immunity which is acquired. It essentially contains immune stimulating potent antigens from infectious agent by means of which the host is sensitized to the infection and starts mounting an immune response against that agent comparable to immune response induced by natural infection. The response is generally humoral in nature

TABLE 16.3: Factors affecting vaccine efficacy

Pathogen factors	Host factors
Intrinsic nature of structural antigens	Population of APCs and cytokine milieu at the site of antigen exposure
Dose and route of administration of antigen	Immune status
Adjuvants	

but can additionally also be cellular, thereby protecting from the infection. The antigens for antifungal vaccines are usually prepared from living or inactivated whole cells, or from one component of fungi such as cell wall components, cytoplasmic extracts, and genetic recombinant proteins which are immunogenic in nature.[8–10]

Development of dermatophyte vaccine is based on isolation, characterization and use of major antigenic determinants able to elicit a specific Th1 response and to stimulate strong memory T-cell responses. Activation of cellular immunity represented by a Th1 response with induction of IL-12 and IFN-γ is required from an effective anti-dermatophyte vaccine.

An ideal anti-dermatophyte vaccine is one with clearly defined composition and immunologic properties, high safety degree and stimulating a strong and long-lasting Th1 response. Certain factors can influence the efficacy of vaccine (**Table 16.3**).

EXISTING VACCINES AGAINST DERMATOPHYTE INFECTIONS IN ANIMALS

Both live attenuated and inactivated vaccines against dermatophyte infections have been developed and marketed for use in animals: cattle, horses and cats. A live attenuated vaccine against *Trichophyton verrucosum* is being used in Norway since 1980 to immunize cattle against dermatophyte infection. This vaccine offers protection by stimulating both humoral and cellular immune responses.[1,2,11]

Inactivated vaccines have the advantage of being both prophylactic and therapeutic with potential use in diseased animals too but their efficacy and the duration of protection offered is doubtful with disappointing observations in cattle and horses.[1,11] Specific antigens from *Trichophyton* species have been used in some recent studies to enhance the prophylactic action of the inactivated antifungal vaccine by stimulating cellular immunity to provide stronger immunization.[1]

A new preparation of vaccine from inactivated *T. mentagrophytes* showed effective prophylaxis and treatment results against dermatophytosis in rabbits with reported long-term protection and a short treatment time.[2]

A polyvalent dermatophyte vaccine has shown promising protective prophylactic action against dermatophytosis, with no or minimal post-vaccination reaction.[11] Recent trend is to develop safer and more efficient subunit or recombinant vaccines against dermatophyte infections.

SUMMARY

Vaccines for dermatophyte infections have seen a very slow progression compared to studies on other mycoses owing to lack of encouraging results in early human studies and due to efficacious systemic antifungal drugs. The emergence of drug resistance and chronic recurrent dermatophytosis cases requiring long-term antifungal therapy has, however, rekindled the scientific interest in development of *Trichophyton* vaccines wherein many potential vaccine candidate antigens have been characterized at the molecular level. Understanding the immunopathogenesis of dermatophytes, especially with respect to factors and pathways associated in host–fungus interaction is essential and still ongoing. Various components of dermatophytes have been evaluated for vaccine development. Amongst existing vaccines for dermatophyte infections in animals, none have a license from a regulatory organization for commercial use. Search continues for a suitable vaccine with good prophylactic and therapeutic activity against dermatophytosis.

RECENT ADVANCES

Functional investigation of fungal genes is now possible: Gene disruption has been achieved via homologous recombination for *T. rubrum* and *M. canis*. RNA interference technology has been used to downregulate the expression of genes coding for Sub3 and Dpp4 in *M. canis*. Expressed sequence tags (ESTs) and high-throughput methods have been developed in *T. rubrum*. These help to analyze transcriptomes, cDNA microarrays and secreted proteomes allowing insight into host–fungus relationship. *Ex vivo* or *in vitro* infection models (RFE) are needed to evaluate role of fungal virulence factors on the innate host immune system. Also, studies focussing on identification of specific pattern recognition receptors (PRRs) involved in dermatophyte keratinocyte interaction are required to expose molecular level detailing of dermatophytic virulence factors. Elucidation of the amino acid sequence of *Trichophyton* antigens allows T-cell epitope mapping using overlapping peptide methodology for defining antigenic determinants associated with protective immune responses. This may play an important role in the development of alternative therapeutic strategies for the treatment of chronic dermatophytosis.

CONCLUSION

Although a vaccine seems to be the answer to surging dermatophytosis, the development of a vaccine against human dermatophytosis needs to be carefully evaluated on medical and economic basis and keeping in mind the challenges in development of the new vaccines (**Box 16.2**).

BOX 16. 2: Challenges in the development of vaccines for dermatophytosis

- Vaccine preparation is expensive, especially new generation recombinant vaccines
- Vaccine may act on the normal flora in the human body
- Possibility of autoimmune response upon using an antigen similar to host antigen
- It is not necessary that a vaccine will induce adequate immunization in some individuals

Key Points

- In the current scenario, control of dermatophyte infections with a vaccine would be an effective therapeutic strategy to prevent the disease burden both in humans and animals globally.
- Hitherto there is no effective vaccine for preventing or treating dermatophytosis in humans.
- Animal vaccination campaigns have been held in western countries with both favorable and contradictory responses.
- Amongst existing vaccine for dermatophyte infections in animals, none has a license from a regulatory organization for commercial use.
- A polyvalent dermatophyte vaccine has shown promising protective prophylactic action against dermatophytosis, with no or minimal post-vaccination reaction.
- Search continues for a suitable vaccine with good prophylactic and therapeutic activity against dermatophytosis.

REFERENCES

1. Mignon B, Tabart J, Baldo A, Mathy A, Losson B, Vermout S. Immunization and dermatophytes. Curr Opin Infect Dis 2008;21(2):134–40.
2. Al-Janabi AAHS, Al-Khikani FHO. Prophylaxis and therapeutic ability of inactivated dermatophytic vaccine against dermatophytosis in the rabbits as an animal model. Turk J Pharm Sci 2021;18(3):326–31.
3. Gudding R, Lund A. Immunoprophylaxis of bovine dermatophytosis. Can Vet J 1995;36(5):302–6.
4. Woodfolk JA. Allergy and dermatophytes. Clin Microbiol Rev 2005;18(1):30–43.
5. Smith JM, Griffin JF. Strategies for the development of a vaccine against ringworm. J Med Vet Mycol 1995;33(2):87–91.
6. Woodfolk JA, Platts-Mills TA. The immune response to dermatophytes. Res Immunol 1998;149(4–5):436–45; discussion 522–3.
7. Sahoo AK, Mahajan R. Management of tinea corporis, tinea cruris, and tinea pedis: A comprehensive review. Indian Dermatol Online J 2016;7(2):77–86.
8. Segal E. Vaccines for the management of dermatophyte and superficial yeast infections. Curr Top Med Mycol 1989;3:36–49.
9. Hussin Z, Smith JM. Vaccination procedures and the infectivity of dermatophyte lesions. Mycopathologia 1983;81(2):71–6.
10. Segal E. Vaccines against fungal infections. Crit Rev Microbiol 1987;14(3):229–71.
11. Abo-Elyazeed H, Soliman R, Hassan H, El-Seedy FR, Aboul-Ella H. Development, preparation, and evaluation of a novel non-adjuvanted polyvalent dermatophytes vaccine. Sci Rep 2023;13(1):157.

Index